T0172891

LIVING WITHOUT AN AMYGDALA

LIVING WITHOUT AN AMYGDALA

EDITED BY

David G. Amaral
Ralph Adolphs

THE GUILFORD PRESS
New York   London

Last digit is print number: 9   8   7   6   5   4   3   2   1

The authors have checked with sources believed to be reliable in their efforts to
provide information that is complete and generally in accord with the standards
of practice that are accepted at the time of publication. However, in view of the
possibility of human error or changes in behavioral, mental health, or medical
sciences, neither the authors, nor the editors and publisher, nor any other party
who has been involved in the preparation or publication of this work warrants
that the information contained herein is in every respect accurate or complete,
and they are not responsible for any errors or omissions or the results obtained
from the use of such information. Readers are encouraged to confirm the
information contained in this book with other sources.

Library of Congress Cataloging-in-Publication Data

Names: Amaral, David, 1950- editor. | Adolphs, Ralph, editor.
Title: Living without an amygdala / edited by David G. Amaral, Ralph Adolphs.
Description: New York : The Guilford Press, [2016] | Includes bibliographical
   references and index.
Identifiers: LCCN 2016016690 | ISBN 9781462525942 (hardback)
Subjects: LCSH: Amygdaloid body. | Affective neuroscience. | Emotions and
   cognition. | Neuropsychology. | BISAC: PSYCHOLOGY / Neuropsychology. |
   MEDICAL / Neuroscience. | PSYCHOLOGY / Emotions. | MEDICAL / Psychiatry /
   General.
Classification: LCC QP376 .L582 2016 | DDC 612.8/23—dc23
LC record available at *https://lccn.loc.gov/2016016690*

To my wonderful wife, Tammy,
who has brought balance to my life and enabled me
to carry out projects such as this

—D. G. A.

To all the human and animal experimental subjects
that have taught us what it is like to live
without an amygdala

—R. A.

About the Editors

David G. Amaral, PhD, is Distinguished Professor of Psychiatry and Neuroscience and Research Director of the UC Davis MIND Institute at the University of California, Davis. His interests include the neurobiology of social behavior and the development, neuroanatomical organization, and plasticity of the primate and human amygdala and hippocampal formation, with a particular focus on understanding the biological bases of autism spectrum disorder. Dr. Amaral is Director of Autism BrainNet, which solicits postmortem brain tissue to facilitate autism research, and Editor-in-Chief of *Autism Research*. He is a past president of the International Society for Autism Research and a Fellow of the American Association for the Advancement of Science, among other honors.

Ralph Adolphs, PhD, is Bren Professor of Psychology and Neuroscience at the California Institute of Technology. He leads a social neuroscience laboratory that investigates the psychological and neurobiological underpinnings of social behavior, with a particular focus on the role of the human amygdala and prefrontal cortex. A major goal is to make comparisons and contrasts across different clinical populations and research techniques. Dr. Adolphs is a past president of the Association for the Scientific Study of Consciousness, a Fellow of the Association for Psychological Science, and a recipient of the Distinguished Investigator Award from the Social and Affective Neuroscience Society, among other honors.

Contributors

Ralph Adolphs, PhD, Division of the Humanities and Social Sciences, California Institute of Technology, Pasadena, California

David G. Amaral, PhD, Department of Psychiatry and Behavioral Sciences and UC Davis MIND Institute, University of California, Davis, Sacramento, California

Adam K. Anderson, PhD, College of Human Ecology, Cornell University, Ithaca, New York

Jocelyne Bachevalier, PhD, Yerkes National Primate Research Center, Department of Psychology, Emory University, Atlanta, Georgia

Eliza Bliss-Moreau, PhD, California National Primate Research Center, University of California, Davis, Davis, California

June-Seek Choi, PhD, Department of Psychology, Korea University, Seoul, South Korea

Justin S. Feinstein, PhD, Department of Psychology and Oxley College of Health Sciences, University of Tulsa, and Laureate Institute for Brain Research, Tulsa, Oklahoma

Andrew S. Fox, PhD, Department of Psychiatry, University of Wisconsin School of Medicine and Public Health, Madison, Wisconsin

René Hurlemann, MD, PhD, Department of Psychiatry and Division of Medical Psychology, University of Bonn, Bonn, Germany

Ned H. Kalin, MD, Department of Psychiatry, University of Wisconsin School of Medicine and Public Health, Madison, Wisconsin

Jeansok J. Kim, PhD, Department of Psychology, University of Washington, Seattle, Washington

Aaron Lee, BS, Department of Psychiatry and Behavioral Sciences and UC Davis MIND Institute, University of California, Davis, Sacramento, California

Hongjoo J. Lee, PhD, Department of Psychology, University of Texas, Austin, Texas

Gilda Moadab, BS, California National Primate Research Center, University of California, Davis, Davis, California

Christopher S. Monk, PhD, Department of Psychology, University of Michigan, Ann Arbor, Michigan

Barak Morgan, PhD, Department of Human Biology, University of Cape Town, Observatory, Cape Town, South Africa

Elisabeth A. Murray, PhD, Laboratory of Neuropsychology, National Institute of Mental Health, Bethesda, Maryland

Jonathan A. Oler, PhD, Department of Psychiatry, University of Wisconsin School of Medicine and Public Health, Madison, Wisconsin

Alexandra Patin, MA, MSc, Department of Psychiatry and Division of Medical Psychology, University of Bonn, Bonn, Germany

Elizabeth A. Phelps, PhD, Department of Psychology, New York University, New York, New York

Daniel S. Pine, MD, Section on Development and Affective Neuroscience, National Institute of Mental Health, Bethesda, Maryland

Jessica Raper, PhD, Yerkes National Primate Research Center, Department of Psychology, Emory University, Atlanta, Georgia

Sarah E. V. Rhodes, PhD, Office of Science Policy, National Institutes of Health, Bethesda, Maryland

Mar Sanchez, PhD, Department of Psychiatry and Behavioral Sciences, School of Medicine, Emory University, Atlanta, Georgia

Emma Sarro, PhD, Department of Child and Adolescent Psychiatry, The Child Study Center at New York University Langone Medical Center, New York, New York

Cynthia M. Schumann, PhD, Department of Psychiatry and Behavioral Sciences and UC Davis MIND Institute, University of California, Davis, Sacramento, California

Alexander J. Shackman, PhD, Department of Psychology, University of Maryland, College Park, College Park, Maryland

Dan J. Stein, PhD, Department of Psychiatry, University of Cape Town, Observatory, Cape Town, South Africa

Shannon B. Z. Stephens, PhD, Yerkes National Primate Research Center, Department of Psychology, Emory University, Atlanta, Georgia

Regina M. Sullivan, PhD, Department of Child and Adolescent Psychiatry, The Child Study Center at New York University Langone Medical Center, New York, New York

David Terburg, PhD, Department of Psychology/Experimental Psychology, Utrecht University, Utrecht, The Netherlands

Helena Thornton, PhD, Department of Psychiatry and Mental Health, University of Cape Town, Observatory, Cape Town, South Africa

Rebecca M. Todd, PhD, Department of Psychology, University of British Columbia, Vancouver, British Columbia, Canada

Daniel Tranel, PhD, Departments of Neurology and Psychology, University of Iowa, Iowa City, Iowa

Jack van Honk, PhD, Department of Psychology/Experimental Psychology, Utrecht University, Utrecht, The Netherlands

Martha V. Vargas, BS, Counseling Division, Transfer Center, Santa Ana College, Novato, California

Kim Wallen, PhD, Yerkes National Primate Research Center, Department of Psychology, Emory University, Atlanta, Georgia

Preface

The amygdala, or more properly the amygdaloid complex, is about 2.0 cm³ on each side of the human brain. If a normal adult brain is approximately 1,300 cm³, then the amygdala makes up about 0.3% of its volume. The human amygdala has about 12 million neurons on each side. This compares to estimates of 100 billion neurons in the entire brain and 20 billion in the cerebral cortex. By any quantitative measure, the amygdala makes up a very small portion of the human brain. Yet there is virtually no psychiatric or neurological disorder in which it has not been suggested to play an important role.

Why is the amygdala so popular in neuropsychiatry? And why edit a book on it? The answer to these questions is that despite its small size, the amygdala is one of the most densely connected structures in the brain. This feature of connectivity, in turn, fits very well with hypotheses about not only psychiatric illnesses (that they are disconnection or misconnection syndromes in many cases), but also the functions that the amygdala is thought to implement. First and foremost among these latter hypotheses is that the amygdala helps orchestrate global organismic states that we call "emotions"—states that are pervasively dysfunctional in psychiatric illness, but that also show considerable variation across individual differences in the healthy population. In short, the reason for interest in the amygdala derives from its pervasive role: In implementing emotional states, it modulates nearly every cognitive function one can think of.

Much of what we know about the function of the amygdala has come from studies in which it is damaged in one way or another, and the resulting alterations of behavior are evaluated. There are dangers in this approach, since it is clear that all behaviors are subserved by many brain regions linked together in multiple functional systems. On the one hand, the brain does not resign itself to the damage of one of the component structures but attempts to reorganize in order to optimize its ability to deal with a complex environment. On the other hand, very convergent story lines for the function of the amygdala emanate from lesion studies in both humans and experimental animals. While the era of permanent lesions is rapidly giving way to strategies for genetically mediated transient inactivation, the hypotheses that are being tested with these new techniques have arisen from lesion studies.

Our goal in this book was to take stock of what has been learned from humans and nonhuman experimental animals that are living their lives without a functioning amygdala. We decided early on to focus primarily on research carried out in human patients and in nonhuman primates. However, it is clear that much of what is known about the amygdala has come from research in rodents. To represent this body of research, Sarro and Sullivan (Chapter 4) summarize their research on the role of the amygdala in the early development of behavior. Kim, Choi, and Lee (Chapter 5) provide an overview of their use of novel approaches toward quantifying fear in rodents in a controlled but naturalistic foraging task.

Since the book is heavily focused on primate studies, Schumann, Vargas, and Lee (Chapter 2) remind us of the complex neuroanatomical organization of the amygdaloid complex. Amaral (Chapter 3) provides a historical summary of the studies carried out in nonhuman primates that played a major part in our current appreciation of the role of the amygdala in emotional regulation. He also discusses the period of psychosurgery in which human patients received bilateral amygdalectomy for control of seizures and unmanageable behavior.

There are a number of chapters related to nonhuman primate research. Bliss-Moreau, Moadab, and Amaral (Chapter 6) and Bachevalier, Sanchez, Raper, Stephens, and Wallen (Chapter 7) describe studies in which rhesus monkeys receive lesions very early in life and are then raised in seminaturalistic environments with their mothers and social groups. These chapters raise the issue of plasticity and change in the effects of these early lesions as the animals mature. The effects of losing amygdala function as an adult in relation to anxiety are discussed by Oler, Fox, Shackman, and Kalin (Chapter 8). Murray and Rhodes (Chapter 9) explore the consequences relative to cognitive and emotional behavior of losing amygdala function in the mature rhesus monkey.

Several chapters in the book focus on patients who have the mysterious Urbach–Wiethe syndrome, which can often result in relatively selective, bilateral damage of the amygdala. Feinstein, Adolphs, and Tranel (Chapter 1) present the human perspective of living without an amygdala through interviews with patient S. M., who has been studied by this group for several decades. Adolphs (Chapter 10) reviews data from several patients with Urbach–Wiethe syndrome and indicates that there are several challenges for the future of this research, including better delineation of the lesions, concurrent neuroimaging to quantify systems-level changes following amygdala lesions, and comparisons across different ages. Van Honk, Terburg, Thornton, Stein, and Morgan (Chapter 12) describe their studies of South African patients with Urbach–Wiethe syndrome and begin to raise the issue of whether alteration of function can be localized to one or more regions of the amygdala based on patients with subnuclear damage. And Patin and Hurlemann (Chapter 11) again raise the issue of compensatory adaptations after damage by studying monozygotic twins who are affected by Urbach–Wiethe syndrome.

There are relatively few individuals who have bilateral lesions of the amygdala due to disease, but unilateral amygdalectomy is still a common practice for the alleviation of epilepsy. Todd, Anderson, and Phelps (Chapter 13) describe one patient who apparently had unilateral damage to the amygdala on one side, then the removal of the opposite amygdala when she was 47 years old for treatment of her seizure disorder. They recount some of the sequelae of this loss of amygdala function in an adult.

The book ends with a synthesis chapter by Monk and Pine (Chapter 14), which delves into the role of the amygdala in psychiatric disorders. The Epilogue by Amaral and Adolphs looks back at what we have learned from lesions of the amygdala, what have been lost opportunities, and where the future of amygdala research may be heading.

We asked the authors to present their material in a way that would be accessible to researchers, clinicians, and the lay audience. Taken together, these chapters provide a glimpse into the worlds of individuals who have lost the ability to detect dangers in their environment and how that impacts their lives. They also tell a story of how the brain compensates for brain damage, particularly when it occurs early in life. However, the adaptation is never complete, and loss of the amygdala, with its unique structure and connections with other brain regions, has a lifelong impact on the individual.

Contents

CHAPTER 1

A Tale of Survival from the World of Patient S. M.

JUSTIN S. FEINSTEIN
RALPH ADOLPHS
DANIEL TRANEL

Patient S. M. is one of the most renowned lesion cases in the history of neuropsychology. Her focal bilateral amygdala damage has led to a host of behavioral impairments that have been well-documented across dozens of research publications. This chapter provides an overview of S. M.'s seminal contributions to the study of brain–behavior relationships, with an emphasis on the role of the human amygdala in the emotion of fear. For the first time, we also provide a detailed exploration of the real-world ramifications of living life without an amygdala. For S. M., the consequences have been severe. Her behavioral deficits and impoverished experience of fear repeatedly lead her back to the very situations she should be avoiding, highlighting the amygdala's indispensable role in promoting survival by compelling the organism away from danger in the external world. In stark contrast, threats arising from the internal world of S. M.'s body are capable of inducing a primal state of fear and panic, even in the absence of a functioning amygdala. The unique case of S. M. reveals that the brain contains specialized circuits for fear and multiple fear pathways, notably, an interoceptive pathway that bypasses the amygdala and an exteroceptive pathway that requires the amygdala. So much of the extant neuroscience research investigating fear has focused almost exclusively on the exteroceptive pathway. If there is one final lesson that S. M. can teach the world, it is that we need to refocus our efforts toward exploring the relatively uncharted terrain of interoceptive fear.

The year was 1968 and the world was in a state of pandemonium. Amid the chaos of wars, protests, and assassinations, a young psychiatrist by the name of Arthur Kling began a series of experiments that had never been tried before, and to this day have never been tried again. The aim was simple: Capture a group of wild monkeys, surgically remove their amygdalae, release them back into the wild, and see if they could survive. In the first experiment (Dicks, Myers, & Kling, 1969), the investigators studied a group of rhesus monkeys on Cayo Santiago, a small island just off the coast of Puerto Rico. Upon their return to the wild, the amygdalectomized monkeys were quickly alienated from their social group, often times attacked and chased into the ocean by the other monkeys. Within 2 weeks, all of the older amygdalectomized monkeys were found dead, either from starvation, attack wounds, or having drowned in the ocean. It was concluded that the amygdalectomized monkeys "appear retarded in their ability to foresee and avoid dangerous confrontations. . . . they are vulnerable to attack and unable to compete for food" (p. 71). Meanwhile, on the other side of the world, Kling carried out another experiment (Kling, Lancaster, & Benitone, 1970), this time in wild vervet monkeys living along the Zambezi River in Africa, only a few miles upstream from the great Victoria Falls. Once released, the amygdalectomized monkeys immediately isolated themselves from the other monkeys by hiding in the low brush or climbing to the high branches of a nearby tree. Despite an abundance of natural food and water nearby, the monkeys were never observed eating or drinking. Within 7 hours, all of the amygdalectomized monkeys were literally lost in the wild, never to be seen again. Years later, Dr. Kling speculated that the amygdalectomized monkeys "had been taken by predators" (Kling, 1986). Both field experiments were over almost as soon as they began. The answer was clear: Living without an amygdala does not bode well for survival.

Around the same time that Dr. Kling's team of observers had given up hope of ever finding the missing amygdalectomized monkeys, an experiment of nature was already under way in America. No monkeys would be required this time, however, since this new experiment was being carried out in a living human being. There would also be no need for any invasive brain surgeries. Instead, the amygdala was naturally and selectively damaged by an extremely rare genetic mutation. The damage would take many years and even decades to unfold. In the winter of 1968, as Dr. Kling was scouring through the forests of Zambia for signs of survival, a young girl who would become known to the world as "Patient S. M." was celebrating her third birthday. Little did S. M. know at the time, but her life would soon be catapulted into a trajectory akin to that of Dr. Kling's amygdalectomized monkeys. A key difference is that somehow, someway, S. M. has managed to stay alive, and in 2015 she celebrated her 50th birthday. This chapter provides a rare glimpse into the life of S. M. and her half-century struggle for survival.

The Case of Patient S. M.

Shortly after birth, the doctors could tell something was amiss. Whereas most babies have no trouble screaming and crying, S. M. could barely emit a muffled whimper. Doctors soon discovered abnormal thickening of the tissue around her vocal cords, as well as characteristic lesions on her skin, leading them to an eventual diagnosis of a rare autosomal recessive genetic condition known as Urbach–Wiethe disease (UWD) or lipoid proteinosis (Hofer, 1973). The rarity of this genetic condition cannot be overstated, as there have only been several hundred reported cases, worldwide, over the past century. S. M.'s genetic diagnosis was officially confirmed by Dr. Wolfram Kunz at the University of Bonn, who sequenced S. M.'s DNA and found a single nucleotide deletion in exon 6 of the gene encoding her extracellular matrix protein 1 (*ECM1*). Her particular genetic mutation (a homozygous 507delT/507delT) predicts a more severe clinical phenotype (Hamada et al., 2003) and, indeed, S. M.'s condition is more severe than most other patients with UWD (see van Honk, Terburg, Thornton, Stein, & Morgan, Chapter 12, and Patin & Hurlemann, Chapter 11, this volume). Hoarseness of voice is one of the disease's cardinal symptoms, and S. M. has spent the bulk of her life being alienated and belittled by her peers for sounding so different. She also has to undergo laser surgery several times a year to ensure that the buildup of hyaline deposits around her vocal cords and throat does not obstruct her airway. The condition has also affected her skin, causing excessive scarring and a waxy appearance that makes her look much older than her actual age. S. M. finds this aspect of her condition to be particularly upsetting and openly admits that her rapidly aging skin has taken a toll on her self-esteem and makes her feel unattractive. In recent years, her overall state of health has been deteriorating, and it appears that her disease is progressing more rapidly as she ages, infiltrating her tongue, gums, teeth, lips, eyelids, tear ducts, and uterus, and causing a host of complications, some of which we discuss later on.

Beyond these widespread systemic effects on S. M.'s body, the disease has also spread into her brain. In one of the most perplexing medical mysteries of our time, mutations in the *ECM1* gene can lead to calcifications that infiltrate the brain and selectively destroy the amygdala, bilaterally, while leaving the rest of the brain largely unaffected. And while there have been some isolated case reports of patients with damage to other brain regions, the disease's predilection for calcifying the amygdala is striking. This is precisely what happened to S. M., who has one of the most complete amygdala lesions ever reported with UWD (Figure 1.1; see Adolphs, Chapter 10, this volume).

On November 7, 1986, Dr. Daniel Tranel met S. M. for the very first time when a neurologist referred her to the Benton Neuropsychology

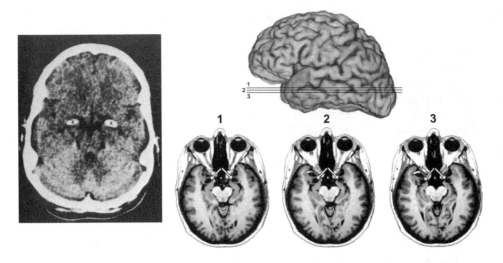

FIGURE 1.1. S. M.'s brain. On the left is the original computed tomography (CT) scan of S. M.'s brain, taken in 1986, when she was 20 years old. By this point in life, her amygdala lesions were clearly present, as evidenced by the bilateral bean-shaped hyperdense signals (X marks the spots). Over 20 years later, much more detailed magnetic resonance imaging (MRI) scans of S. M.'s brain reveal circumscribed bilateral amygdala lesions appearing as vacant black holes underneath the white arrows. The lesions affect not only gray matter in the local vicinity but also fibers of passage and tissue immediately adjacent to the amygdala, including the anterior entorhinal cortex. Both the hippocampus and parts of the extended amygdala (e.g., bed nucleus of the stria terminalis) appear to be intact. Other key neural structures related to emotion also appear to be intact, including the insular cortices, the ventromedial prefrontal cortices, and the hypothalamus and brainstem (including the periaqueductal gray).

Clinic at the University of Iowa. She was 20 years old, and what started as a simple neuropsychological evaluation quickly turned into a lifelong project. S. M. was subsequently inducted into the Iowa Neurological Patient Registry established at the University of Iowa by Drs. Antonio and Hanna Damasio. The registry has now accrued over 3,000 lesion patients, but at the time of her induction, S. M. was patient number 46.

After viewing S. M.'s first brain scan (Figure 1.1), it was evident that her focal and symmetrical amygdala lesions were unlike anything that had been seen before. It was not uncommon to test patients with unilateral amygdala lesions stemming from stroke or neurosurgical resection. On rare occasions, we might test a patient with bilateral amygdala lesions secondary to herpes simplex encephalitis, but their damage would invariably impact other brain structures outside of the amygdala. S. M.

was the first patient we had ever met with bilateral amygdala lesions that appeared to be largely confined to the amygdala.

Dr. Tranel immediately began testing S. M. to illuminate the impairments that could arise from such a circumscribed lesion. The results of her initial neuroimaging and neuropsychological tests were published a few years later (Tranel & Hyman, 1990), in what would be the first in a long line of S. M.-related publications. Hundreds of experiments over the course of nearly three decades of testing have made S. M. one of the best-characterized neuropsychological case studies of all time. The corpus of research built around S. M. has led to a host of discoveries across a broad range of domains (Table 1.1). The implications of this body of work have been far-reaching, impacting not just the fields of neuropsychology and neuroscience, but also philosophy, sociology, law, economics, and anthropology. And of perhaps greatest importance, the field of psychiatry has benefited immensely from this research as the case of S. M. has contributed important clues about the etiology of a number of different conditions, especially along the spectrums of anxiety and autism.

For more details about published research on S. M., the reader is pointed to several review chapters that have been written on this topic (Adolphs & Tranel, 2000; Adolphs & Tranel, 2004; Buchanan, Tranel, & Adolphs, 2009; see Adolphs, Chapter 10, this volume). Two of these chapters (Adolphs & Tranel, 2000; Buchanan et al., 2009) also contain detailed descriptions of S. M.'s neuropsychological profile, which has remained generally stable over the years, and in line with expectations given her educational and occupational background. Most of her test performances are within the normal range on standardized measures of IQ, memory, language, and perception, with some noted weaknesses on tests tapping nonverbal visual memory and phonemic fluency. In recent years, we have found signs of decline in her verbal memory, but not yet near the scope or severity that would be indicative of dementia. Overall, her cognitive functioning remains relatively preserved, and she continues to live independently. In terms of occupational functioning, S. M. has spent the majority of her adult life unemployed and surviving off of government assistance in the form of monthly disability checks. The only exception was a 3-year period during the late 1990s when S. M. worked as a security guard, a job she specifically chose as part of a welfare-to-work program. She claims to have enjoyed working as a security guard but was laid off when her employer closed down the building where she worked.

The case of S. M. provides a compelling example of the functional consequences of living life without an amygdala. The other chapters in this book highlight additional cases with bilateral amygdala damage, providing the most comprehensive picture to date of the various behavioral manifestations that can develop following focal disruption to the core

TABLE 1.1. A List of Peer-Reviewed Publications That Tested Patient S. M.

Domain	Authors (year)	Journal	Citations
Background assessment	Tranel & Hyman (1990)	*Archives of Neurology*	228
	Boes et al. (2011)	*Social Cognitive and Affective Neuroscience*	7
Emotion recognition	Adolphs et al. (1994)	*Nature*	2,103
	Adolphs et al. (1995)	*Journal of Neuroscience*	1,169
	Adolphs et al. (1999b)	*Neuropsychologia*	812
	Adolphs & Tranel (1999)	*Neuropsychologia*	181
	Adolphs et al. (2005a)	*Nature*	1,000
	Atkinson et al. (2007)	*Neuropsychologia*	59
	Gosselin et al. (2007)	*Neuropsychologia*	148
	Spezio et al. (2007)	*Journal of Neuroscience*	142
	Tsuchiya et al. (2009)	*Nature Neuroscience*	137
Emotional memory	Adolphs et al. (1997)	*Learning and Memory*	411
	Adolphs et al. (2005b)	*Nature Neuroscience*	227
	Bechara et al. (1995)	*Science*	1,318
	Bechara et al. (2003)	*Annals of the New York Academy of Sciences*	450
Emotional experience and arousal	Adolphs et al. (1999a)	*Psychological Science*	238
	Feinstein et al. (2011)	*Current Biology*	156
	Feinstein et al. (2013)	*Nature Neuroscience*	79
	Glascher & Adolphs (2003)	*Journal of Neuroscience*	309
	Tranel et al. (2006)	*Cognitive Neuropsychiatry*	69
Neuroeconomics and decision making	Bechara et al. (1999)	*Journal of Neuroscience*	1,640
	De Martino et al. (2010)	*Proceedings of the National Academy of Sciences USA*	178
	Hampton et al. (2007)	*Neuron*	68
	Shiv et al. (2005)	*Psychological Science*	394
Social cognition and behavior	Adolphs et al. (1998)	*Nature*	1,238
	Adolphs et al. (2002)	*Journal of Cognitive Neuroscience*	449
	Birmingham et al. (2011)	*Social Neuroscience*	18
	Heberlein & Adolphs (2004)	*Proceedings of the National Academy of Sciences USA*	137
	Kennedy & Adolphs (2010)	*Neuropsychologia*	49
	Kennedy et al. (2009)	*Nature Neuroscience*	171
	Paul et al. (2010)	*Journal of Neurodevelopmental Disorders*	38
	Wang et al. (2015)	*Social Cognitive and Affective Neuroscience*	8

Note. The studies are broken down into the different domains that were tested. The number of citations was calculated in December of 2015, using *Google Scholar*.

circuitry of the amygdala. When comparing different cases, it is important to recognize that a multitude of factors can fundamentally alter the behavioral manifestations of a lesion, including the etiology and developmental time course of the lesion, the extent of damage, the brain's compensation following the damage, and the unique personality and set of life experiences of each individual lesion case (see Adolphs, Chapter 10, and Patin & Hurlemann, Chapter 11, this volume). S. M.'s amygdala lesion is developmental in nature, likely emerging around the age of 10 and slowly progressing over the course of adolescence and adulthood (Feinstein, Adolphs, Damasio, & Tranel, 2011). Due to the critical involvement of the amygdala in emotional learning, the behavioral presentation of a developmental lesion may differ from that of an adult-onset lesion (Bechara, Damasio, & Damasio, 2003; Hamann et al., 1996), and this certainly appears to be the case for S. M. (e.g., see Figure 1.2). Even when directly comparing S. M. to other developmental lesion cases with the same etiology, there may still be fundamental behavioral differences related to the greater extent of amygdala damage found in S. M.'s brain (see Van Honk et al., Chapter 12, this volume). The borders of S. M.'s lesion appear to extend slightly beyond the amygdala, encroaching on tissue in the anterior entorhinal cortex and adjacent white matter, and in recent years, there is emerging evidence of small additional lesions outside of the medial temporal lobe (Feinstein et al., 2011). It is also worth reiterating that the lesion likely includes fibers of passage within the amygdala—in this respect, when compared to nonhuman animals, S. M.'s lesion is more comparable to aspiration-type lesions rather than ibotenic acid lesions (Meunier, Bachevalier, Murray, Málková, & Mishkin, 1999). The severity of her lesion presentation is consistent with the severity of her clinical phenotype, and both of these factors are likely playing a role in S. M.'s unique behavioral presentation. As previously discussed, UWD is a systemic condition, and it is plausible that certain somatic symptoms (e.g., hoarseness of voice and aging skin) may have affected S. M.'s social behavior independently of her amygdala damage. These points notwithstanding, rare lesion patients, such as S. M., offer the opportunity to elucidate the "neurobiological" definition of concepts such as emotion, fear, and psychiatric disease. This book and its fascinating collection of lesion cases provide an invaluable road map for deciphering the critical behavioral functions of the amygdala.

Exteroceptive Fear

When it comes to survival, no other emotion is as imperative as fear. Across humanity, fear is universally recognized and experienced, and across the animal kingdom, fear-like behaviors such as freezing and withdrawal are

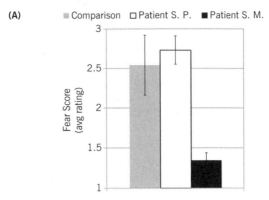

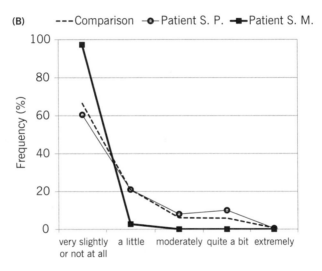

FIGURE 1.2. Fear following developmental versus adult-onset bilateral amygdala damage. S. M. (developmental lesion) reported experiencing considerably less fear than patient S. P. (adult-onset lesion), a woman with bilateral amygdala lesions stemming from a right medial temporal lobectomy (at the age of 48), along with reactive gliosis of unknown extent in her left amygdala (see Todd, Anderson, & Phelps, Chapter 13, this volume). Both patients completed state and trait versions of the Positive and Negative Affect Schedule (PANAS; Watson, Clark, & Tellegen, 1988). Data for S. P. and 20 healthy comparison participants were reported in Anderson and Phelps (2002), in which a "fear score" was computed using five PANAS items (afraid, scared, nervous, jittery, and distressed). We computed the same fear score for S. M. (A) Trait fear: Mean trait fear in S. M. and S. P. on a scale ranging from 1 ("very slightly or not at all") to 5 ("extremely"). Means were derived by averaging the scores across multiple administrations of the trait version of the PANAS; S. M. completed seven administrations over a 3-year period, and S. P. completed three administrations over a 1-year period. All error bars represent the standard error of the mean. (B) State fear: Frequency distribution of state fear ratings in S. M. and S. P., reflecting how often each patient reported experiencing different magnitudes of the five fear-related items on the PANAS. S. M. completed the state version of the PANAS multiple times a day over a 3-month period, and S. P. completed it daily over a 30-day period.

ubiquitous (Anderson & Adolphs, 2014). Consequently, fear is the most extensively studied emotion in all of science, and the field of neuroscience is no exception (Adolphs, 2013; Feinstein, 2013). In this regard, one of S. M.'s most seminal contributions has been the remarkable selectivity of her emotional deficits to the realm of "exteroceptive fear," which encompasses all manner of environmental threats conveyed to the brain via the *external senses* of vision, hearing, smell, and touch.

The first discovery came in 1994, when we found that S. M. was unable to recognize the emotion of fear in another person's face (Adolphs, Tranel, Damsio, & Damasio, 1994, 1995; Adolphs et al., 1999b). In contrast, her recognition of other facial expressions was generally intact, with the exception of some difficulty recognizing surprise, an emotion that contains many of the same facial features as fear. Control tests showed that S. M.'s profound impairment in the realm of fear recognition could not be accounted for by a basic perceptual impairment (e.g., she is able to accurately discriminate and recognize the identity of faces) or conceptual impairment (e.g., she understands the concept of fear and has intact knowledge of what the word "fear" means; Adolphs et al., 1994, 1995; Feinstein et al., 2011). Follow-up experiments revealed that a major reason for S. M.'s difficulty in recognizing fear in faces is because she fails to orient her attention to the eyes, which in the case of fear are opened wide with upper eyelids raised— the telltale sign that a person is scared (Adolphs et al., 2005a). Interestingly, S. M.'s fear recognition deficit extends into the social domain, where she is severely impaired at judging the approachability and trustworthiness of other people, often rating the most unsavory characters as both approachable and trustworthy (Adolphs, Tranel, & Damasio, 1998). S. M. also has no sense of personal space and feels no discomfort or unease when other people are standing in close proximity, even during the highly awkward situation of standing nose-to-nose with a total stranger (Kennedy, Gläscher, Tyszka, & Adolphs, 2009). Consistent with lesion work in nonhuman animals, S. M. has a severe impairment in fear conditioning through both visual and auditory channels (Bechara et al., 1995). In contrast, she is able to mount a normal skin conductance response (SCR) to unconditioned stimuli, such as a 100 decibel boat horn (Bechara et al., 1995). On the Iowa Gambling Task, S. M. failed to generate anticipatory SCRs prior to making disadvantageous choices, and she also failed to generate SCRs in response to monetary rewards and punishments (Bechara, Damasio, Damasio, & Lee, 1999), a finding that may partially explain her notable lack of loss aversion when making monetary gambles (De Martino, Camerer, & Adolphs, 2010). Taken together, these studies suggest that S. M. has great difficulty accurately recognizing and processing exteroceptive information that is conducive to survival. She also appears to be impaired in generating the appropriate response to this exteroceptive information, irrespective of whether the response is physiological (e.g., a conditioned SCR), cognitive (e.g., judging the trust-worthiness of a person), or behavioral (e.g., regulating interpersonal distance).

Given S. M.'s diverse array of fear-related deficits detected in the laboratory, we became very interested in learning about how such deficits might manifest in the real world. In 2003, we started an in-depth case study of S. M. that lasted for the better part of a decade. Beyond just exploring her behavior in everyday life, we were also intrigued by the prospect of assessing her emotional experience (Tranel, Gullickson, Koch, & Adolphs, 2006). In particular, we wanted to know whether her amygdala damage had in some way impaired her ability to feel fear. While lesion studies in nonhuman animals have been largely confined to the examination of "threat-induced defensive reactions" (LeDoux, 2013), S. M. provided the unique opportunity to examine fear as a conscious emotional experience. This was an exciting new avenue of research, but it came with a host of challenges. "Feelings," by definition, are subjective, and hidden within the vaults of consciousness. There are no objective indices that can definitively reveal the content of another person's conscious experience of emotion, and currently the only way to validly and reliably determine how someone is feeling is by asking them (Barrett, 2004; Watson, 2000). Unfortunately, self-report has its own set of limitations, the least of which are the inherent demand characteristics of the experiment and the possibility that a person is not accurately portraying how he or she really feels. To date, there have only been two other studies that attempted to measure the subjective experience of emotion in patients with amygdala damage (Sprengelmeyer et al., 1999; Anderson & Phelps, 2002). Both studies relied on a single self-report questionnaire for assessing fear (e.g., Figure 1.2), and neither study directly exposed the patient to any fear-inducing stimuli.

From the outset, we decided to take a more comprehensive and systematic approach to answering the question as to whether or not S. M. was capable of feeling fear (Figure 1.3). Instead of relying on a single measure of self-report, we had S. M. complete a battery of eight different fear measures, multiple times over the course of several years, with questions probing a wide range of different fear experiences from both a state and trait perspective. We also used experience sampling to capture S. M.'s emotional experience in real time as it unfolded in her natural environment. S. M. was provided with a small handheld computer that she took with her everywhere she went over the course of a 3-month period. At three random times each day, an alarm in the computer would ring, prompting S. M. to rate her current emotional state across a set of 50 different emotion terms, covering a whole spectrum of different emotional experiences, including fear. In order to mitigate the risks of relying solely on self-report, we also collected detailed behavioral observations while

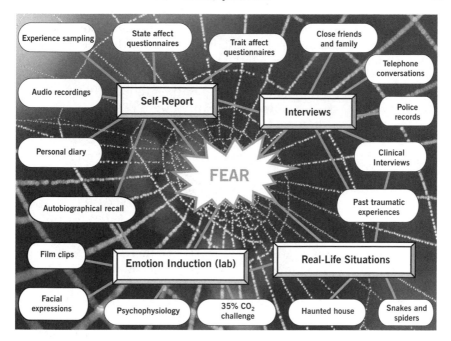

FIGURE 1.3. Assessing the tangled web of fear in S. M. There are a multitude of methods for assessing the expression and experience of fear, both inside and outside the laboratory. This diagram provides an overview of the various methods we utilized in our case study of S. M. Rather than viewing any single method as being conclusive in and of itself, we looked for consistency across methods. This comprehensive approach allows for a more fine-grained analysis of how fear is expressed and experienced in different contexts and time frames, while greatly enhancing the overall ecological validity.

directly exposing S. M. to realistic and ecologically valid inducers of fear, including 10 different horror films, real live snakes and tarantulas, and a world-famous haunted house. Finally, we spent many hours querying S. M. about her past, searching for any experiences that may have induced fear. We also scoured through her personal diary, spoke with close friends and family members, and examined police records. In 2011, the results from this in-depth case study were published in *Current Biology* (Feinstein et al., 2011).

Across the wide range of different tasks and approaches, S. M. consistently experienced a marked absence of fear, even when directly exposed to fear-provoking stimuli. The large selection of horror films all failed to induce fear, yet S. M. had no difficulty expressing or experiencing a range of other emotions when viewing a different set of films, including sadness, happiness, anger, disgust, and surprise. More than just a loss of fear, her behavior was conspicuously lacking in avoidance, and instead featured an excess of exploratory approach. For example, at the haunted house, S. M. voluntarily anointed herself the leader of our group, excitedly guiding five strangers and two researchers down dark hallways and into scare traps. S. M. would continually run ahead of the group, yelling, "This way guys, follow me!" as she summoned us with a wave of her arm before jetting down another dark passageway. The whole experience felt as if we were being led into battle. Yet, if this were a real battle, our group would not have survived very long. There was no caution or hesitation in S. M.'s approach. She always seemed to take the most direct path into harm's way. When an elaborately dressed actor would suddenly appear from behind a wall to scare us, the rest of the group would jump backwards and scream. S. M. never screamed. She never jumped backwards. She never flinched. The repeated attempts at scaring her all failed, and with the exception of a very loud explosion, she was never startled either. Instead, she would gaze with amusement at the monstrous creatures, smiling or laughing at them, and in one instance, even scaring an actor dressed as Hellraiser when she poked him in the head because she was "curious" as to what the mask would feel like. Throughout the haunted house, she explicitly denied feeling any fear, but did report a high level of excitement and enthusiasm on par with how she remembered feeling while riding a rollercoaster. S. M. has also told us, on a number of occasions, that she really wants to try skydiving. While these observations insinuate a high-level of "sensation seeking," it is worth noting that in everyday life S. M. rarely engages in purposeful risk-taking behavior, perhaps due to her inability to afford such activities.

Based on the results from the case study (Feinstein et al., 2011), it became apparent that S. M.'s experience of fear was lacking. During the 3-months of experience sampling, she rated all of the fear terms at the lowest possible level. Likewise, she reported an impoverished experience of fear across the entire battery of fear measures. In contrast to her paucity of fear as an adult, S. M. remembers experiencing several fearful incidents as a young child, all occurring before the age of 10 and likely before the onset of her amygdala damage (Feinstein et al., 2011). One incident involved a large and vicious Doberman pinscher that trapped her in a corner and caused her to feel "gut-wrenching scared," suggesting that S. M. understands, at an experiential level, what fear is supposed to feel like. As an adult, S. M. denies experiencing any intense states of fear despite the fact that she has faced numerous situations that would be considered fear-inducing or even traumatic in nature. It is evident that she has great difficulty detecting looming threats in her environment and learning to avoid dangerous situations, features of her behavior that have in all likelihood contributed to her high incidence of life-threatening encounters.

Quite strikingly, during the aftermath of a traumatic event, S. M. reports no signs of avoidance, hyperarousal, or emotional reexperiencing. Indeed, S. M. appears to be largely immune to the devastating effects of posttraumatic stress. Interestingly, a group of war veterans who survived penetrating brain injuries during battle that damaged their amygdalae also failed to develop posttraumatic stress disorder (PTSD; Koenigs et al., 2008). Without fear, S. M.'s distress lacks the deep heartfelt intensity endured by most survivors of trauma. Such an interpretation is consistent with a previous study (Tranel et al., 2006), in which two experienced clinical psychologists interviewed S. M. without having any knowledge of her condition. To the psychologists, S. M. came across as a "survivor," as being "resilient" and even "heroic" in the way that she has dealt with adversity in her life. Taken together, these findings suggest that the amygdala is a critical site for triggering a state of fear when an individual encounters threatening stimuli in the external environment. Many different cognitive, autonomic, and behavioral changes comprise a state of fear, and the induction of such a state is required in order to experience a feeling of fear. Thus, we view S. M.'s lack of experienced fear as a direct consequence of her failure to mount a normal fear response to external threats.

Survival in "the Wild"

Far from the fringing forests of Zambia and the ocean shores of Cayo Santiago lies the American Midwest, where S. M. was born and raised, and where she lives to this very day. While certainly not *wild* in the traditional sense of the word, S. M.'s environment has been challenging, to say the least. Given her striking deficits in the realm of exteroceptive fear, we have often wondered how S. M. has managed to survive, especially in light of the fact that she has spent her entire adult life living on her own. When Dr. Kling's amygdalectomized monkeys were let back into the wild, it was only a matter of days, and sometimes weeks, before they met their demise, often related to starvation, social abandonment, assault, or being attacked by a predator (Dicks et al., 1969; Kling et al., 1970). As it turns out, S. M. has faced her fair share of all these predicaments. Below, we discuss each of these situations in more detail. The details were gathered over the course of hundreds of hours of observation and conversation with S. M. across a range of different contexts, including the laboratory, her home, and over the phone.

Food and Money

Living in a poor area of the country and sustaining herself with government assistance, S. M. has repeatedly found herself in need of food.

Interestingly, these dry periods fail to trigger the sort of desperation that one might expect. In a manner reminiscent of amygdalectomized monkeys, S. M. does not seem very motivated to find food during times of hunger, adding further support to the notion that the amygdala plays an important role in the regulation of feeding behavior (Cai, Haubensak, Anthony, & Anderson, 2014). In this context, it is important to emphasize that she is by no means anorexic, and she will gladly eat food if it is easily accessible. However, her food preferences are rather discriminative, mostly limited to sugary treats (e.g., chocolate and artificially sweetened juices and soda) and foods that can be easily chewed and swallowed (e.g., pasta and mashed potatoes). Her lack of motivation for food is primarily evident during those times when she is out of food *and* out of money. During these dry periods, she has gone entire days without eating, and typically only asks for assistance once her hunger has reached rather extreme levels. What's more, many of these episodes of hunger could have easily been prevented had she made wiser decisions on how she spent her money, a likely consequence of her deficit in loss aversion (De Martino et al., 2010). For S. M., money comes and goes very quickly, with little forethought about the consequences. Left on her own, S. M. will habitually spend her money on frivolous items that are clearly not necessary for survival. For example, one month, with only a few dollars remaining, S. M. decided to purchase a "ring back" tone for her phone, an entirely useless feature that allows the caller to hear a song being played instead of the traditional ring tone. Similarly, S. M. will often buy very expensive food for her pets, even at the expense of not being able to eat herself. It is evident that S. M. does not have a good conceptual understanding about the value of money, and despite repeated attempts, she appears incapable of spending her money wisely, perhaps a by-product of her disturbed circuitry in the ventromedial prefrontal cortex (Boes et al., 2011; Hampton, Adolphs, Tyszka, & O'Doherty, 2007). In order to help remedy her repeated financial dilemmas, we have now requested that a payee help manage all of her money. For the most part, this new arrangement has succeeded in ensuring that S. M. always has money available to buy food. Sadly, without this extra help, starvation would not have been outside the realm of possibility.

Social Relationships and Prosocial Behavior

S. M. has never been able to maintain a long-term relationship, intimate or otherwise, and this includes members of her own family. She raised three children as a single mother, but rarely speaks to any of her children (all of whom are now adults). Her first child was conceived at the age of 18 with her first sexual partner, a man who quickly abandoned S. M. as soon as he discovered she was pregnant. In her early 20s, S. M. had an unstable relationship with an abusive man who was the biological father of her other two children, and who left her while she was pregnant with her last child. In her mid-20s, she was married to a man for less than a year, a marriage that ended in a divorce following a harrowing incident (described later in the chapter). Since the divorce, S. M. has not been in any other serious romantic relationships.

Part of S. M.'s difficulty in maintaining a long-term relationship stems from her overly trusting nature and lack of interpersonal space (Adolphs et al., 1998; Kennedy et al., 2009), leaving her unable to discern when someone is trying to take advantage of her and unable to understand the social etiquette of how to build a relationship slowly over time. Another part stems from S. M.'s personality and her "tendency to be somewhat coquettish and disinhibited" during social interactions (Tranel & Hyman, 1990). For example, during conversations S. M. has a tendency to speak in hypersexual undertones, which can leave the uninitiated feeling somewhat uncomfortable (of note, we have never witnessed overt hypersexual behavior). Sadly, most people, including her own family members, have great difficulty accepting S. M. for who she is (i.e., the way she speaks, the way she looks, and all her behavioral eccentricities).

Over the years, we have witnessed many friendships develop, only to fall apart. The typical pattern goes as follows: (1) When a stranger first meets S. M., it is not uncommon for her to divulge very personal details and discuss intimate topics, leaving the stranger with the impression that he or she is having a conversation with someone they have known for a very long time; (2) if the stranger reciprocates, he or she will quickly be swept up as S. M.'s new best friend, and asked to perform myriad favors, such as helping her with chores, giving her rides, and being willing to chat at all hours of the day; and (3) when the newly anointed friend is not willing to conform to S. M.'s rapid pace and all of her requests, and asks for some space, S. M. has a tendency to take it very personally and the friendship usually dissolves shortly thereafter. S. M.'s lack of a social circle is in line with recent work showing that greater amygdala volume is correlated with a larger social network (Bickart, Wright, Dautoff, Dickerson, & Barrett, 2010), and is also consistent with the reduced social network found in another bilateral amygdala lesion patient, B. G. (Becker et al., 2012; Patin & Hurlemann, Chapter 11). Based on these observations, it appears that one outcome of living life without an amygdala is abandonment and social isolation, conditions that conflict with S. M.'s extraverted nature. In the first article ever written about S. M., it was noted that she "has occasionally reported depressive symptomatology, related to difficult situational exigencies" (Tranel & Hyman, 1990, p. 350). For S. M., there is nothing more difficult than the loneliness of having no social circle and the feeling of being abandoned by the people who you love the most.

This should in no way insinuate that S. M. is not a good friend. In fact, she will do almost anything to help a friend in need. She once helped care for an older adult lady (Miss B.) who lived all by herself and needed some extra help due to her obesity and severe diabetic neuropathy. Every week S. M. would walk several miles to take Miss B. her groceries, help her out around the house, and keep her company. It was obvious that S. M. received great joy knowing that someone else needed her. One evening, as we were speaking to S. M. on the phone, a severe thunderstorm came rolling into her town, with warnings of a possible tornado. The thunder was so loud that we could hear it over the phone, shaking S. M.'s building. A few minutes later, while we were still on the phone, Miss B. called S. M. on her other line and told her that the power had just gone out at her house and she needed help. Before we had time to persuade her otherwise, S. M. was outside in the middle of the storm, walking over to Miss B.'s house. When we spoke to her later that night to make sure she was okay, S. M. told us that the storm was quite intense, with a heavy downpour of rain, strong winds, and streaks of lightning flashing everywhere. It was evident from her voice that she found the whole experience to be quite exciting. Remarkably, she denied feeling scared, even by the loud booms of thunder. The fact that she was voluntarily walking outside during such a vicious storm supports her assertion. When queried, S. M. was well aware of the dangers of being outside but reported being glad to have gone because, when she finally arrived, she found Miss B. huddled in the corner of her home crying. Even S. M. was able to recognize how scared Miss B. was. It took a while to calm her down, but eventually she fell asleep in S. M.'s arms, the fearless holding the fearer. The storm finally passed.

At this juncture, it is worth taking a moment to comment on an important observation: S. M. is *not* a psychopath. Case in point is her selfless and compassionate behavior toward Miss B. And while many psychopaths may indeed have amygdalar dysfunction and a lack of exteroceptive fear (Blair, 2008; Marsh, 2013), S. M. reveals that these factors may not be the causal ingredients driving the psychopathic behavior. Certainly, an outright lesion of the amygdala is not the correct neurological model for psychopathy. Such a model would fail to account for the fact that S. M. appears to have a keen sense of empathy and hates to see others suffer, especially those who are downtrodden and alone. For example, she once saw a homeless man shivering on the sidewalk during the middle of winter and immediately took him to the local Salvation Army and bought him a coat with the little money she had left to spend that month. It is also worth noting that throughout her life, S. M. has never intentionally broken the law or committed any crimes, though she has been the victim of numerous crimes. It turns out, S. M. is actually quite averse to breaking the law, and part of this stems from the fact that she does not like getting in trouble. Some may call this a fear of punishment, but it may actually have more to do with her personality and compensatory strategies. Perhaps as a consequence of her amygdala damage, she often views rules and laws in a very black-and-white manner, and has trouble seeing shades of gray. She also has a preserved, yet rigid, understanding of basic concepts such as good and bad, and right and wrong; consequently, her behavior is rarely reckless and typically conforms to societal standards. Instances in which she fails to conform usually involve benevolent acts that transcend social barriers. For many years, S. M. attended a church where she was the only white person in a crowd of all black people. Even though there were other churches nearby that catered to a white audience, S. M. actually preferred the black church, and enjoyed the festive nature of the gathering, especially the music and singing. She adamantly denied feeling any sense of discomfort being the only white person in attendance. As S. M. explains, "In my eyes, we're all the same. I don't look at people differently. We all bleed the same color red." This point is made even more poignant by the fact that many of the crimes committed against S. M. involved a perpetrator who was black. Despite these negative encounters, S. M. always viewed them as isolated incidents and has never developed any distrust or racism toward African Americans.

Response to Social Threat

The sacrifice and courage that S. M. displays in the face of her own demise will often come out whenever other people are in danger. S. M. frequently tells a story about a "6 foot 5 neighbor lady" who slapped S. M.'s eldest son when he was a young boy. Without hesitation, S. M. confronted this much larger woman and a pushing match ensued. Things quickly escalated as the neighbor lady's entire family came running outside and surrounded S. M., threatening to attack her as a group. Other neighbors called the police, who quickly arrived and managed to break up the tussle before it escalated further. This was documented in police records that we were able to obtain. These same records helped verify another claim that S. M. has made for many years: Several other neighbors (and their associates) had explicitly threatened to kill S. M. on multiple occasions. Apparently, when S. M.'s son found a small bag of crack cocaine in the backyard, S. M. quickly took the bag to the police and told them exactly which neighbors she thought were dealing the drugs. When the police followed up on S. M.'s tip, unaddressed letters started appearing on S. M.'s doorstep, detailing elaborate plans to kill her if she did not stop speaking to the cops. Such threats did not alter S. M.'s determination to make sure that her kids were not exposed to drugs. When her son found more drugs in the backyard, S. M. immediately went back to the police to file another report. Once again, her motherly instincts prevailed over her own safety.

Around the same period of time when she was receiving all the death threats, S. M. remembers an incident while standing by herself outside her apartment. A large man (whom S. M. claims to have never seen before) suddenly appeared from behind a corridor, holding a gun in his hand. Without saying a word, he walked up to S. M., put the gun to her head, and yelled at the top of his lungs, "BAM!" before running away, never to be seen again. S. M. remembers finding the whole experience "strange" and seemed perplexed as to why someone would do something like that, apparently not connecting the dots between the man with the gun and all the recent death threats she had received. She has no recollection of feeling afraid, even when the gun was put to her head. Later that day, S. M. was back in her apartment and received a knock at her door. It was a local police officer. He sounded concerned and asked S. M. if everything was okay. She replied that she was doing just fine and inquired as to why he was there. The officer, a bit confused at this point, told S. M. that they had received a call from a neighbor who was quite disturbed and reported that she witnessed a man putting a gun to S. M.'s head. S. M. explained to the officer that this did indeed happen, but nothing ever came of it and the man had left the scene.

The striking disconnect between S. M.'s reaction to threats against her own life versus threats against other people's lives warrants more attention and investigation. At the very least, S. M.'s behavior suggests that she has great difficulty responding and appropriately reacting to threats against her own life, while at the same time, reacting quickly—and even somewhat overreacting—to threats that could harm others. Why she would contact the police during the latter situations but not the former is quite perplexing. When queried, S. M. does not have a clear explanation for her behavior. In the absence of such an explanation, it can be inferred that external threats to her own life often fail to induce fear and consequently do not leave much of an impression. On the other hand, external threats to other people's lives, especially loved ones, reflexively engage S. M.'s protective motherly instincts, a social form of threat detection that apparently can be deployed by circuitry outside of the amygdala.

Finally, even though S. M. is not living in the jungle with wild rhesus monkeys, she does live in a fairly dangerous area that harbors human predators. An incident in which a drugged-out man put a knife to her throat and threatened to kill her is a perfect example (Feinstein et al., 2011). There are many other traumatic incidents, some of which paint a rather grim picture of the human race and all its unsavory characters. One incident that really highlights the dangers of living without an amygdala involved a middle-aged man whom S. M. described as "tall and skinny with glasses." One day this stranger pulled up beside S. M. in his aquamarine pickup truck. The man struck up a conversation and told S.

M. that he knew one of her friends and wanted to take her out on a date to shoot some pool. Not surprisingly, S. M. immediately trusted this man and gladly took him up on his offer.

When they arrived at the pool hall, it was closed and would not be open for another hour. They decided to go for a drive through the countryside as they waited for the pool hall to open. The man eventually pulled up to an old abandoned barn and asked S. M. if she wanted to go outside and explore the barn. Interestingly, S. M. reported being hesitant to get out of the pickup. When asked to elaborate, S. M. claims that she was worried that they were on private property and could get in trouble for trespassing (a good example of her black-and-white thinking about rules and laws). Never once did she report feeling threatened by this strange man she had just met or the isolated environment to which he had surreptitiously guided her. After a little more prodding, the man eventually convinced S. M. to get out of the truck and they started walking toward the barn.

As they stepped inside the barn, the man quickly came up from behind S. M. and tackled her to the ground. He proceeded to flip her over and pull at her shirt, exposing her breasts. S. M. started yelling, "Take me home! Take me home!" The man started to unbuckle her belt and tried to remove her pants. S. M. continued yelling, her hoarse voice screeching through the sky. When retrospectively asked how she was feeling at the time, she denied feeling scared, but did report feeling extremely angry. Suddenly a dog appeared at the abandoned barn, attracted by all the commotion. When the man saw the dog, he quickly stood up, perhaps scared that the dog's owner was not far behind. He nonchalantly dusted himself off, asked S. M. if she was all right, and offered to help her up. S. M., still very upset, picked herself up from the ground and again yelled for the man to take her home. She proceeded to get back into the pickup truck on her own, and the man drove her home without saying another word about the events that had just transpired.

Hearing S. M. recount this incident was shocking to everyone in the laboratory. While we fully understood her deficit in the realm of trust and approachability of strangers, here was a clear-cut example of someone who had just attempted to rape her, yet, she got back in the car with him! Why would she do this? Why not run to the nearest farm and ask for help? Why not demand that the man leave without her? What if the man decided to take her to a more isolated location instead of taking her home? These were the questions that echoed through the minds of those with a functioning amygdala. Apparently, none of these thoughts crossed S. M.'s mind. She clearly did not accurately appraise the danger of the situation or the danger of this man. Instead, she thought that if he left her at the abandoned barn, she would have difficulty getting home, since they were quite far away from any town. While most people presented with this same situation would have preferred being stranded than having to spend another moment with such a savage, S. M. apparently did not feel this way.

On the way back home, S. M. directed the man to her apartment complex, seemingly unconcerned that he would now know where she was living. Upon arriving, the man nonchalantly asked S. M. if she wanted to do something later that night. S. M. said no thanks, got out of the car, and walked up to her apartment. She did not even take the time to remember or write down the number on the man's license plate. As soon as we learned about what had happened, we directed S. M. to immediately call the police. Unfortunately, she had no defining details to provide them. No license plate, no name or model for the pickup, no last name of the perpetrator, just a vague description of some middle-aged man and his aquamarine pickup truck. The police were unable to offer her any help. We implored her to be cautious, since the man knew where she lived, and to run away quickly if she should ever see this man again. S. M. reported feeling *violated*, *worthless*, and *lower than dirt*, and remained upset for several days afterward. These negative feelings, however, were not enough to stop her from reengaging with the world outside. Later that same day, S. M. was back outside on her typical walk, putting herself at great risk of encountering this predator once again.

Survival with the Wild

A recent study that involved collecting human intracranial recordings of amygdala neurons found that cells in the right amygdala have a high rate of response to pictures of animals, even more so than pictures of people (Mormann et al., 2011). Other amygdala neurons seem to be selective for emotional facial expressions such as fear (Wang, Tudusciuc, et al., 2014). Likewise, functional neuroimaging has found significantly higher levels of amygdala activation in response to pictures of threatening animals and people versus pictures of threatening objects, such as guns (Yang, Bellgowan, & Martin, 2012). These data suggest that the amygdala hones in on detecting various forms of life in the animal kingdom (humans, as well as other species), with somewhat of a predilection for animals that are dangerous. Beyond mere detection of animate life, the data from nonhuman animals further suggest that the amygdala plays a critical role in rapidly constructing the defense barriers we erect when confronted with an unfamiliar animal, halting our approach behavior and minimizing interspecies interaction. Consequently, amygdala damage can manifest as a striking lack of avoidance of innately feared stimuli, as borne out by rats with amygdala lesions who approach cats (Blanchard & Blanchard, 1972) or a predator-like robot (Choi & Kim, 2010), or by monkeys with amygdala lesions that readily approach humans (e.g., Weiskrantz, 1956) or snakes (e.g., Meunier et al., 1999). The conspicuous reduction in avoidance and defense responses when confronted with potentially dangerous animals is one of the most well-replicated findings in nonhuman animals with amygdala lesions (in this volume, see Amaral, Chapter 3; chapter, Kim, Choi, & Lee, Chapter 5; Bachevalier, Sanchez, Raper, Stephens, & Wallen, Chapter 7; Oler, Fox, Shackman, & Kalin, Chapter 8). Since nonhuman animals are unable to report verbally on their internal subjective experience, we became interested in learning how S. M. felt about other animals, especially species that are commonly feared by humans.

To our surprise, S. M. has repeatedly told us that she "hates" snakes. Given the aforementioned findings in nonhuman animals, we were rather bewildered by this revelation. It is possible that S. M.'s snake aversion developed as a child. She remembers an incident when she was very young and out on a hike through the woods with her father. Some loose brush covered a hole in the ground, and when she walked over this brush, it gave way, and she fell several feet into the hole. To S. M.'s dismay, the hole contained a nest of young snakes that quickly started to slither up her legs. She recalls screaming for her father to help and finding the whole experience extremely upsetting. While her amygdala damage likely emerged later in life, the memory for this event remained and probably contributed to her hatred for snakes.

Taking her word at face value, we assumed that S. M. would naturally avoid snakes when confronted with them in real life. Moreover, the fact that S. M. would repeatedly tell us, year after year, how much she disliked snakes, led us to believe that she might even have a mild form of ophidiophobia. In order to examine this possibility further, we arranged for a visit to an exotic pet store containing a large collection of different snakes of various sizes and colors (Feinstein et al., 2011). The store also contained more traditional pets, such as hamsters, birds, and puppies. Upon arrival, we asked S. M. if she wanted to go inside the pet store and check it out. Given her love for animals, she was more than happy to comply. Our goal was simply to observe her behavior around this large collection of animals. We had envisioned that she would probably focus most of her attention on animals she liked, such as the puppies. Since it was an exotic pet store, we also thought she might occasionally look at the snakes from afar, and perhaps she would even go near their housing so we could assess whether her reported level of fear changed at different proximities. As soon as we entered the store, however, we quickly realized that our expectations were way off base. Instead of observing the snakes from afar, S. M. was spontaneously drawn to them and strongly captivated by their presence. Simply looking at them was not enough. She needed to touch them. A store employee took notice and brought out a snake for S. M. to handle. As it wrapped around her hands, S. M. was mesmerized. She started rubbing the snake's leathery scales while closely inspecting all aspects of its body. The flicking tongue really grabbed her attention and she started gently touching it with her fingertips, spontaneously commenting, "This is so cool!" After 3 minutes of interacting with the snake, she was ready to move on, except now she desperately wanted to "touch" and "poke" the larger and more dangerous snakes, asking the store employee 15 different times if this would be possible, despite the employee repeatedly telling her that the larger snakes were not safe and could potentially bite her. In the past, S. M. has also told us about her aversion to spiders, yet at the exotic pet store, she tried to touch a very large and hairy tarantula and once again had to be stopped because of the high risk of being bitten. S. M.'s compulsive desire to approach snakes and spiders at the pet store is highly reminiscent of the behavior of monkeys with Klüver–Bucy syndrome (Klüver & Bucy, 1939). It is also worth noting that S. M.'s behavior was not merely the result of feeling comfortable in the relatively safe environment of a pet store, since we later learned (from a family member) that S. M. once encountered a very large snake outdoors and behaved in a similar manner (see Supplemental Data in Feinstein et al., 2011).

Throughout the whole experience at the pet store, S. M. was clearly overcome with "curiosity," which is exactly what she would tell us every time we asked why she would want to touch or hold something that she claims to hate. It was as if her amygdala damage had created a disconnect between cognition and behavioral control. Cognitively, she hates snakes, and to this very day she continues to hate them. Yet, while in their presence, she is compelled to touch them. Such a striking dissociation between cognition and behavior highlights the perils of relying solely on self-report, and the importance of observing behavior as it unfolds in the real world. Even though S. M.'s cognitive aversion to snakes is strong, it clearly is not strong enough to win the battle over behavioral control. Is winning this battle perhaps a key function of the amygdala? Each moment, as we navigate an uncertain world with unfettered curiosity and appetitive motivation, the amygdala acts as a powerful opposing force that inhibits our exploratory behavior, provoking both caution and avoidance in the face of danger. Such an explanation is corroborated by the rich set of behavioral observations in nonhuman animals with amygdala lesions (in this volume, see Amaral, Chapter 3; chapter, Kim et al., Chapter 5; Bachevalier et al., Chapter 7; Oler et al., Chapter 8). The case of S. M. further suggests that much of this battle over behavioral control occurs at an unconscious level, far outside the jurisdiction of reason and rational thinking.

One of the most readily observable forms of behavior is avoidance, which serves many functions beyond its critical role in fear. For example, disgust also features a core aspect of behavioral avoidance, and a burgeoning body of functional neuroimaging work indicates that the amygdala is highly responsive to disgusting stimuli (e.g., Lindquist, Wager, Kober, Bliss-Moreau, & Barrett, 2012; Stark et al., 2003). It is quite possible that another reason S. M. reports hating snakes is because she cognitively believes they are disgusting (e.g., she has, on occasion, used the word "gross" to describe snakes). She also finds cockroaches to be quite "gross" and "icky"; nevertheless, when S. M. found a cockroach scurrying about her apartment floor, she reported capturing it with her bare hands and systematically pulling off its body parts. Curiosity prevailed once again, and when asked to explain her discrepant behavior, she said, "I wanted to find out what made it tick, what it looked like inside." Viewed in this light, S. M.'s deficits in avoidance may extend beyond the realm of fear and into the domain of disgust. However, the overlap is only partial, for there are a variety of situations and objects that induce disgust in S. M. and prompt behavioral avoidance. Most of these revolve around consumption. For example, when we showed her a short video clip of a person eating dog feces from the film *Pink Flamingos*, she found it to be extremely disgusting (Feinstein et al., 2011). Likewise, there are many different foods and liquids that S. M. finds disgusting (e.g., most vegetables), and as a consequence she refuses to consume them. One morning, shortly after drinking some milk, S. M. became sick to her stomach and started vomiting. For the next week, she refused to drink any milk, even though her neighbor drank out of the same container of milk and showed no signs of illness. This suggests that S. M.'s conditioned aversion to taste is preserved, and further suggests that gustatory stimuli (which stimulate an interoceptive, rather than exteroceptive, sensory channel) are capable of triggering avoidance in the absence of an amygdala. Clearly, more research is needed to explore the boundaries between fear-induced and disgust-induced avoidance in order to provide a more parsimonious explanation of the amygdala's core function.

Interoceptive Fear

After many years of unsuccessful attempts using external threats to scare S. M., we decided to shift course. Unfortunately, almost the entire arsenal of paradigms and techniques currently employed to study fear use exteroceptive stimuli, typically processed through visual and auditory channels. Options for safely triggering internally induced states of fear are far more limited, but one such method that has been well-studied involves the inhalation of an air mixture containing 35% carbon dioxide (CO_2). To put this amount in perspective, we are talking about a quantity of CO_2 that is 875 times greater than that in the air we typically breathe. Given such high concentrations, the subject only takes a single vital capacity inhalation of the mixture, triggering a brief hypercapnic state that is typically resolved within 30 seconds. During this time period, chemoreceptors in both the central and peripheral nervous system are activated, driving physiological responses, especially breathing. The most commonly reported side effect of this experiment is a profound sense of air hunger that is felt almost immediately after the inhalation and lasts for about a minute. Interestingly, oxygen levels are typically unaffected, so the manipulation is actually triggering an illusion of air hunger. Despite its illusory nature, the feeling is very real and capable of inducing fear, and even panic, in up to one-fourth of healthy individuals who undergo this challenge (Colasanti, Esquivel, Schruers, & Griez, 2012). In patients with a history of panic disorder, the manipulation readily produces full-blown panic attacks that closely parallel those occurring in everyday life (Colasanti et al., 2012; Schruers, Van de Mortel, Overbeek, & Griez, 2004).

The aversive nature of CO_2 appears to be evolutionarily hardwired into our physiological system. For example, *Drosophila* fruit flies have specialized olfactory sensory neurons that are able to detect minute changes in levels of CO_2 in the environment, and rapidly trigger a change in flight pattern in order to avoid that area of space (Suh et al., 2004). Climbing up the evolutionary ladder, it has been shown that the amygdala in mice has the ability to directly detect changes in CO_2 and acidosis through acid-sensing ion channels, leading to CO_2-evoked fear behaviors (Ziemann et al., 2009). Given this finding in mice, in addition to S. M.'s remarkable absence of fear in response to the diverse array of previously discussed exteroceptive threats, and the fact that several prominent theories highlight a central role for the amygdala in the generation of panic (Coplan & Lydiard, 1998; Gorman, Kent, Sullivan, & Coplan, 2000), we hypothesized that S. M.'s bilateral amygdala lesions would reduce her level of CO_2-evoked fear. In collaboration with Dr. John Wemmie at the University of Iowa, we arranged for S. M. to undergo a 35% CO_2 challenge, marking the first time we had ever directly exposed S. M. to an interoceptive threat.

Immediately following the inhalation of 35% CO_2, S. M. began breathing at a rapid pace and gasping for air. Her physiological response to the CO_2 was clearly intact. Approximately 8 seconds following the inhalation, she started waving her right hand frantically near the air mask. By this point, S. M. was clearly in a state of distress. At 14 seconds post-inhalation, S. M. gestured with her right hand toward the mask and exclaimed, "Help me!" The experimenter immediately removed the mask from S. M.'s face. As this was happening, her body became rigid, her toes curled, and her fingers on both hands were flexed toward the ceiling. As soon as the mask was removed, S. M. grabbed the experimenter's hand and in a relieved tone said, "Thank you." The skin on her face was flushed, her nostrils were flared, and her eyes were opened wide. At 30 seconds post-inhalation, S. M. let go of the experimenter's hand and said, "I'm all right." However, she was not all right, at least not yet. Her breathing remained slightly belabored, and we could hear her on occasion trying to pull extra air in through her nose. Approximately 2 minutes later, one of the experimenters was going through a list of the various symptoms that people might feel during a panic attack. Just as she was asking S. M. about whether she had experienced the sensation of choking, S. M. suddenly stopped answering the questions. She started waving her right arm again as she struggled to communicate. She whispered, "I can't," as her right hand started tapping her throat. We asked if she was okay. S. M. shook her head no and with all her willpower gasped, "I can't breathe."

S. M. had just experienced the first panic attack of her life. The whole episode, from inhalation to her eventual recovery, lasted a total of 5 minutes (considerably longer than most other CO_2-induced panic attacks, which usually last on the order of 1–2 minutes). Every experimenter in the room was shocked. S. M. had actually felt fear. She called it the "worst" fear she had ever felt. In all likelihood, it was probably the first time she had experienced fear since childhood. Her response was unlike anything we had seen before. After many years of attempting to scare S. M., we had finally found her kryptonite: carbon dioxide.

In one breath, we immediately learned that the amygdala could not be the brain's quintessential and sole "fear center." Plasticity of function is certainly a possibility. Without a functioning amygdala, S. M. was still able to experience an intense and prolonged state of fear. If anything, her fear response was actually exaggerated. To test whether this result was reproducible, we collaborated with Dr. René Hurlemann, who identified monozygotic twin sisters (A. M. and B. G.) who both have focal bilateral amygdala lesions secondary to UWD (see Patin & Hurlemann Chapter 11, this volume). The twins were flown to Iowa from their home in Germany and administered the same testing protocol that S. M. had completed. Replicating the finding in S. M., CO_2 triggered panic attacks in both twins (Feinstein et al., 2013). The rate of CO_2-evoked panic attacks in the patients with amygdala lesions was significantly higher than that observed in a matched sample of neurologically intact comparison participants (Figure 1.4). This paradoxical finding suggests that instead of inducing panic, the amygdala is integrally involved in inhibiting panic. Such an inhibitory role might help explain how another patient with an amygdala lesion developed spontaneous panic attacks (Wiest, Lehner-Baumgartner, & Baumgartner, 2006), as well as provide a plausible account for the significant amygdalar atrophy found in patients with panic disorder (Hayano et al., 2009; Massana et al., 2003). In both scenarios, the amygdala pathology could conceivably lead to disinhibition of downstream panic circuits given that the output from the central nucleus of the amygdala is gamma-aminobutyric acid (GABA)ergic (Ciocchi et al., 2010) and projects to brainstem nuclei that have been implicated in producing panic-like behavior (Del-Ben & Graeff, 2009).

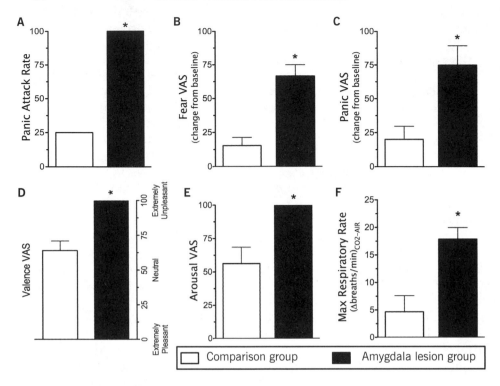

FIGURE 1.4. Results from the CO_2 experiment (Feinstein et al., 2013). A single vital capacity inhalation of 35% CO_2 triggered a panic attack (A) in all of the patients with amygdala lesions but only one-fourth of the comparison subjects. There were no significant differences between the patients with amygdala lesions and those comparison subjects who did panic. However, in relation to the comparison subjects who did not panic, the patients with amygdala lesions reported experiencing significantly higher levels of fear (B), panic (C), unpleasantness (D), and arousal (E). They also exhibited a significantly higher rate of respiration to the CO_2 challenge (F). * $p < .05$; all error bars represent the standard error of the mean. VAS, visual analogue scale.

The results from the CO_2 experiment (Figure 1.4) showed that a single inhalation of air containing 35% CO_2 triggered a panic attack in all of the patients with amygdala lesions, characterized by an intense feeling of suffocation, high levels of self-reported fear and panic, heightened physiological arousal (including hyperventilation and gasping for air), prominent signs of escape behavior, and concomitant thoughts of dying (Feinstein et al., 2013). This latter observation was particularly poignant, since it highlights that the type of fear we evoked was tapping into a very primal and existential system in the brain. Evidently, our fear of death, and the brain systems that allow this fear to permeate our consciousness, does not require the amygdala.

If not the amygdala, then what other brain regions could be responsible for generating such a primal experience of fear in S. M. and the other patients with amygdala lesions? While a definitive answer to this question will require further research, certain observations from the CO_2 experiment provide some important clues. During debriefing, all of the patients reported that the fear induced by the CO_2 was clearly linked to the feeling of suffocation. This observation appears to support Donald Klein's (1993, p. 306) suffocation false alarm theory of spontaneous panic, which hypothesizes that "a physiologic misinterpretation by a suffocation monitor misfires an evolved suffocation alarm system. This produces sudden respiratory distress followed swiftly by a brief hyperventilation, panic, and the urge to flee. Carbon dioxide hypersensitivity is seen as due to the deranged suffocation alarm monitor." Our data suggest that patients with bilateral amygdala lesions have a deranged suffocation alarm monitor that is hypersensitive to CO_2. An important follow-up question is to elucidate the precise location of this suffocation monitor, since it is the likely source of the fear and panic experienced by S. M. Although it is too early to know for sure, we predict that the suffocation monitor is embedded deep within the circuitry of the brainstem and hypothalamus, inside a cluster of closely connected nuclei that are adept at detecting changes in CO_2 and respiration, and rapidly inducing a state of fear and panic when the changes surpass a certain threshold. The critical nuclei likely include the periaqueductal gray, parabrachial nucleus, nucleus of the solitary tract, retrotrapezoid nucleus, locus coeruleus, raphe nucleus, and the dorsomedial and perifornical nuclei of the hypothalamus (Davenport & Vovk, 2009; Deakin & Graeff, 1991; Guyenet & Abbott, 2013; Grove, Coplan, & Hollander, 1996; Johnson et al., 2011; Nattie, 1999). Additionally, the experience of suffocation likely recruits higher-order brain regions, including the insula and anterior cingulate cortices (Banzett et al., 2000; Evans et al., 2002; Liotti et al., 2001). The truth is, we know very little about how the human brain instantiates fear from interoceptive signals. It will be incumbent on future research to unravel the neural basis of interoceptive fear, and this is currently an active area of investigation in our laboratory.

Interestingly, in S. M., fear was only one part of the experience that was activated by CO_2. After the experiment was over, S. M. told us that during her panic attack she had a flashback to a traumatic event. In the early 1990s, S. M. was married for a short period of time. She soon discovered that her husband was cheating on her. She approached him about the infidelity and asked him to move out of the house. The conversation quickly escalated into a fight that ended with the husband on top of S. M., strangling her. She remembers blacking out for a short period of time. By that point, he had let her go, left the house, and never returned again. When S. M. recalls this event, she denies ever feeling scared, even at the time of the assault, but she readily admits that she was extremely angry and also devastated that the man she loved would do this to her. The memory of the episode was on her mind for many months and even years after the event had taken place. Eventually, however, she moved on, and rarely ever thought about the event. It is quite remarkable that 16 years later a single inhalation of CO_2 caused S. M. to relive this traumatic memory.

Much of our understanding about the neural basis of emotional memory revolves around the amygdala and the important role that it plays in the consolidation of emotional memory, especially for arousing events (Hamann, 2001; LaBar & Cabeza, 2006). While S. M.'s emotional memory for exteroceptive events (i.e., events she sees, hears, or smells) is generally deficient (Adolphs, Cahill, Schul, & Babinsky, 1997; Adolphs et al., 2005b; Buchanan, Tranel, & Adolphs, 2003), her emotional memory for interoceptive events appears, at least anecdotally, to be much better. The feeling of suffocation while being strangled by her unfaithful husband likely induced a strong state of arousal in S. M. and, in the process, created an indelible memory trace that was reactivated by the closely associated feeling of suffocation induced by CO_2. This suggests that emotional memories for arousing interoceptive events may not require the amygdala. If this is true, then we would expect S. M.'s memory for the CO_2-induced panic attack to also be enhanced. Sure enough, more than 2 years after the CO_2 experiment, we were on the phone with S. M. discussing the possibility of an upcoming research visit. Without ever mentioning anything about the CO_2, S. M. spontaneously remarked, "That test with the gas. I don't want to do it no more. It makes me very uncomfortable. It brought back memories of when my husband strangled me." Not only had she remembered her experience with the CO_2, but she also remembered the memory that was reactivated by the experience. What's more, her preserved emotional memory was accompanied by a preserved avoidance response. She had absolutely no interest in ever inhaling CO_2 again and was averse to the very idea of it. This suggests that emotional memories for arousing interoceptive events can be encoded, consolidated, and retrieved without a functioning amygdala.

Such observations made us wonder whether there are other interoceptive events that S. M. experienced that might have induced states of fear and arousal leading to enhanced emotional memory and preserved avoidance behavior. So far, we have been able to identify two potent examples, both of which involve painful medical procedures related to her disease.

As previously mentioned, S. M. has a rather severe form of UWD, and the calcifications have infiltrated many different systems throughout her body. Recently, her tear ducts have become calcified, causing a buildup of tears in her eyes. To help correct this, an ophthalmologist placed small artificial tubes in her tear ducts, but these would frequently fall out after a short period of time. Finally, he decided to try a rather invasive procedure to keep the tubes in place by creating a small incision in her nasal bone and threading the tubes through this incision. Apparently no anesthesia was used during the procedure, causing S. M. extreme pain. After the procedure was over, S. M. remembers crying the entire way home. To this day, she still vividly remembers the pain. Eventually the tubes fell out again, but she refused to go back to the doctor even though the excessive tearing caused her to have blurry vision. Further questioning revealed that she was scared he would perform the same painful procedure again, and she did not want to risk having to endure the pain. The situation was eventually resolved when the doctor promised to put her under general anesthesia. Nevertheless, the day before the procedure, S. M. called us, extremely worried about what would happen if the doctor did not follow through on his promise to use anesthesia. Her voice was filled with apprehension, and she said that she had been worried all week long, dreading the procedure. We had never observed such anticipatory anxiety relative to any of the other surgical procedures that she typically undergoes several times a year, and that have been commonplace throughout her life. In this instance, her anxiety was clearly a by-product of the intense interoceptive pain experienced during the original procedure, combined with her preserved emotional memory for the painful experience.

S. M.'s disease also adversely affects her gums and teeth. Several years ago, we noticed that her teeth were falling out. We asked S. M. what her dentist was doing to help maintain her teeth, and she proceeded to tell us that she does not have a dentist and has no interest in seeing one. We started probing deeper to figure out what was behind her resistance to seeing a dentist. Apparently, 15–20 years ago, S. M. reported that she had all four of her wisdom teeth removed, but the dentist failed to use a sufficient amount of anesthesia during the surgery. In S. M.'s own words, "I felt everything. Every pull, every tug, I felt it all. And I couldn't tell him because he had my mouth propped open. And I tried to stop him with my hands and he had the nurse hold my hands down. He said to me that if you do that again, I may slip and I might hurt you. And in the back of my mind I was like you are hurting me now, stop!" The pain was excruciating, and ever since this incident she has been afraid to go back to the dentist. The mere thought of a drill makes her cringe. We did not know it at the time, but we later learned that S. M. had purposefully avoided going to the dentist for over 15 years. She said that she would rather lose her teeth than see another dentist. True to her word, last year S. M. lost her very last tooth.

A Tale of Two Fears

What appears to be emerging is a tale of two very different worlds inside our brain: the internal world of our body, and the external world in which that body lives. Each waking moment, the brain is in constant flux, attempting to pair what is happening on the outside with what is happening on the inside. At the interface between these two worlds lies the amygdala, a critical gatekeeper that is responsible for helping to merge these worlds together so that the next time they collide, the body will be better prepared to cope with the challenges posed by the external environment. The case of S. M. reveals that the amygdala does not provide a two-way street between these disparate worlds. Whereas external threats traverse the amygdala in order to induce a state of fear, internal threats are capable of bypassing the amygdala altogether. The amygdala's role in processing internal threats appears to be more regulatory in nature, inhibiting panic centers in the brainstem and hypothalamus, while scouring the external environment to find a plausible source that can explain, and subsequently predict, the internal disturbance.

Ultimately, the amygdala is not the quintessential source of fear in the brain (Janov, 2013). The neuroanatomical arrangement is such that only the internal fear pathway has direct access to the body, and the amygdala must communicate through this pathway in order for external stimuli to induce a state of fear. Sensory and association cortices required for representing external stimuli are intact in S. M.'s brain, as are the brainstem and hypothalamic circuitry necessary for orchestrating the action program of a fear response. S. M.'s amygdala lesions in effect disconnect these two components, making it improbable, if not impossible, for external sensory representations to trigger full-blown fear responses, leading to S. M.'s profound deficits in the realm of exteroceptive fear. On the other hand, interoceptively conveyed sensory information can directly stimulate the brainstem and hypothalamus, triggering a fear response that culminates in S. M.'s conscious experience of fear and panic. In comparison to exteroceptively-induced fear, it can be argued that interoceptive fear is more central to survival; consequently, the neural circuitry responsible for its induction may be more resilient to brain injury.

In the end, the life of S. M. has been a struggle from the very beginning. From an abusive upbringing to constant ridicule as a child, through failed relationships, and poverty, and pain, and death threats, and near-death experiences, S. M. has lived through it all. She has experienced a lifetime of adversity, with many more trials and tribulations likely to come. What is remarkable is that throughout this struggle, S. M. has maintained her composure and positive outlook on life, a steadfast resilience that endures to this day (see Box 1.1). In essence, the horrors of life

BOX 1.1. A Selection of Quotes from S. M. Obtained from Diary Entries, Interviews, and Conversations

"I struggle with this question all the time. What is my purpose? What is my purpose in life? I truly have no clue."

"I have no idea why I keep on going. Why haven't I just given up? Tossed in the towel?"

"I have no place to go, no one to go to, no money in my pocket. The old saying goes 'history repeats itself.' It's true!"

"I'm now getting evicted. Well here I am, the story of my life. All by myself, no one to turn to. No money. I'm back to square one. But hey, I will be just fine. I ain't going down without a good fight!"

"I'm the type of lady that can and will handle anything that comes my way! I can stand on my own two feet. I can and will survive."

"I try to be a tough woman. I try to take the whole world on by myself . . . I ain't going down without a fight."

"As you know, I have been through a lot! I will always keep a positive attitude, and will always have a smile no matter how hard life is!"

"I'm sitting here. It's a beautiful day, sunny, warm as can be. I haven't been outside yet. And I'm so lonesome that I could just cry. I am. I swear to God, I am."

"In my lifetime I hardly ever had any close friends. Friends to me are just like family members. I always get close to them and it's like one minute they're there, and the next minute they're nowhere to be found."

"The way I look at life, I was a loner when I was growing up. I didn't have many friends. I was always picked on. I was always by myself. I'm still alone now. . . . I don't want to be alone for the rest of my life."

"And this condition I have, with my skin and everything, kind of puts me down. Seems like every single day I get up in the mornings, I look in the mirror and I look 10, 15 years older than I am. And that kind of brings me down, too. I mean, I'm 43 and I look like I'm 55 or 60. . . . Seriously, I look like I'm an old lady!"

"I just wish, pray, that someone would come up with a cure for this."

"My life has been nothing but a lot of hurt, pain, and hateful people. My life has also been joy, love, and most of all, survival. I am thankful for my life and what kind of woman it made me. I am strong, very hard-headed, stubborn, very loving, caring, very passionate. But most of all, I am very thankful for having a good heart."

(continued)

Diary question: What have your life experiences taught you about what it means to survive?

S. M.: *It has taught me to be able to stand on my own two feet and take all the punches that life throws and still be able to stand and to keep right on going. It taught me to be strong, never give up. It taught me that I can not count on anyone but myself to take care of business. My life experiences are what made me the woman I am today. To be honest, loving, caring, understanding, nonjudgmental, to accept any situation that comes my way. Most of all, this may sound strange, but it also taught me never to hate!*

Experimenter: Your son is now a soldier in Afghanistan, right? Are you worried about him?

S. M.: *Yes, I am.*

Experimenter: What are you worried about?

S. M.: *I am worried about him being hurt, having bad things happening to him. Someone can be holding a gun to my son right now.*

Experimenter: There's something interesting there. You basically say that if someone held a gun to you, you wouldn't be afraid. But if someone did that to your son then you would be afraid?

S. M.: *I am not afraid. I just don't want that for him. What you need to understand is that I am worried, but not afraid.*

Experimenter: What do you think is the difference between "being worried" about something and "being afraid" of something?

S. M.: *"Afraid" means being frightened. Being scared. And "worried" means not wanting something to happen. I have always been worried about things, but I am never afraid. If I could stand between my son and the bullet, I would do that because I am not afraid.*

seem unable to penetrate her emotional core and stamp their traumatic imprint. Like Dr. Kling's amygdalectomized monkeys, S. M. repeatedly finds herself in precarious circumstances. Unlike Dr. Kling's monkeys, S. M. has somehow managed to stay alive all of these years. Whether this reveals something important about the evolution of the human race or the necessity of fear for survival in modern society is open for debate. What is not debatable is that we owe S. M. a tremendous debt of gratitude for her unwavering support of brain research and all of the incredible insights she has provided to the scientific community. As the science of fear advances to new levels of understanding, the case of S. M. lives on, her star shining brightly in the night sky, helping to lead the way.

REFERENCES

Adolphs, R. (2013). The biology of fear. *Current Biology, 23*(2), R79–R93.

Adolphs, R., Baron-Cohen, S., & Tranel, D. (2002). Impaired recognition of social emotions following amygdala damage. *Journal of Cognitive Neuroscience, 14*(8), 1264–1274.

Adolphs, R., Cahill, L., Schul, R., & Babinsky, R. (1997). Impaired declarative memory for emotional material following bilateral amygdala damage in humans. *Learning and Memory, 4*(3), 291–300.

Adolphs, R., Gosselin, F., Buchanan, T. W., Tranel, D., Schyns, P., & Damasio, A. R. (2005a). A mechanism for impaired fear recognition after amygdala damage. *Nature, 433*(7021), 68–72.

Adolphs, R., Russell, J. A., & Tranel, D. (1999a). A role for the human amygdala in recognizing emotional arousal from unpleasant stimuli. *Psychological Science, 10*(2), 167–171.

Adolphs, R., & Tranel, D. (1999). Intact recognition of emotional prosody following amygdala damage. *Neuropsychologia, 37*(11), 1285–1292.

Adolphs, R., & Tranel, D. (2000). Emotion recognition and the human amygdala. In J. P. Aggleton (Ed.), *The Amygdala: A functional analysis* (pp. 587–630). New York: Oxford University Press.

Adolphs, R., & Tranel, D. (2004). Emotion. In M. Rizzo & P. J. Eslinger (Eds.), *Principles and practice of behavioral neurology and neuropsychology* (pp. 457–474). Philadelphia: Elsevier/Saunders.

Adolphs, R., Tranel, D., & Buchanan, T. W. (2005b). Amygdala damage impairs emotional memory for gist but not details of complex stimuli. *Nature Neuroscience, 8*(4), 512–518.

Adolphs, R., Tranel, D., & Damasio, A. R. (1998). The human amygdala in social judgment. *Nature, 393*(6684), 470–474.

Adolphs, R., Tranel, D., Damasio, H., & Damasio, A. (1994). Impaired recognition of emotion in facial expressions following bilateral damage to the human amygdala. *Nature, 372*(6507), 669–672.

Adolphs, R., Tranel, D., Damasio, H., & Damasio, A. R. (1995). Fear and the human amygdala. *Journal of Neuroscience, 15*(9), 5879–5891.

Adolphs, R., Tranel, D., Hamann, S., Young, A. W., Calder, A. J., Phelps, E. A., et al. (1999b). Recognition of facial emotion in nine individuals with bilateral amygdala damage. *Neuropsychologia, 37*(10), 1111–1117.

Anderson, A. K., & Phelps, E. A. (2002). Is the human amygdala critical for the subjective experience of emotion?: Evidence of intact dispositional affect in patients with amygdala lesions. *Journal of Cognitive Neuroscience, 14*(5), 709–720.

Anderson, D. J., & Adolphs, R. (2014). A framework for studying emotions across species. *Cell, 157*(1), 187–200.

Atkinson, A. P., Heberlein, A. S., & Adolphs, R. (2007). Spared ability to recognise fear from static and moving whole-body cues following bilateral amygdala damage. *Neuropsychologia, 45*(12), 2772–2782.

Banzett, R. B., Mulnier, H. E., Murphy, K., Rosen, S. D., Wise, R. J., & Adams, L. (2000). Breathlessness in humans activates insular cortex. *NeuroReport, 11*(10), 2117–2120.

Barrett, L. F. (2004). Feelings or words?: Understanding the content in self-report ratings of experienced emotion. *Journal of Personality and Social Psychology, 87*(2), 266–281.

Bechara, A., Damasio, H., & Damasio, A. R. (2003). Role of the amygdala in decision-making. *Annals of the New York Academy of Sciences, 985*(1), 356–369.

Bechara, A., Damasio, H., Damasio, A. R., & Lee, G. P. (1999). Different contributions of the human amygdala and ventromedial prefrontal cortex to decision-making. *Journal of Neuroscience, 19*(13), 5473–5481.

Bechara, A., Tranel, D., Damasio, H., Adolphs, R., Rockland, C., & Damasio, A. R. (1995). Double dissociation of conditioning and declarative knowledge relative to the amygdala and hippocampus in humans. *Science, 269*(5227), 1115–1118.

Becker, B., Mihov, Y., Scheele, D., Kendrick, K. M., Feinstein, J. S., Matusch, A., et al. (2012). Fear processing and social networking in the absence of a functional amygdala. *Biological Psychiatry, 72*(1), 70–77.

Bickart, K. C., Wright, C. I., Dautoff, R. J., Dickerson, B. C., & Barrett, L. F. (2010). Amygdala volume and social network size in humans. *Nature Neuroscience, 14*(2), 163–164.

Birmingham, E., Cerf, M., & Adolphs, R. (2011). Comparing social attention in autism and amygdala lesions: Effects of stimulus and task condition. *Social Neuroscience, 6*(5–6), 420–435.

Blair, R. J. R. (2008). The amygdala and ventromedial prefrontal cortex: Functional contributions and dysfunction in psychopathy. *Philosophical Transactions of the Royal Society B: Biological Sciences, 363*(1503), 2557–2565.

Blanchard, D. C., & Blanchard, R. J. (1972). Innate and conditioned reactions to threat in rats with amygdaloid lesions. *Journal of Comparative and Physiological Psychology, 81*(2), 281–290.

Boes, A. D., Mehta, S., Rudrauf, D., Van Der Plas, E., Grabowski, T., Adolphs, R., et al. (2011). Changes in cortical morphology resulting from long-term amygdala damage. *Social Cognitive and Affective Neuroscience, 7*(5), 588–595.

Buchanan, T. W., Tranel, D., & Adolphs, R. (2003). A specific role for the human amygdala in olfactory memory. *Learning and Memory, 10*(5), 319–325.

Buchanan, T. W., Tranel, D., & Adolphs, R. (2009). The human amygdala in social function. In P. J. Whalen & E. A. Phelps (Eds.), *The human amygdala* (pp. 289–318). New York: Guilford Press.

Cai, H., Haubensak, W., Anthony, T. E., & Anderson, D. J. (2014). Central amygdala PKC-δ+ neurons mediate the influence of multiple anorexigenic signals. *Nature Neuroscience, 17*(9), 1240–1248.

Choi, J. S., & Kim, J. J. (2010). Amygdala regulates risk of predation in rats foraging in a dynamic fear environment. *Proceedings of the National Academy of Sciences, 107*(50), 21773–21777.

Ciocchi, S., Herry, C., Grenier, F., Wolff, S. B., Letzkus, J. J., Vlachos, I., et al.

(2010). Encoding of conditioned fear in central amygdala inhibitory circuits. *Nature, 468*(7321), 277–282.

Colasanti, A., Esquivel, G., J Schruers, K., & Griez, E. J. (2012). On the psychotropic effects of carbon dioxide. *Current Pharmaceutical Design, 18*(35), 5627–5637.

Coplan, J. D., & Lydiard, R. B. (1998). Brain circuits in panic disorder. *Biological Psychiatry, 44*(12), 1264–1276.

Davenport, P. W., & Vovk, A. (2009). Cortical and subcortical central neural pathways in respiratory sensations. *Respiratory Physiology and Neurobiology, 167*(1), 72–86.

Deakin, J. W., & Graeff, F. G. (1991). 5-HT and mechanisms of defence. *Journal of Psychopharmacology, 5*(4), 305–315.

Del-Ben, C. M., & Graeff, F. G. (2009). Panic disorder: is the PAG involved? *Neural Plasticity, 108135*, 1–9.

De Martino, B., Camerer, C. F., & Adolphs, R. (2010). Amygdala damage eliminates monetary loss aversion. *Proceedings of the National Academy of Sciences, 107*(8), 3788–3792.

Dicks, D., Myers, R. E., & Kling, A. (1969). Uncus and amygdala lesions: Effects on social behavior in the free-ranging rhesus monkey. *Science, 165*(3888), 69–71.

Evans, K. C., Banzett, R. B., Adams, L., McKay, L., Frackowiak, R. S., & Corfield, D. R. (2002). BOLD fMRI identifies limbic, paralimbic, and cerebellar activation during air hunger. *Journal of Neurophysiology, 88*(3), 1500–1511.

Feinstein, J. S. (2013). Lesion studies of human emotion and feeling. *Current Opinion in Neurobiology, 23*(3), 304–309.

Feinstein, J. S., Adolphs, R., Damasio, A., & Tranel, D. (2011). The human amygdala and the induction and experience of fear. *Current Biology, 21*(1), 34–38.

Feinstein, J. S., Buzza, C., Hurlemann, R., Follmer, R. L., Dahdaleh, N. S., Coryell, W. H., et al. (2013). Fear and panic in humans with bilateral amygdala damage. *Nature Neuroscience, 16*(3), 270–272.

Gläscher, J., & Adolphs, R. (2003). Processing of the arousal of subliminal and supraliminal emotional stimuli by the human amygdala. *Journal of Neuroscience, 23*(32), 10274–10282.

Gorman, J. M., Kent, J. M., Sullivan, G. M., & Coplan, J. D. (2000). Neuroanatomical hypothesis of panic disorder, revised. *American Journal of Psychiatry, 157*(4), 493–505.

Gosselin, N., Peretz, I., Johnsen, E., & Adolphs, R. (2007). Amygdala damage impairs emotion recognition from music. *Neuropsychologia, 45*(2), 236–244.

Grove, G., Coplan, J. D., & Hollander, E. (1996). The neuroanatomy of 5-HT dysregulation and panic disorder. *The Journal of Neuropsychiatry and Clinical Neurosciences, 9*(2), 198–207.

Guyenet, P. G., & Abbott, S. B. (2013). Chemoreception and asphyxia-induced arousal. *Respiratory Physiology and Neurobiology, 188*(3), 333–343.

Hamada, T., Wessagowit, V., South, A. P., Ashton, G. H., Chan, I., Oyama, N., et al. (2003). Extracellular matrix protein 1 gene (*ECM1*) mutations in lipoid proteinosis and genotype–phenotype correlation. *Journal of Investigative Dermatology, 120*(3), 345–350.

Hamann, S. (2001). Cognitive and neural mechanisms of emotional memory. *Trends in Cognitive Sciences, 5*(9), 394–400.

Hamann, S. B., Stefanacci, L., Squire, L. R., Adolphs, R., Tranel, D., Damasio, H., et al. (1996). Recognizing facial emotion. *Nature, 379*(6565), 497.

Hampton, A. N., Adolphs, R., Tyszka, J. M., & O'Doherty, J. P. (2007). Contributions of the amygdala to reward expectancy and choice signals in human prefrontal cortex. *Neuron, 55*(4), 545–555.

Hayano, F., Nakamura, M., Asami, T., Uehara, K., Yoshida, T., Roppongi, T., et al. (2009). Smaller amygdala is associated with anxiety in patients with panic disorder. *Psychiatry and Clinical Neurosciences, 63*(3), 266–276.

Heberlein, A. S., & Adolphs, R. (2004). Impaired spontaneous anthropomorphizing despite intact perception and social knowledge. *Proceedings of the National Academy of Sciences USA, 101*(19), 7487–7491.

Hofer, P. A. (1973). Urbach–Wiethe disease (lipoglycoproteinosis; lipoid proteinosis; hyalinosis cutis et mucosae). A review. *Acta Dermato-Venereologica, 53*(Suppl. 71), 1–52.

Janov, A. (2013). The origins of anxiety, panic and rage attacks. *Activitas Nervosa Superior, 55*(1–2), 51–66.

Johnson, P. L., Fitz, S. D., Hollis, J. H., Moratalla, R., Lightman, S. L., Shekhar, A., et al. (2011). Induction of c-Fos in "panic/defence"-related brain circuits following brief hypercarbic gas exposure. *Journal of Psychopharmacology, 25*(1), 26–36.

Kennedy, D. P., & Adolphs, R. (2010). Impaired fixation to eyes following amygdala damage arises from abnormal bottom-up attention. *Neuropsychologia, 48*(12), 3392–3398.

Kennedy, D. P., Gläscher, J., Tyszka, J. M., & Adolphs, R. (2009). Personal space regulation by the human amygdala. *Nature Neuroscience, 12*(10), 1226–1227.

Klein, D. F. (1993). False suffocation alarms, spontaneous panics, and related conditions: An integrative hypothesis. *Archives of General Psychiatry, 50*(4), 306–317.

Kling, A., Lancaster, J., & Benitone, J. (1970). Amygdalectomy in the free-ranging vervet (*Cercopithecus aethiops*). *Journal of Psychiatric Research, 7*(3), 191–199.

Kling, A. S. (1986). Neurological correlates of social behavior. *Ethology and Sociobiology, 7*(3), 175–186.

Klüver, H., & Bucy, P. C. (1939). Preliminary analysis of functions of the temporal lobes in monkeys. *Archives of Neurology and Psychiatry, 42*(6), 979–1000.

Koenigs, M., Huey, E. D., Raymont, V., Cheon, B., Solomon, J., Wassermann, E. M., & Grafman, J. (2008). Focal brain damage protects against post-traumatic stress disorder in combat veterans. *Nature Neuroscience, 11*(2), 232–237.

LaBar, K. S., & Cabeza, R. (2006). Cognitive neuroscience of emotional memory. *Nature Reviews Neuroscience, 7*(1), 54–64.

LeDoux, J. E. (2013). The slippery slope of fear. *Trends in Cognitive Sciences, 17*(4), 155–156.

Lindquist, K. A., Wager, T. D., Kober, H., Bliss-Moreau, E., & Barrett, L. F. (2012). The brain basis of emotion: A meta-analytic review. *Behavioral and Brain Sciences, 35*(03), 121–143.

Liotti, M., Brannan, S., Egan, G., Shade, R., Madden, L., Abplanalp, B., et al.

(2001). Brain responses associated with consciousness of breathlessness (air hunger). *Proceedings of the National Academy of Sciences, 98*(4), 2035–2040.

Marsh, A. A. (2013). What can we learn about emotion by studying psychopathy? *Frontiers in Human Neuroscience, 7*(181), 1–13.

Massana, G., Serra-Grabulosa, J. M., Salgado-Pineda, P., Gastó, C., Junqué, C., Massana, J., et al. (2003). Amygdalar atrophy in panic disorder patients detected by volumetric magnetic resonance imaging. *NeuroImage, 19*(1), 80–90.

Meunier, M., Bachevalier, J., Murray, E. A., Málková, L., & Mishkin, M. (1999). Effects of aspiration versus neurotoxic lesions of the amygdala on emotional responses in monkeys. *European Journal of Neuroscience, 11*(12), 4403–4418.

Mormann, F., Dubois, J., Kornblith, S., Milosavljevic, M., Cerf, M., Ison, M., et al. (2011). A category-specific response to animals in the right human amygdala. *Nature Neuroscience, 14*(10), 1247–1249.

Nattie, E. (1999). CO_2, brainstem chemoreceptors and breathing. *Progress in Neurobiology, 59*(4), 299–331.

Paul, L. K., Corsello, C., Tranel, D., & Adolphs, R. (2010). Does bilateral damage to the human amygdala produce autistic symptoms? *Journal of Neurodevelopmental Disorders, 2*(3), 165–173.

Schruers, K. R. J., Van de Mortel, H., Overbeek, T., & Griez, E. (2004). Symptom profiles of natural and laboratory panic attacks. *Acta Neuropsychiatrica, 16*(2), 101–106.

Shiv, B., Loewenstein, G., Bechara, A., Damasio, H., & Damasio, A. R. (2005). Investment behavior and the negative side of emotion. *Psychological Science, 16*(6), 435–439.

Spezio, M. L., Huang, P. Y. S., Castelli, F., & Adolphs, R. (2007). Amygdala damage impairs eye contact during conversations with real people. *Journal of Neuroscience, 27*(15), 3994–3997.

Sprengelmeyer, R., Young, A. W., Schroeder, U., Grossenbacher, P. G., Federlein, J., Buttner, T., et al. (1999). Knowing no fear. *Proceedings of the Royal Society of London B: Biological Sciences, 266*(1437), 2451–2456.

Suh, G. S., Wong, A. M., Hergarden, A. C., Wang, J. W., Simon, A. F., Benzer, S., et al. (2004). A single population of olfactory sensory neurons mediates an innate avoidance behaviour in *Drosophila. Nature, 431*(7010), 854–859.

Stark, R., Schienle, A., Walter, B., Kirsch, P., Sammer, G., Ott, U., et al. (2003). Hemodynamic responses to fear and disgust-inducing pictures: An fMRI study. *International Journal of Psychophysiology, 50*(3), 225–234.

Tranel, D., Gullickson, G., Koch, M., & Adolphs, R. (2006). Altered experience of emotion following bilateral amygdala damage. *Cognitive Neuropsychiatry, 11*(3), 219–232.

Tranel, D., & Hyman, B. T. (1990). Neuropsychological correlates of bilateral amygdala damage. *Archives of Neurology, 47*(3), 349–355.

Tsuchiya, N., Moradi, F., Felsen, C., Yamazaki, M., & Adolphs, R. (2009). Intact rapid detection of fearful faces in the absence of the amygdala. *Nature Neuroscience, 12*(10), 1224–1225.

Wang, S., Tsuchiya, N., New, J., Hurlemann, R., & Adolphs, R. (2015). Preferential attention to animals and people is independent of the amygdala. *Social Cognitive and Affective Neuroscience, 10*(3), 371–380.

Wang, S., Tudusciuc, O., Mamelak, A. N., Ross, I. B., Adolphs, R., & Rutishauser, U. (2014). Neurons in the human amygdala selective for perceived emotion. *Proceedings of the National Academy of Sciences, 111*(30), E3110–E3119.

Watson, D. (2000). *Mood and temperament.* New York: Guilford Press.

Watson, D., Clark, L. A., & Tellegen, A. (1988). Development and validation of brief measures of positive and negative affect: the PANAS scales. *Journal of Personality and Social Psychology, 54*(6), 1063–1070.

Weiskrantz, L. (1956). Behavioral changes associated with ablation of the amygdaloid complex in monkeys. *Journal of Comparative and Physiological Psychology, 49*(4), 381–391.

Wiest, G., Lehner-Baumgartner, E., & Baumgartner, C. (2006). Panic attacks in an individual with bilateral selective lesions of the amygdala. *Archives of Neurology, 63*(12), 1798–1801.

Yang, J., Bellgowan, P. S., & Martin, A. (2012). Threat, domain-specificity and the human amygdala. *Neuropsychologia, 50*(11), 2566–2572.

Ziemann, A. E., Allen, J. E., Dahdaleh, N. S., Drebot, I. I., Coryell, M. W., Wunsch, A. M., et al. (2009). The amygdala is a chemosensor that detects carbon dioxide and acidosis to elicit fear behavior. *Cell, 139*(5), 1012–1021.

CHAPTER 2

A Synopsis of
Primate Amygdala Neuroanatomy

CYNTHIA M. SCHUMANN
MARTHA V. VARGAS
AARON LEE

The amygdala is a medial temporal lobe structure that occupies barely 0.3% of the volume of the human brain. Despite its size, it has been associated with more neurodevelopmental and psychiatric disorders than perhaps any other brain region. This may be because the amygdala is part of a system focused on detecting danger in the environment, processing cortical sensory input via the more lateral nuclei, and orchestrating the subsequent response via the central and more medial nuclei. If this system becomes dysfunctional, inappropriate social behavior or anxiety may arise, as is observed in many, often debilitating, disorders. Thus, treatment approaches for several common neuropsychiatric disorders may be facilitated by a precise understanding of the cellular composition and structural development of the amygdala. The amygdala is, in fact, a complex region made up of at least 13 nuclei and cortical areas in the primate brain. There are approximately 13 million neurons in the adult human amygdala (in each hemisphere), with more than 50% residing in the lateral and basal nuclei. The lateral nucleus is the largest of the nuclei, occupying one third of total amygdala volume. In this chapter, we provide a brief synopsis of the cytoarchitecture and the intrinsic and extrinsic connectivity of nuclei in the primate amygdala. A precise understanding of the typically developing primate amygdala provides a vital baseline for which to compare cellular alterations associated with psychiatric disorders in humans and in the nonhuman primate models.

The amygdaloid complex, or more commonly the amygdala, is an almond-shaped structure that comprises 13 individual nuclei located in the anterior portion of the medial temporal lobe (Figure 2.1). It occupies barely 0.3% (2 cm³ on each side) of the volume of the human brain. Despite

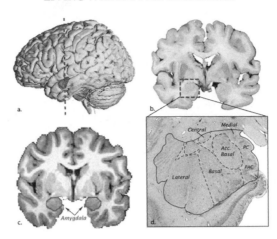

FIGURE 2.1. Neuroanatomy of the human amygdala. (a) Lateral view of a three-dimensional reconstruction of an MRI (dashed line represents location of coronal slice in (b)); (b) MRI coronal image with amygdala outlined; (c) coronal section of brain tissue (box around amygdala); (d) Nissl-stained section of amygdala nuclei. PAC, periamygdaloid cortex. Adapted from Amaral, Schumann, and Nordahl (2008). Copyright 2008 by Elsevier, Inc. Adapted by permission.

its small size, it has been associated with more neurodevelopmental and psychiatric disorders than perhaps any other brain region (Schumann, Bauman, & Amaral, 2011). Therefore, establishing a clear understanding of typical human and nonhuman primate amygdala anatomical structure and development is critical for evaluating pathology that may have profound effects on behavior. In this brief chapter, we provide an overview of primate amygdala neuroanatomy, including ontogeny and developmental trajectory across the lifespan, macroscopic and microscopic neuroanatomy, and intrinsic and extrinsic connectivity.

Basics of Amygdala Neuroanatomy

The amygdala can be globally identified on magnetic resonance imaging (MRI) scans of both human (Schumann et al., 2004) and nonhuman primates (Figure 2.2). The rostral extent (Figures 2.2a and 2.2b) of the amygdala is bordered laterally by temporal lobe white matter and dorsomedially by the medial surface of the brain. The entorhinal cortex is present along the ventromedial border, separated by a thin band of white matter, and the temporal horn of the lateral ventricle forms the ventral border. At the midstrocaudal level (Figures 2.2c and 2.2d), the dorsal surface of the hippocampus forms the ventral border of the amygdala, separated by a thin white-matter band referred to as the alveus. At this point, the ventral claustrum is present along the dorsolateral border. Caudally (Figures 2.2e and 2.2f), the amygdala is bordered dorsally by the substantia innominata and fibers of the anterior commissure, laterally by the putamen, and ventrally by the temporal horn of the lateral ventricle. At the most caudal extent, the medial surface of the amygdala abuts the optic tract, the putamen is present along the dorsolateral border, and the temporal horn of the lateral ventricle separates the hippocampus from the amygdala along the ventral surface. In the macaque monkey, the global definition is quite similar to that of the human (Schumann et al., 2004), with the exception of a less defined dorsolateral border with the ventral putamen and tail of the caudate in the caudal extent of the monkey amygdala (Figures 2.2e′ and 2.2f′).

Adopting nomenclature outlined by Amaral and colleagues (Amaral & Bassett, 1989; Amaral & Insausti, 1992), all 13 nuclei of the amygdala can be organized under the following three categories: the deep nuclei, the superficial nuclei, and the remaining nuclei. The "deep nuclei" consist of the lateral nucleus, basal nucleus, accessory basal nucleus, and paralaminar nucleus. The "superficial nuclei" include the anterior cortical nucleus, medial nucleus, nucleus of the lateral olfactory tract, periamygdaloid cortex, and posterior cortical nucleus. Finally, the "remaining nuclei" include the anterior amygdaloid area, central nucleus, amygdalohippocampal area, and intercalated nuclei.

Amygdala Developmental Trajectory

Early in prenatal development in primates, the amygdala is derived from the germinal layer of the ganglionic eminence contiguous with the hippocampus and closely related to the striatum (Kordower, Piecinski, & Rakic, 1992; Müller & O'Rahilly, 2006). Neuroblasts that are to become amygdala neurons migrate along radial glia around the fifth month of gestation (Humphrey, 1968, Ulfig, Setzer, & Bohl, 2003, Müller & O'Rahilly, 2006). The more superficial nuclei of the amygdala, such as the medial and central nuclei, become identifiable and begin to undergo synaptogenesis, as evidenced by the presence of growth-associated protein (GAP-43) immunolabeling, during the fifth month of gestation. However, the deeper nuclei, such as lateral and basal nuclei, do not show evidence of synaptogenesis until around the seventh month (Humphrey, 1968; Ulfig, Setzer, & Bohl, 2003). Neuronal migration and synaptogenesis is essentially complete by the end of the eighth month of gestation (Ulfig et al., 1998; Setzer & Ulfig, 1999; Ulfig et al., 1999, 2003) to form 13 well-defined nuclei that make up the "amygdaloid complex" (Amaral & Insausti, 1992; Schumann & Amaral, 2005; Freese & Amaral, 2009).

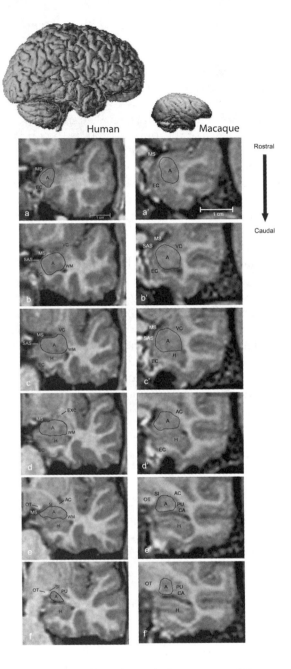

FIGURE 2.2. Representative slices through the rostrocaudal extent of the amygdala and surrounding regions. Structures noted are as follows: amygdala (A), hippocampus (H), entorhinal cortex (EC), white matter (WM), medial surface of the brain (MS), ventral claustrum (VC), optic tract (OT), substantial inominata (SI), semiannular sulcus (SAS), anterior commissure (AC), putamen (PU), and caudate (CA). Human sections (slides a–f) are based on Schumann et al. (2004).

Therefore, the basic cellular architecture of the amygdala appears to be well established at the time of birth in primates. Neurotransmitter systems, such as serotonin and opiate receptors, show a distribution similar to that seen in adults (Bauman & Amaral, 2005). The pathways of amygdalocortical connectivity are also relatively well developed, although processes such as myelination continue through early childhood (Emery & Amaral, 2000). Both cytoarchitectural and MRI studies demonstrate rapid postnatal enlargement of the nonhuman primate amygdala between birth and 3 months of age (Payne, Machado, Bliwise, & Bachevalier, 2010; Chareyron, Lavenex, Amaral, & Lavenex, 2012).

Surprisingly, MRI studies indicate that the human and nonhuman primate amygdala continues to undergo substantial postnatal growth throughout childhood and well into adolescence (nonhuman primates: Schumann, Scott, Lee, Fletcher, Buonocore, et al., in preparation; humans: Giedd et al., 1996; Giedd, Castellanos, Rajapakse, Vaituzis, & Rapoport, 1997; Schumann et al., 2004; Uematsu et al., 2012). The dramatic increase in amygdala volume observed over this time period is in striking contrast to what is seen throughout much of the rest of the cortex, which actually contracts in size during this period. Several independent cross-sectional MRI studies have found that the amygdala increases in size by ~40% from 5 years of age to adulthood in typically developing males (Giedd et al., 1996, 1997; Schumann et al., 2004; Ostby, Tamnes, Fjell, Westlye, Due-Tønnessen, & Walllhovd, 2009). There appear to be sex differences in this remarkable growth trajectory, with female children and adolescents showing somewhat earlier enlargement than males (Giedd et al., 1996, 1997). The underlying neurobiology that produces the extended developmental trajectory of postnatal amygdala growth into adolescence in humans is currently under investigation. In a stereological study of the nonhuman primate amygdala, individual nuclei were found to exhibit different developmental profiles (Chareyron et al., 2012). The lateral, basal, and accessory basal nuclei exhibit a large increase in volume from birth to 3 months, followed by a slower growth beyond 1 year of age. The medial nucleus is near adult size at birth. In both human and nonhuman primate studies, the central nucleus exhibits significant age-related growth beyond childhood and into adulthood (Schumann & Amaral, 2005; Chareyron et al., 2012). Neuronal somal size and number, and astrocyte number, do not appear to change during postnatal development. However, oligodendrocyte number increases substantially in parallel with amygdala volume after 3 months of age in nonhuman primates (Chareyron et al., 2012).

As we discuss later in more detail, the mature amygdala establishes a dense network of connections with many other regions of the brain. Information typically enters the amygdala via the lateral and, to some extent, basal nuclei from both higher-order sensory and association cortices. Prominent among these regions are "social brain" components such as the orbitofrontal cortex, superior temporal gyrus, medial prefrontal cortex, anterior cingulate cortex, and fusiform face area (for reviews, see Amaral, Schumann, & Nordahl, 2008; Adolphs, 2009; Freese & Amaral, 2009). From the lateral and basal nucleus, in general, information is either returned via reciprocal connections to cortical regions to modulate social and emotional processes or flows medially to the central and medial nuclei for output to subcortical and brainstem regions. Via these regions, the amygdala modulates the autonomic nervous system, which is involved in preparing the body for action in response to novel or often fearful stimuli.

Cytoarchitecture and Intrinsic Connectivity of Amygdala Nuclei

The 13 nuclei of the human (Figure 2.3) and nonhuman primate (Figure 2.4) amygdala are distinguishable from each other by cytoarchitectural features, neurochemistry, as well as characteristic intrinsic and extrinsic connectivity. The nuclei and their subdivisions are summarized in Table 2.1 for human (Sorvari, Soininen, Paljärvi, Karkola, & Pitkänen, 1995) and nonhuman (Amaral & Bassett, 1989; Pitkänen & Amaral, 1998) primates. Very little information is available on the connectivity of the human amygdala due to several limitations inherent to human studies; therefore, the amygdala of the nonhuman primates, such as the macaque monkey, have been used extensively as a model due to the homology between the two species (Sorvari et al., 1995; Sorvari, Soininen, & Pitkänen, 1996a, 1996b; Pitkänen & Kemppainen, 2002). Specifically, anterograde and retrograde tracers displaying connectivity of brain regions with amygdala nuclei performed on the nonhuman primate brain can be useful to predict how these regions are connected in the human brain. The major intrinsic connections of the amygdala are summarized in Figure 2.5. Below we summarize the cytoarchitecture and intrinsic connectivity of the following deep nuclei: lateral nucleus, basal nucleus, and accessory basal nucleus, as well as the central nucleus. The superficial nuclei are summarized in Table 2.2, and the remaining nuclei as well as the paralaminar nucleus are summarized in Table 2.3.

Lateral Nucleus

The lateral nucleus spans the entire width of the human and nonhuman primate amygdala. As it is the most lateral of the amygdala nuclei, it serves as the outer boundary of the amygdala along the lateral, dorsal, and ventral surface. The medial border of the lateral nucleus is defined by the fiber tract referred to as the lateral medullary lamina, which is

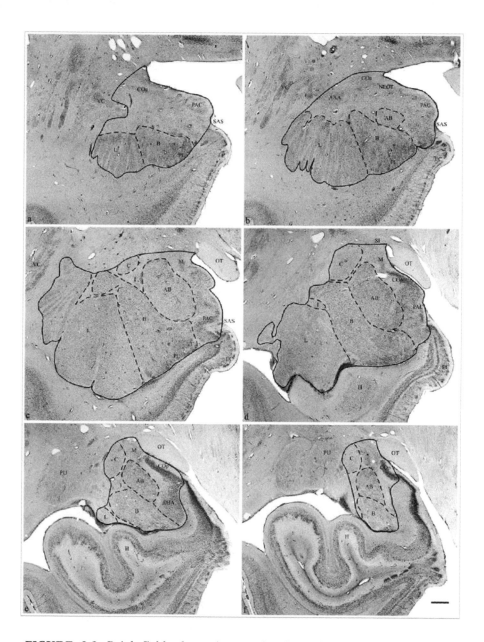

FIGURE 2.3. Brightfield photomicrograph of Nissl-stained coronal section through (a, b) rostral, (c, d) midrostrocaudal, and (e, f) caudal amygdaloid complex. AAA, anterior amygdaloid area; AB, accessory basal nucleus; AHA, amygdalohippocampal area; B, basal nucleus; C, central nucleus; COa, anterior cortical nucleus; COp, posterior cortical nucleus; EC, entorhinal cortex; H, hippocampus; I, intercalated nuclei; L, lateral nucleus; M, medial nucleus; NLOT, nucleus of the lateral olfactory tract; OT, optic tract; PAC, periamygdaloid cortex; PL, paralaminar nucleus; PU, putamen; SAS, semiannular sulcus; VC, ventral claustrum. Scale bar: 2 mm.

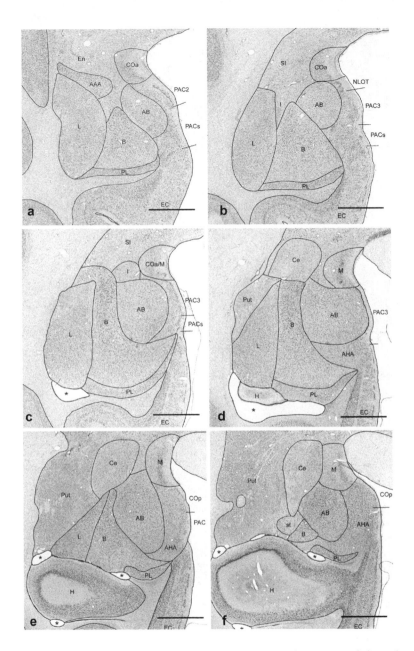

FIGURE 2.4. Photomicrograph of Nissl-stained coronal sections of the primate amygdala from rostral (a) to caudal (f). The sections are 720 μm apart. AAA, anterior amygdaloid area; AB, accessory basal nucleus; AHA, amygdalohippocampal area; B, basal nucleus;, Ce, central nucleus; Coa, anterior cortical nucleus; Cop, posterior cortical nucleus; EC, entorhinal cortex; En, endopiriform nucleus; H, hippocampus; I, intercalated nuclei; L, lateral nucleus; M, medial nucleus; NLOT, nucleus of the lateral olfactory tract; PAC, periamygdaloid cortex; PL, paralaminar nucleus; Put, putamen; SI, substantia innominata; St, stria terminalis. Scale bar = 2 mm. Adapted from Freese and Amaral (2009). Copyright 2009 by The Guilford Press. Adapted by permission.

TABLE 2.1. Summary of Nuclei of the Amygdaloid Complex and Divisions

	Human subdivisions	Monkey subdivisions
	Deep nuclei	
Lateral nucleus (L)	Medial Lateral	Dorsal (Ld) Dorsal intermediate (Ldi) Ventral (Lv) Ventral intermediate (Lvi)
Basal nucleus (B)	Magnocellular (Bmc) Intermediate (Bi) Pavicellular (Bpc)	Magnocellular (Bmc) Intermediate (Bi) Parvicellular (Bpc)
Accessory basal nucleus (AB)	Magnocellular (ABmc) Parvicellular (ABpc) Ventromedial (ABvm)	Magnocellular (ABmc) Parvicellular (ABpc) Ventromedial (ABvm)
Paralaminar nucleus	Medial Lateral	None noted
	Superficial nuclei	
Medial nucleus (M)	No subdivisions	None noted
Anterior cortical nucleus (Coa)	No subdivisions	None noted
Posterior cortical nucleus (Cop)	No subdivisions	None noted
Nucleus of the lateral olfactory tract (NLOT)	None noted	None noted
Periamygdaloid cortex (PAC)	PACo PAC1 PAC3 PACs	PAC2 PAC3 PACs
	Remaining nuclei	
Anterior amygdaloid area (AAA)	None noted	None noted
Central nucleus (CE)	Medial (CEm) Lateral (CEl)	Medial (CEm) Lateral (CEl)
Amygdalohippocampal area (AHA)	Medial Lateral	None noted
Intercalated nuclei (I)	None noted	None noted

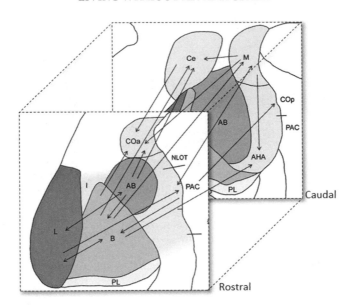

FIGURE 2.5. Intrinsic amygdala connectivity. A sample of the major intrinsic amygdaloid projections depicted between two primate amygdala sections. Corresponding nuclei between the two sections are shaded the same. AB, accessory basal nucleus; AHA, amygdalohippocampal area; B, basal nucleus; Ce, central nucleus; Coa, anterior cortical nucleus; Cop, posterior cortical nucleus; I, intercalated nuclei; L, lateral nucleus; M, medial nucleus; NLOT, nucleus of the lateral olfactory tract; PAC, periamygdaloid cortex; PL, paralaminar nucleus.

present between the lateral and basal nuclei. In general, neurons in the lateral nucleus are medium to large in size relative to other nuclei and slightly smaller relative to basal nucleus neurons (Figure 2.6).

The lateral nucleus is subdivided into lateral and medial regions in the human (Sorvari et al., 1995), and into dorsal (Ld), dorsal intermediate (Ldi), ventral (Lv), and ventral intermediate (Lvi) divisions in the nonhuman primate (Price, Russchen, & Amaral, 1987; Pitkänen & Amaral, 1998). The cytoarchitectural subdivisions can be visualized based on cell size, shape, and density with the aid of different histological staining techniques. A sample of distinguishing characteristics between subdivisions of the lateral nucleus in the nonhuman primate is presented in Table 2.4.

The lateral nucleus is highly interconnected within its subdivisions and is thought to project to all other nuclei in the amygdaloid complex, as summarized in Table 2.4. Yet it receives very few reciprocal projections back from other amygdaloid nuclei, with minor connections primarily received from the basal, accessory basal, and central nuclei (Price & Amaral, 1981; Aggleton, 1985).

TABLE 2.2. Summary of Superficial Nuclei

Nuclei	Location	Distinguishing features	Nuclei intrinsic afferents	Nuclei intrinsic efferents
Medial nucleus (M)	Dorsomedial portion, caudal to the anterior cortical nucleus	• Dense narrow band of layer II cells • Large portion of cells are gamma-aminobutyric acid-ergic (GABAergic)	Strongest: • Lateral nucleus Other: • Basal nucleus • Accessory basal nucleus • Periamygdaloid cortex References: Aggleton (1985); Gloor (1997)	Moderately: • Anterior cortical nuclei • Periamygdaloid cortex • Central nucleus • Amygdalohippocampal area Lightly: • Basal nucleus • Accessory basal nucleus References: Aggleton (1985); Gloor (1997)
Anterior cortical nucleus (Coa)	Along the dorsomedial edge, rostral to medial nucleus	• Layer I: wide and cell free • Layer II: thick, with low concentrations of cells • Layer III: density of cells are lower than layer II	• Lateral nucleus • Accessory basal nucleus • Medial nucleus • Central nucleus References: Pitkänen & Amaral (1998); Price & Amaral (1981); Price et al. (1987)	• No efferent projections have yet been reported
Posterior cortical nucleus (Cop)	Caudomedial portion, dorsal to AAA	Two layers:s • Layer I: thin • Layer II: thicker than layer I, with medium-sized neurons	• Lateral nucleus • Accessory basal nucleus • Periamygdaloid cortex References: Pitkänen & Amaral (1998); Price & Amaral (1981); Van Hoesen (1981)	• Potentially, as the amygdalohippocampal area was included in these studies • Accessory basal nucleus • Medial nucleus • Periamygdaloid cortex References: Price et al. (1987); Amaral & Insausti (1992)
Nucleus of the lateral olfactory tract (NLOT)	Rostral half, ventral to Coa, dorsal to PAC	• Dense layer II • Stains strongly for AChE	• Light projection from lateral and basal nuclei Reference: Pitkänen & Amaral (1998)	• No efferent projections have yet been reported
Periamygdaloid cortex (PAC)	Anteromedial surface, ventral to COa or NLOT rostrally, medial to AB nuclei	PAC2: • Layer II: thin, dense layer of darkly Nissl-stained cells • Layer III: less dense layer, lightly Nissl-stained cells PAC3: • Layer II: lightly Nissl-stained cells • PACs: layers II and II are not easily distinguishable	• Lateral nucleus • Basal nucleus • Accessory basal nucleus • Medial nucleus • Central nucleus References: Aggleton (1985); Pitkänen & Amaral (1998); Price & Amaral (1981)	• Basal nucleus • Accessory basal nucleus • Medial nucleus • Posterior cortical nucleus • Central nucleus References: Price & Amaral (1981); Price et al. (1987); Van Hoesen (1981)

Note. Adapted from Freese and Amaral (2009). Copyright 2009 by The Guilford Press. Adapted by permission.

TABLE 2.3. Summary of Remaining Nuclei and Paralaminar Nucleus

Nuclei	Location	Distinguishing features	Nuclei intrinsic afferents	Nuclei intrinsic efferents
Anterior amygdaloid area (AAA)	Rostral half of amygdala, dorsal to L nucleus, ventrolateral to the COa	• Low levels of AChE • Medium- to small-sized cells (Nissl)	• Lateral nucleus • Central nucleus References: Aggleton (1985); Pitkänen & Amaral (1998)	• No efferent projections have been reported to date
Amygdalohippocampal area (AHA)	Caudal portion of amygdala, ventromedial to the basal and accessory basal nuclei, ventrolateral to the PAC	Rostral portion: • Lightly packed and lightly stained cells (Nissl) Caudal portion: • Densely packed and darkly stained cells (Nissl)	• Lateral nucleus • Basal nucleus • Accessory basal nucleus • Medial nucleus • Central nucleus References: Aggleton (1985); Pitkänen & Amaral (1998)	• All tracer injections included the posterior cortical nucleus, so these are potential connections • Accessory basal nucleus • Medial nucleus • Periamygdaloid cotex Reference: Amaral & Insausti (1992)
Intercalated nuclei (I)	Location varied through amygdala, primarily surround rostral half of B and AB of the amygdala	• Made of dopamine-D1 and μ-opioid receptor-rich GABAergic interneurons References: Millhouse (1986); Nitecka & Ben-Ari (1987); Busti et al. (2011)	• Lateral nucleus • Accessory basal nucleus References: Aggleton (1985); Pitkänen & Amaral (1998)	• No efferent projections have been reported to date in primates
Paralaminar nucleus (PL)	Most ventral portion of amygdala, ventral to the B nucleus	• Cells are densely packed • High concentration of glial cells • AChE poor References: Fudge & Tucker (2009); de Campo & Fudge (2012)	• Lateral nucleus Reference: Pitkänen & Amaral (1998)	• Basal nucleus • Central nucleus References: Fudge & Tucker (2009); Amaral & Insausti (1992); Pitkänen & Amaral (1991)

Note. Adapted from Freese and Amaral (2009). Copyright 2009 by The Guilford Press. Adapted by permission.

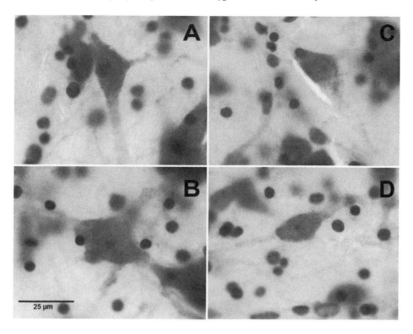

FIGURE 2.6. Examples of tissue at a 40× magnification. This shows differences in neuron size among adjacent nuclei. (A) Lateral nucleus; (B) basal nucleus; (C) accessory basal nucleus; (D) central nucleus. Scale bar = 25 µm in B (applies to A–D).

TABLE 2.4. Distinguishing Features of Lateral Nucleus Subdivisions

	Ld	Ldi	Lv	Lvi
Cell size (Nissl)	Medium to large	Varied	Varied	Large
Cell shape (Nissl)	Modified and pyramidal	Varied	Varied	Round
Cell density	Low	Low	High	High
Parvalbumin	Dense	Dense	Light	Dense; >Lvi
Calbindin-D28K	High density	Low density	Low density	High density
Acetylcholinesterase (AChE)	Light	Light	Light	Heavy
Density of serotonergic fibers	Medium/low	Medium/low	Low	Medium

Note. Data from Pitkänen and Amaral (1998).

Basal Nucleus

The basal nucleus is medial to the lateral nucleus through most of the amygdala (Amaral and Insausti, 1992, Schumann and Amaral, 2005). Therefore, the lateral nucleus, separated by the lateral medullary lamina, serves as its lateral border. Medially, the intermediate medullary lamina clearly separates the accessory basal nucleus from the basal nucleus, primarily defining its medial border. In addition, the basal nucleus can be further distinguished from the surrounding lateral, accessory basal, and central nuclei due to its characteristically large neurons (Figure 2.6). It is divided into mangocellular, intermediate, and parvicellular subdivisions in both the human and nonhuman primate (Price et al., 1987; Amaral & Bassett, 1989). Table 2.5 provides a sample of cytoarchitectonic characteristics distinguishing subdivisions of the basal nucleus (Price et al., 1987; Amaral & Bassett, 1989; Pitkänen & Amaral, 1993; Bauman & Amaral, 2005; Buckwalter, Schumann, & Van Hoesen, 2008).

The strongest basal nucleus projections flow from dorsal to ventral (Price et al., 1987). The lateral nucleus projects strongly to the entire basal nucleus, while the accessory basal nucleus, paralaminar, medial, periamygdaloid cortex, and the central nucleus project lightly (Price & Amaral, 1981; Van Hoesen, 1981; Pitkänen & Amaral, 1991, 1998). A sample of the basal nucleus efferent projections is provided in Table 2.6 with the strongest projections indicated in bold (Price & Amaral, 1981; Pitkänen & Amaral, 1998).

TABLE 2.5. Distinguishing Features of Basal Nucleus Subdivisions

	Magnocellular	Intermediate	Parvicellular
Cell size (Nissl)	Large, darkly stained	Large, lightly stained, less densely packed	Small lightly stained
Stain intensity (Nissl)	Dark	Light	Light
Acetylcholinesterase (AChE)	High	High	High
Parvalbumin	High immunoreactivity	High immunoreactivity	Low immunoreactivity
Density of serotonergic fibers	Medium/high	Medium/low	Not uniform, medium/high

TABLE 2.6. Lateral, Basal, Accessory Basal, and Central Nuclei Efferent Projections

Nuclei	Termination of projection
Lateral nucleus	**Basal nucleus** **Accessory basal nucleus** **Periamygdaloid cortex** Paralaminar nucleus Medial nucleus Anterior cortical nucleus Posterior cortical nucleus Nucleus of the lateral olfactory tract Anterior amygdaloid area Central nucleus Amygdalohippocampal area Intercalated nuclei
Basal nucleus	**Medial nucleus** **Central nucleus** **Anterior cortical nucleus** **Amygdalohippocampal area** Lateral nucleus Accessory basal nucleus Nucleus of the lateral olfactory tract Periamygdaloid cortex
Accessory basal nucleus	**Central nucleus** Medial nucleus Anterior cortical nucleus Posterior cortical nucleus Periamygdaloid cortex Amygdalohippocampal area Intercalated nucleus Lateral nucleus Basal nucleus
Central nucleus	Anterior cortical nucleus Periamygdaloid cortex Anterior amygdaloid area Amygdalohippocampal area Lateral nucleus Basal nucleus Accessory basal nucleus

Note. The strongest projections are in **bold.**

Accessory Basal Nucleus

The accessory basal nucleus is the most medial of the deep nuclei. Laterally, it is separated from the basal nucleus by the intermediate medullary lamina. The medial medullary lamina is present along the medial edge and separates it from the superficial cortical nuclei. The accessory basal nucleus is subdivided into the magnocellular, parvicellular, and ventromedial divisions in the human and nonhuman primate model (Price et al., 1987; Sorvari et al., 1995; Freese & Amaral, 2009). Table 2.7 provides a sample of distinguishing characteristics between each subdivision in the nonhuman primate (Price et al., 1987; Pitkänen & Amaral, 1993; Bauman & Amaral, 2005; Freese & Amaral, 2009).

The accessory basal nucleus receives strong connections from the lateral nucleus and minor inputs from the basal nucleus, medial nucleus, periamygdaloid cortex, and central nucleus (Price & Amaral, 1981; Aggleton, 1985; Pitkänen & Amaral, 1998; Freese & Amaral, 2009). The intrinsic efferent projections of the accessory basal nucleus are summarized in Table 2.6 with the strongest projections bolded (Price & Amaral, 1981; Aggleton, 1985; Gloor, 1997).

Central Nucleus

The central nucleus is located in the caudal half of the amygdala, bordered by the basal and accessory basal nuclei ventrally. It is a major recipient of intrinsic inputs from other nuclei of the amygdala, as well as the amygdala's major extrinsic output nucleus (Fudge & Tucker, 2009). The central nucleus is divided into lateral and medial divisions in both human and nonhuman primates based on cytoarchitectural differences,

TABLE 2.7. Distinguishing Features of Accessory Basal Nucleus Subdivisions

	Magnocellular	Parvicellular	Ventromedial
Cell size (Nissl)	Medium to large	Small	Medium
Stain intensity (Nissl)	Dark	Light	Medium
Acetylcholinesterase (AChE)	Moderate to high	Low	High
Parvalbumin	Medium immunoreactivity	Medium immunoreactivity	Medium immunoreactivity
Density of serotonergic fibers	Medium	Very low	Medium

TABLE 2.8. Distinguishing Features of Central Nucleus Subdivisions

	Medial	Lateral
Cell size (Nissl)	Small to medium	Small
Stain intensity (Nissl)	Light	Dark
Acetylcholinesterase (AChE)	Moderate	Low
Parvalbumin	Low	Low
Density of serotonergic fibers	High	High

as summarized in Table 2.8 (Price et al., 1987; Pitkänen & Amaral, 1993; Sorvari et al., 1995; Bauman & Amaral, 2005; Fudge & Tucker, 2009).

While most regions in the amygdala project to the central nucleus, including the lateral nucleus, medial nucleus, and periamygdaloid cortex, the major afferents are from the basal and accessory basal nuclei (Price & Amaral, 1981; Van Hoesen, 1981; Aggleton, 1985; Price et al., 1987; Pitkänen & Amaral, 1998; Fudge & Tucker, 2009). The central nucleus's intrinsic efferent projections are summarized in Table 2.6 (Price & Amaral, 1981; Aggleton, 1985; Freese & Amaral, 2009).

Superficial Nuclei, Remaining Nuclei, and the Paralaminar Nucleus

Tables 2.2 and 2.3 (pp. 49 and 50) provide of summary of the intrinsic connectivity of the superficial nuclei, the remaining nuclei, and the paralaminar nucleus.

Extrinsic Connectivity of the Amygdala

The extrinsic connectivity of the amygdala is summarized in Figure 2.7.

Amygdala Connectivity to Other Subcortical Structures

The amygdala is interconnected with many subcortical regions including the striatum, bed nucleus of the stria terminalis, basal forebrain, thalamus, hypothalamus, midbrain, and hindbrain. A synopsis of these connections has been briefly presented in Table 2.9.

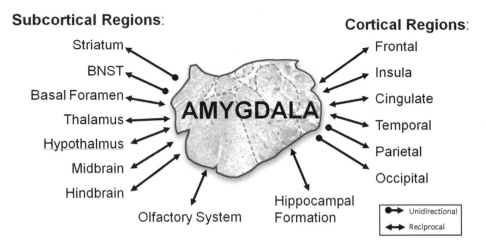

FIGURE 2.7. Extrinsic amygdala connectivity.

Amygdala Connectivity to the Olfactory System

In the nonhuman primate, the olfactory bulb, located along the ventromedial extent of the frontal lobe, has established connections with several of the superficial amygdala nuclei, including the anterior cortical nucleus, nucleus of the lateral olfactory tract, and periamygdaloid nucleus (Turner, Gupta, & Mishkin, 1978). The lateral olfactory tract, as well as the periamygdaloid nucleus, in turn, send reciprocal connections to the olfactory bulb (Amaral, Price, Pitkänen, & Carmichael, 1992). The piriform cortex, another region involved in olfaction, projects into the same amygdala subregions as the olfactory bulb (Amaral et al., 1992).

Amygdala Connectivity to Cortical Structures

Studies utilizing neuroanatomical tracers in the nonhuman primate reveal widespread connectivity between the amygdala and cerebral cortex. These cortical structures include the frontal, insular, cingulate, temporal, parietal, and occipital cortices. These connections primarily originate and terminate in deep nuclei, including the lateral, basal, and accessory basal nuclei. Most of these cortical structures generate projections back to the amygdala, with the exception of parietal and occipital cortices, where the flow of information is thought to be unidirectional.

TABLE 2.9. Summary of Subcortical Connectivity

	Striatum	Bed nucleus of the stria terminalis (BNST)	Basal forebrain	Thalamus	Hypothalamus	Midbrain	Hindbrain
Description	Consists of the caudate, putamen, and nucleus accumbens	Located dorsal to anterior commissure	Located ventral to the striatum	Located superior to midbrain	Located ventral and anterior to thalamus	Located between hindbrain and thalamus	Contains the medulla oblongata, pons, and cerebellum
Amygdala afferents	No projections have been shown	No projections have been shown	**B, NLOT**, L, B, AB, PAC, CE References: Amaral & Bassett (1989); Price et al. (1987)	B, M, CE, L, and AB References: Aggleton & Mishkin (1984); Aggleton et al. (1980); Amaral et al. (1992); Mehler (1980)	CE, B, AB, M, PAC, NLOT, AAA, Coa, Cop References: Amaral et al. (1982); Mehler (1980)	L, M, AB, CE References: Aggleton et al. (1980); Amaral & Insausti (1992); Jones et al. (1976); Mehler (1980)	CE, B References: Mehler (1980); Price et al. (1987)
Amygdala efferents	**B, AB**, L, AHA, CE, M, PAC, Coa, Cop References: Cho et al. (2013); Fudge et al. (2002); Nauta (1962); Parent et al. (1983); Russchen et al. (1985b)	B, AB, M, Cop, AHA, CE References: Price & Amaral (1981); Price et al. (1987)	B, AB, CE References: Price & Amaral (1981); Russchen et al. (1985a)	B, L, AB, PAC, AHA, M, CE References: Aggleton & Mishkin (1984); Price & Amaral (1981)	M, Coa, AB, AHA, Cop, B, CE References: Price & Amaral (1981); Price et al. (1987); Price (1986)	CE References: Hopkins (1975); Price & Amaral (1981); Price et al. (1987); Price (1986)	CE References: Price & Amaral (1981); Price et al. (1987)

Note. The stronger projections are in **bold**.

Frontal Cortex

The amygdala is highly interconnected with the frontal lobe. These connections are visually summarized in Figure 2.8. The amygdala afferent connections are more numerous than efferent ones; however, a general trend observed in the interconnectivity of the two structures is that projections to and from the amygdala have a higher density from the caudal aspects of the frontal cortex (Amaral & Price, 1984; Carmichael & Price, 1995; Barbas & De Olmos, 1990; Ghashghaei & Barbas, 2002; Stefanacci & Amaral, 2002).

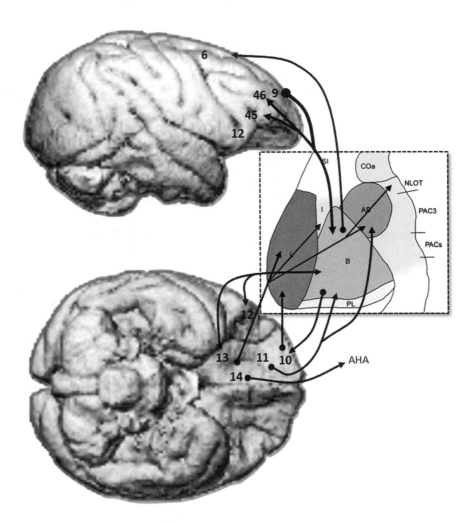

FIGURE 2.8. A representation of notable connections between the amygdala and regions of the frontal lobe including the medial (Brodman area 14), dorsolateral (45, 46, 6), and orbitofrontal (10, 11, 12, and 13) cortical regions.

The orbitofrontal cortex (OFC; Brodmann areas 11, 13, and parts of areas 10, 12, 14, and 24) receives projections from the basal nucleus with additional, minor projections from the lateral and accessory basal nuclei (Porrino, Crane, & Goldman-Rakic, 1981; Amaral & Price, 1984; Barbas and De Olmos, 1990; Morecraft, Geula, & Mesulam, 1992; Baylis, Rolls, & Baylis, 1995; Carmichael & Price, 1995; Cavada, Compañy, Tejedor, Cruz-Rizzolo, & Reinoso-Suárez, 2000; Ghashghaei & Barbas, 2002). While the caudal aspects of the OFC have projections to the nucleus of the lateral olfactory tract (NLOT), anterior amygdaloid area, and intercalated nuclei, the rostral portions of the prefrontal cortex have light projections to the basal nucleus (Amaral & Cowan, 1980; Amaral & Insausti, 1992; Van Hoesen, 1981; Carmichael & Price, 1995; Cavada et al., 2000; Stefanacci & Amaral, 2000, 2002; Ghashghaei & Barbas, 2002). The densest projections terminate within the magnocellular division of the basal nucleus, but other nuclei also receive projections, such as the accessory basal and lateral nuclei (Amaral & Cowan, 1980; Amaral & Insausti, 1992; Van Hoesen, 1981; Carmichael & Price, 1995; Cavada et al., 2000; Stefanacci & Amaral, 2000, 2002; Ghashghaei & Barbas, 2002).

The medial prefrontal cortex (mPFC) receives projections from the basal nucleus, along with minor contributions from the accessory basal nucleus, medial nucleus, anterior and posterior cortical nuclei (Porrino et al., 1981; Amaral & Price, 1984; Barbas & De Olmos, 1990; Carmichael & Price, 1995; Ghashghaei & Barbas, 2002). In conjunction with the OFC, it has projections to the lateral, basal, accessory basal, and medial nuclei, as well as the amygdalohippocampal area. Additionally, the mPFC has projections to the anterior and posterior cortical nuclei, the periamygdaloid cortex, as well as the central nucleus (Aggleton, Burton, & Passingham, 1980; Van Hoesen, 1981; Amaral & Insausti, 1992; Carmichael & Price, 1995; Cavada et al., 2000; Stefanacci & Amaral, 2000, 2002; Ghashghaei & Barbas, 2002; Cho, Ernst, & Fudge, 2013).

The lateral prefrontal cortex (regions 8, 45, and 46 as well as parts of Brodmann areas 9 and 12) has light reciprocated projections with the basal nucleus (Amaral & Price, 1984; Barbas & De Olmos, 1990; Amaral & Insausti, 1992; Ghashghaei & Barbas, 2002). The premotor cortex also has light reciprocal connections with the basal nucleus (Avendaño, Price, & Amaral, 1983; Amaral & Price, 1984)

Insular Cortex

The insular cortex and the amygdala are strongly interconnected, because almost all amygdala nuclei receive inputs of varying strengths (Mufson, Mesulam, & Pandya, 1981; Van Hoesen, 1981; Friedman, Murray, O'Neill, & Mishkin, 1986; Amaral & Insausti, 1992; Carmichael & Price, 1995; Stefanacci & Amaral, 2002). Most of these projections originate from the agranular (Ia), dysgranular (Id), and granular insular (Ig) regions (Mufson et al., 1981; Amaral & Price, 1984; Carmichael & Price, 1995). The parainsular cortex and frontoparietal operculum are also reciprocally connected to the amygdala.

The majority of the amygdala efferent connections terminates at the Ia and rostral portion of Id, and originate in the lateral nucleus, basal nucleus, accessory basal nucleus, medial nucleus, anterior cortical nucleus, periamygdaloid cortex, and the anterior amygdaloid area (Mufson et al., 1981; Amaral & Price, 1984, Friedman et al., 1986; Carmichael & Price, 1995). The most dense and strongest insular projections originate in the Ia and rostral aspects of Id, and terminate at the dorsal intermediate portion of the lateral nucleus, parvicellular portion of the basal, and central nucleus (Aggleton et al., 1980; Turner, Mishkin, & Knapp, 1980; Mufson et al., 1981; Van Hoesen, 1981; Friedman et al., 1986; Amaral & Insausti, 1992; Carmichael & Price, 1995; Stefanacci & Amaral, 2000, 2002). Additionally, the Ia and rostral aspect of Id also project to the rest of the lateral and basal nuclei, the accessory basal nucleus, medial nucleus, anterior cortical nucleus, nucleus of the lateral olfactory tract, periamygdaloid cortex, and the anterior amygdaloid area (Aggleton et al., 1980; Turner et al., 1980; Mufson et al., 1981; Van Hoesen, 1981; Friedman et al., 1986; Amaral & Insausti, 1992; Carmichael & Price, 1995; Stefanacci & Amaral, 2000, 2002).

The basal and the accessory basal nuclei, and to a lesser extent the lateral nuclei, originate projections that terminate within the caudal portion of Id and Ig (Mufson et al., 1981; Amaral & Price, 1984). In turn, the Ig and the caudal portion of Id lightly project to the dorsal intermediate portion of the lateral nucleus and central nucleus (Aggleton et al., 1980; Turner et al., 1980; Mufson et al., 1981; Van Hoesen, 1981; Friedman et al., 1986; Amaral & Insausti, 1992; Carmichael & Price, 1995; Stefanacci & Amaral, 2000, 2002).

The frontoparietal operculum and peri-insular cortex receive weak projections from the basal and accessory basal nuclei (Amaral & Price, 1984). In terms of amygdala afferent connections, the lateral, basal, and accessory basal nuclei receive additional inputs from the parainsular cortex (Aggleton et al., 1980; Amaral & Insausti, 1992; Stefanacci & Amaral, 2000). The frontoparietal operculum has only been found to project to the lateral nucleus (Van Hoesen, 1981).

Cingulate Cortex

The amygdala strongly projects to both the superficial and deep layers of rostral cingulate areas. These projections originate primarily from the basal nucleus, with additional minor projections generated by the lateral and accessory basal nuclei (Porrino et al., 1981; Amaral & Price, 1984; Vogt & Pandya, 1987). There is additional evidence that the basal nucleus also has efferent connections to the retrosplenial cortex, as well as Brodmann area 31 (Buckwalter et al., 2008). Reciprocal connections arising from the rostral cingulate cortex terminate in the lateral and basal nuclei, with minor projections terminating in the accessory basal nucleus, anterior amygdaloid area, and central nucleus (Pandya, Van Hoesen, & Domesick, 1973; Van Hoesen, 1981; Amaral & Insausti, 1992; Stefanacci & Amaral, 2000, 2002). No projections from caudal cingulate areas to the amygdala have been found (Pandya et al., 1973; Van Hoesen, 1981; Amaral & Insausti, 1992; Stefanacci & Amaral, 2000, 2002).

Temporal Cortex

The amygdala has a vast array of projections within the temporal cortex that communicate with areas that process both unimodal and multimodal information (summarized in Figure 2.9; Freese & Amaral, 2009). Through the temporo-occipital amygdalocortical pathway (TOACP), the magnocellular and intermediate divisions of the basal nucleus, with lesser contributions from the parvicellular division of the basal nucleus, the lateral nucleus, as well as the accessory basal nucleus, give rise to strong connections to the visual cortical area TE located on the ventral aspect of the temporal lobe as well as occipital area V1 (Amaral & Price, 1984; Webster, Ungerleider, & Bachevalier, 1991; Amaral, Behniea, & Kelly, 2003; Freese & Amaral, 2005). These connections are strong ipsilaterally, and there is evidence of light projections to the contralateral area TE (Iwai & Yukie, 1987; Webster et al., 1991). Both magnocellular and intermediate divisions of the basal nucleus project to visual area TEO, located along the caudal ventral temporal lobe, as well as to caudal portions of the temporal lobe, such as TC and TAc. The lateral, basal, and accessory basal nuclei send projections to TA (Webster et al., 1991, Kosmal, Malinowska, & Kowalska, 1997; Stefanacci & Amaral, 2000, 2002, Yukie, 2002).

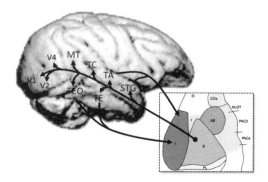

FIGURE 2.9. A representation of connections between the amygdala and other regions within the temporal lobe.

Area TE projects to the lateral nucleus, basal nucleus, accessory basal nucleus, and anterior amygdaloid area (Jones & Powell, 1970; Van Hoesen & Pandya, 1975; Herzog & Van Hoesen, 1976; Aggleton et al., 1980; Turner et al., 1980; Van Hoesen, 1981; Iwai & Yukie, 1987; Iwai, Yukie, Suyama, & Shirakawa, 1987; Webster et al., 1991; Amaral & Insausti, 1992; Cheng, Saleem, & Tanaka, 1997; Stefanacci & Amaral, 2000,2002; Ghashghaei & Barbas, 2002). Area TEO has minor connections to the lateral and basal nuclei, whereas rostral areas of TA projects to the lateral part of the middle and caudal aspects of the lateral nucleus (Webster et al., 1991; Kosmal et al., 1997; Stefanacci & Amaral, 2000, 2002: Yukie, 2002).

The superior temporal gyrus is also reciprocally connected with the amygdala, projecting specifically to the accessory basal nucleus, anterior amygdaloid area, anterior cortical nucleus, nucleus of lateral olfactory tract, periamygdaloid cortex, and medial nucleus (Herzog & Van Hoesen, 1976; Aggleton et al., 1980; Van Hoesen, 1981; Amaral & Price, 1984; Amaral & Insausti, 1992; Stefanacci & Amaral, 2000; Ghashghaei & Barbas, 2002).

The perirhinal cortex receives many connections from the amygdala. It receives strong projections from the lateral nucleus, basal nucleus, accessory basal nucleus, and periamygdaloid cortex, with lesser projections originating from the medial, posterior cortical, and anterior cortical nuclei (Amaral & Price, 1984; Iwai & Yukie, 1987; Morán, Mufson, & Mesulam, 1987; Stefanacci, Suzuki, & Amaral, 1996; Yukie, 2002). In return, the perirhinal cortex originates projections that target the lateral nucleus, basal nucleus, magnocellular division of the accessory basal, medial nucleus, anterior and posterior cortical nuclei, as well as the periamygdaloid cortex (Van Hoesen & Pandya, 1975; Herzog & Van Hoesen, 1976; Aggleton et al., 1980; Turner et al., 1980; Van Hoesen, 1981; Iwai & Yukie, 1987; Amaral & Insausti, 1992; Stefanacci et al., 1996; Stefanacci & Amaral, 2000, 2002; Ghashghaei and Barbas, 2002).

The ventral portions of the parahippocampal cortex also receive connections from the amygdala. The magnocellular division of the basal nucleus is the major propagator of these connections, with lesser projections from the intermediate and parvicellular divisions of the basal nucleus, the lateral nucleus, the accessory basal nucleus, the periamygdaloid cortex, and anterior amygdaloid area (Amaral & Price, 1984; Stefanacci et al., 1996). The parahippocampal cortex in turn has weak projections to the lateral nucleus (Amaral & Insausti, 1992; Stefanacci et al., 1996; Stefanacci & Amaral, 2000).

Hippocampal Formation

The hippocampal formation includes the dentate gyrus, hippocampus proper, the subiculum, and the entorhinal cortex. There are no projections from the amygdala to the dentate gyrus.

Hippocampus Proper

The amygdala has two major pathways to influence hippocampal functioning, one via connections directly to the hippocampus proper and another set of connections to the entorhinal cortex (Freese & Amaral, 2009). Projections from the basal nucleus and posterior cortical nucleus target areas along the entire rostrocaudal portions of the CA1, CA2, CA3 hippocampal regions (Amaral & Cowan, 1980; Aggleton, 1986; Amaral, 1986; Saunders, Rosene, & Van Hoesen, 1988). The parvicellular division of the basal nucleus projects to the CA1–subicular border. Hippocampal-amygdala projections are fewer than the opposite direction and mostly originate from the rostral hippocampus. Though there is no current evidence that the CA2 and CA3 fields have any projections to the amygdala, CA1 is known to have projections to the basal nucleus, accessory basal nucleus, paralaminar nucleus, periamygdaloid nucleus, as well as the anterior and posterior cortical nuclei (Rosene & Van Hoesen, 1977; Aggleton, 1986; Saunders et al., 1988).

Subiculum

The rostrocaudal extent of the subiculum is strongly interconnected with the amygdala. The major contribution comes from the parvicellular portion of the basal nucleus, but the magnocellular portion of the basal, the accessory basal, and the cortical nuclei also generate minor outputs to the subiculum (Aggleton, 1986; Saunders et al., 1988). In return, the subiculum strongly projects to the parvicellular division of the basal nucleus and periamygdaloid cortex (Aggleton, 1986; Saunders et al., 1988). Minor projections terminate in the lateral nucleus, cortical nuclei, and the intermediate and magnocellular portions of the basal nucleus receive more minor inputs (Aggleton, 1986; Saunders et al., 1988).

Entorhinal Cortex

The interconnectivity between the amygdala and the entorhinal cortex is a secondary pathway for the amygdala to have an impact on hippocampal function, because the entorhinal cortex in turn projects to every hippocampal field (Witter & Amaral, 1991). The lateral nucleus constitutes the most significant projection from the amygdala to the entorhinal cortex, but additional minor inputs arise from the basal nucleus, accessory basal nucleus, the paralaminar nucleus, medial nucleus, anterior cortical nucleus, periamygdaloid cortex, and the anterior amygdaloid area (Aggleton, 1986; Amaral, 1986; Insausti, Amaral, & Cowan, 1987; Pitkanen, Kelly, & Amaral, 2002; Saunders & Rosene, 1988). In turn, the entorhinal cortex projects to the lateral nucleus, basal nucleus, and periamygdaloid cortex of the amygdala (Van Hoesen, 1981; Aggleton, 1986; Stefanacci & Amaral, 2000).

Parietal Cortex

In the nonhuman primate, connectivity between the amygdala and parietal cortical areas is sparse and one-directional. The basal and accessory basal nuclei generate light projections to Brodmann area 7 of the parietal cortex (Amaral & Price, 1984). Furthermore, the magnocellular division of the basal nucleus projects to the medial superior temporal visual area (Iwai & Yukie, 1987). Studies have not yet demonstrated projections from the parietal cortex to the amygdala (Aggleton et al., 1980; Turner et al., 1980; Stefanacci & Amaral, 2000, 2002).

Occipital Cortex

As seen with the parietal cortex, connections between the amygdala and the occipital cortex are thought to be unidirectional. The magnocellular division of the basal nucleus is the only region of the amygdala with efferent connections to the occipital cortex, targeting areas V1, V2, V3, V4, and the middle temporal visual area (Mizuno et al., 1981; Tigges et al., 1982; Tigges, Walker, & Tigges, 1983; Amaral & Price, 1984; Iwai & Yukie, 1987; Weller, Steele, & Kaas, 2002; Amaral et al., 2003; Freese & Amaral, 2005). No evidence has suggested that the occipital cortex has projections to the amygdala (Aggleton et al., 1980; Turner et al., 1980; Iwai & Yukie, 1987; Stefanacci & Amaral, 2000).

Conclusions

As described in this chapter, much of what we know about the neuroanatomy and connectivity of the primate amygdala is from nonhuman primate tracer studies of the macaque monkey. New imaging techniques such as diffusion tensor imaging (DTI) and functional connectivity MRI (fcMRI) provide some insight into the human amygdala connectivity and function which, although limited, generally corroborate findings in the monkey (Catani, Jones, Donato, & Ffytche, 2003). DTI holds some promise for defining amygdaloid subnuclei (Solano-Castiella et al., 2010; Saygin, Osher, Augustinack, Fischl, & Gabrieli, 2011). In fcMRI, coactivation between regions may also elucidate knowledge about both the direct and the indirect flow in information between the amygdala and other brain regions (Bzdok, Laird, Zilles, Fox, & Eickhoff, 2013; Gabard-Durnam et al., 2014; Mishra, Rogers, Chen, & Gore, 2014).

Although very similar in cytoarchitecture and connectivity, there are some important distinctions between the human and monkey amygdalae to be considered. In fact, the lateral nucleus in the human amygdala is considerably larger than would be expected for a primate of comparable brain size (Barger, Stefanacci, & Semendeferi, 2007). The human lateral nucleus contains nearly 60% more neurons than would be predicted from nonhuman primate data, suggesting that an emphasis on the lateral nucleus is the main characteristic of amygdala specialization and expansion over the course of human evolution (Barger et al., 2012), which may represent an important distinction between human and nonhuman primate social and emotional behavior (Hrvoj-Mihic, Bienvenu, Stefanacci, Muotri, & Semendeferi, 2013).

Last, we believe that the future of primate amygdala neuroanatomy may lie in combining traditional histological analyses with modern gene expression profiling to delineate specific nuclei and cell types (Hawrylycz et al., 2012). Characterizing the transcriptomic architecture of the human and nonhuman primate amygdala during fetal development, and throughout lifespan, will provide critical information for discerning the neuroanatomical abnormalities underlying many psychiatric and neuro-developmental disorders.

REFERENCES

Adolphs, R. (2009). The social brain: Neural basis of social knowledge. *Annual Review of Psychology, 60*, 693–716.

Aggleton, J. P. (1985). A description of intra-amygdaloid connections in old world monkeys. *Experimental Brain Research, 57*, 390–399.

Aggleton, J. P. (1986). A description of the amygdalo–hippocampal interconnections in the macaque monkey. *Experimental Brain Research, 64*, 515 –526.

Aggleton, J. P., Burton, M. J., & Passingham, R. E. (1980). Cortical and subcortical afferents to the amygdala of the rhesus monkey (*Macaca mulatta*). *Brain Research, 190*, 347–368.

Aggleton, J. P., & Mishkin, M. (1984). Projections of the amygdala to the thalamus in the cynomolgus monkey. *Journal of Comparative Neurology, 222*, 56–68.

Amaral, D. G. (1986). Amygdalohippocampal and amygdalocortical projections in the primate brain. *Advances in Experimental Medicine and Biology, 203*, 3–17.

Amaral, D. G., & Bassett, J. L. (1989). Cholinergic innervation of the monkey amygdala: An immunohistochemical analysis with antisera to choline acetyltransferase. *Journal of Comparative Neurology, 281*, 337–361.

Amaral, D. G., Behniea, H., & Kelly, J. L. (2003). Topographic organization of projections from the amygdala to the visual cortex in the macaque monkey. *Neuroscience, 118*, 1099–1120.

Amaral, D. G., & Cowan, W. M. (1980). Subcortical afferents to the hippocampal formation in the monkey. *Journal of Comparative Neurology, 189*, 573–591.

Amaral, D. G., & Insausti, R. (1992). Retrograde transport of D-[^{3}H]-aspartate injected into the monkey amygdaloid complex. *Experimental Brain Research, 88*, 375–388.

Amaral, D. G., & Price, J. L. (1984). Amygdalo-cortical projections in the monkey (*Macaca fascicularis*). *Journal of Comparative Neurology, 230*, 465–496.

Amaral, D. G., Price, J. L., Pitkänen, A., & Carmichael, S. T. (1992). Anatomical organization of the primate amygdaloid complex. In J. P. Aggelton (Ed.), *The amygdala: Neurobiological aspects of emotion, memory, and mental dysfuntion* (pp. 1–66). New York: Wiley-Liss.

Amaral, D. G., Schumann, C. M., & Nordahl, C. W. (2008) Neuroanatomy of autism. *Trends in Neurosciences, 31,* 137–145.

Amaral, D. G., Veazey, R. B,, & Cowan, W. M. (1982). Some observations on hypothalamo–amygdaloid connections in the monkey. *Brain Research, 252,* 13–27.

Avendaño, C., Price, J. L., & Amaral, D. G. (1983). Evidence for an amygdaloid projection to premotor cortex but not to motor cortex in the monkey. *Brain Research, 264,* 111–117.

Barbas, H., & De Olmos, J. (1990). Projections from the amygdala to basoventral and mediodorsal prefrontal regions in the rhesus monkey. *Journal of Comparative Neurology, 300,* 549–571.

Barger, N., Stefanacci, L., Schumann, C. M., Sherwood, C. C., Annese, J., Allman, J. M., et al. (2012). Neuronal populations in the basolateral nuclei of the amygdala are differentially increased in humans compared with apes: A stereological study. *Journal of Comparative Neurology, 520,* 3035–3054.

Barger, N., Stefanacci, L., & Semendeferi, K. (2007). A comparative volumetric analysis of the amygdaloid complex and basolateral division in the human and ape brain. *American Journal of Physical Anthropology, 134,* 392–403.

Bauman, M. D., & Amaral, D. G. (2005). The distribution of serotonergic fibers in the macaque monkey amygdala: An immunohistochemical study using antisera to 5-hydroxytryptamine. *Neuroscience, 136,* 193–203.

Baylis, L. L., Rolls, E. T., & Baylis, G. C. (1995). Afferent connections of the caudolateral orbitofrontal cortex taste area of the primate. *Neuroscience, 64,* 801–812.

Buckwalter, J. A., Schumann, C. M., & Van Hoesen, G. W. (2008). Evidence for direct projections from the basal nucleus of the amygdala to retrosplenial cortex in the macaque monkey. *Experimental Brain Research, 186,* 47–57.

Busti, D., Geracitano, R., Whittle, N., Dalezios, Y., Mańko, M., Kaufmann, W., et al. (2011). Different fear states engage distinct networks within the intercalated cell clusters of the amygdala. *Journal of Neuroscience, 31,* 5131–5144.

Bzdok, D., Laird, A. R., Zilles, K., Fox, P. T., & Eickhoff, S. B. (2013). An investigation of the structural, connectional, and functional subspecialization in the human amygdala. *Human Brain Mapping, 34,* 3247–3266.

Carmichael, S. T., & Price, J. L. (1995). Limbic connections of the orbital and medial prefrontal cortex in macaque monkeys. *Journal of Comparative Neurology, 363,* 615–641.

Catani, M., Jones, D. K., Donato, R., & Ffytche, D. H. (2003). Occipito-temporal connections in the human brain. *Brain, 126,* 2093–2107.

Cavada, C., Compañy, T., Tejedor, J., Cruz-Rizzolo, R. J., & Reinoso-Suárez, F. (2000). The anatomical connections of the macaque monkey orbitofrontal cortex: A review. *Cerebral Cortex, 10,* 220–242.

Chareyron, L. J., Lavenex, P. B., Amaral, D. G., & Lavenex, P. (2012). Postnatal development of the amygdala: A stereological study in macaque monkeys. *Journal of Comparative Neurology, 520,* 1965–1984.

Cheng, K., Saleem, K. S., & Tanaka, K. (1997) Organization of corticostriatal and corticoamygdalar projections arising from the anterior inferotemporal area TE of the macaque monkey: A *Phaseolus vulgaris* leucoagglutinin study. *Journal of Neuroscience, 17,* 7902–7925.

Cho, Y. T., Ernst, M., & Fudge, J. L. (2013). Cortico-amygdala-striatal circuits are organized as hierarchical subsystems through the primate amygdala. *Journal of Neuroscience, 33,* 14017–14030.

deCampo, D. M., & Fudge, J. L. (2012). Where and what is the paralaminar nucleus?: A review on a unique and frequently overlooked area of the primate amygdala. *Neuroscience and Biobehavioral Reviews, 36,* 520–535.

Emery, N. J., & Amaral, D. G. (2000). The role of amygdala in primate social cognition. In R. D. Land & L. Nadel (Eds.), *Cognitive neuroscience of emotion* (pp. 156–191). London: Oxford University Press.

Freese, J. L., & Amaral, D. G. (2005). The organization of projections from the amygdala to visual cortical areas TE and V1 in the macaque monkey. *Journal of Comparative Neurology, 486,* 295–317.

Freese, J. L., & Amaral, D. G. (2009). Neuoranatomy of the primate amygdala. In P. J. Whalen & E. A. Phelps (Eds.), *The human amygdala* (pp. 3–42). New York: Guildford Press.

Friedman, D. P., Murray, E. A., O'Neill, J. B., & Mishkin, M. (1986). Cortical connections of the somatosensory fields of the lateral sulcus of macaques: Evidence for a corticolimbic pathway for touch. *Journal of Comparative Neurology, 252,* 323–347.

Fudge, J. L., Kunishio, K., Walsh, P., Richard, C., & Haber, S. N. (2002). Amygdaloid projections to ventromedial striatal subterritories in the primate. *Neuroscience, 110,* 257–275.

Fudge, J. L., & Tucker, T. (2009). Amygdala projections to central amygdaloid nucleus subdivisions and transition zones in the primate. *Neuroscience, 159,* 819–841.

Gabard-Durnam, L. J., Flannery, J., Goff, B., Gee, D. G., Humphreys, K. L., Telzer, E., et al. (2014). The development of human amygdala functional connectivity at rest from 4 to 23 years: A cross-sectional study. *NeuroImage, 95,* 193–207.

Ghashghaei, H. T., & Barbas, H. (2002). Pathways for emotion: Interactions of prefrontal and anterior temporal pathways in the amygdala of the rhesus monkey. *Neuroscience, 115,* 1261–1279.

Giedd, J. N., Castellanos, F. X., Rajapakse, J. C., Vaituzis, A. C., & Rapoport, J. L. (1997). Sexual dimorphism of the developing human brain. *Progress in Neuropsychopharmacology and Biological Psychiatry, 21,* 1185–1201.

Giedd, J. N., Vaituzis, A. C., Hamburger, S. D., Lange, N., Rajapakse, J. C., Kaysen, D., et al. (1996). Quantitative MRI of the temporal lobe, amygdala, and hippocampus in normal human development: Ages 4–18 years. *Journal of Comparative Neurology, 366,* 223–230.

Gloor, P. (1997). The amygdaloid system. In P. Gloor (Ed.), *The temporal lobe and limbic system* (pp. 591–721). New York: Oxford University Press.

Hawrylycz, M. J., Lein, E. S., Guillozet-Bongaarts, A. L., Shen, E. H., Ng, L., Miller, J. A., et al. (2012). An anatomically comprehensive atlas of the adult human brain transcriptome. *Nature, 489,* 391–399.

Herzog, A. G., & Van Hoesen, G. W. (1976). Temporal neocortical afferent connections to the amygdala in the rhesus monkey. *Brain Research, 115,* 57–69.

Hopkins, D. A. (1975). Amygdalotegmental projections in the rat, cat and rhesus monkey. *Neuroscience Letters, 1,* 263–270.

Hrvoj-Mihic, B., Bienvenu, T., Stefanacci, L., Muotri, A. R., & Semendeferi, K. (2013). Evolution, development, and plasticity of the human brain: From molecules to bones. *Frontiers of Human Neuroscience, 7,* 707.

Humphrey, T. (1968). The development of the human amygdala during early embryonic life. *Journal of Comparative Neurology, 132,* 135–165.

Insausti, R., Amaral, D. G., & Cowan, W. M. (1987). The entorhinal cortex of the monkey: II. Cortical afferents. *Journal of Comparative Neurology, 264*(3), 356–395.

Iwai, E., & Yukie, M. (1987). Amygdalofugal and amygdalopetal connections with modality-specific visual cortical areas in macaques (*Macaca fuscata, M. mulatta,* and *M. fascicularis*). *Journal of Comparative Neurology, 261,* 362–387.

Iwai, E., Yukie, M., Suyama, H., & Shirakawa, S. (1987). Amygdalar connections with middle and inferior temporal gyri of the monkey. *Neuroscience Letters, 83,* 25–29.

Jones, E. G., Burton, H., Saper, C. B., & Swanson, L. W. (1976). Midbrain, diencephalic and cortical relationships of the basal nucleus of Meynert and associated structures in primates. *Journal of Comparative Neurology, 167,* 385–419.

Jones, E. G., & Powell, T. P. (1970). An anatomical study of converging sensory pathways within the cerebral cortex of the monkey. *Brain, 93,* 793–820.

Kordower, J. H., Piecinski, P., & Rakic, P. (1992). Neurogenesis of the amygdaloid nuclear complex in the rhesus monkey. *Brain Resresearch: Developmental Brain Research, 68,* 9–15.

Kosmal, A., Malinowska, M., & Kowalska, D. M. (1997). Thalamic and amygdaloid connections of the auditory association cortex of the superior temporal gyrus in rhesus monkey (*Macaca mulatta*). *Acta Neurobiologiae Experimentalis (Warsaw), 57,* 165–188.

Mehler, W. R. (1980). Subcortical afferent connections of the amygdala in the monkey. *Journal of Comparative Neurology, 190,* 733–762.

Millhouse, O. E. (1986). The intercalated cells of the amygdala. *Journal of Comparative Neurology, 247,* 246–271.

Mishra, A., Rogers, B. P., Chen, L. M., & Gore, J. C. (2014). Functional connectivity-based parcellation of amygdala using self-organized mapping: A data driven approach. *Human Brain Mapping, 35,* 1247–1260.

Mizuno, N., Uchida, K., Nomura, S., Nakamura, Y., Sugimoto, T., & Uemura-Sumi, M. (1981). Extrageniculate projections to the visual cortex in the macaque monkey: an HRP study. *Brain Research, 212,* 454–459.

Morán, M. A., Mufson, E. J., & Mesulam, M. M. (1987). Neural inputs into the temporopolar cortex of the rhesus monkey. *Journal of Comparative Neurology, 256,* 88–103.

Morecraft, R. J., Geula, C., & Mesulam, M. M. (1992). Cytoarchitecture and neural afferents of orbitofrontal cortex in the brain of the monkey. *Journal of Comparative Neurology, 323,* 341–358.

Mufson, E. J., Mesulam, M. M., & Pandya, D. N. (1981). Insular interconnections with the amygdala in the rhesus monkey. *Neuroscience, 6,* 1231–1248.

Müller, F., & O'Rahilly, R. (2006). The amygdaloid complex and the medial and lateral ventricular eminences in staged human embryos. *Journal of Anatomy, 208,* 547–564.

Nauta, W. J. (1962). Neural associations of the amygdaloid complex in the monkey. *Brain, 85*, 505–520.

Nitecka, L., & Ben-Ari, Y. (1987). Distribution of GABA-like immunoreactivity in the rat amygdaloid complex. *Journal of Comparative Neurology, 266*, 45–55.

Ostby, Y., Tamnes, C. K., Fjell, A. M., Westlye, L. T., Due-Tønnessen, P., & Walhovd, K. B. (2009). Heterogeneity in subcortical brain development: A structural magnetic resonance imaging study of brain maturation from 8 to 30 years. *Journal of Neuroscience, 29*, 11772–11782.

Pandya, D. N., Van Hoesen, G. W., & Domesick, V. B. (1973). A cingulo-amygdaloid projection in the rhesus monkey. *Brain Research, 61*, 369–373.

Parent, A., Mackey, A., & De Bellefeuille, L. (1983). The subcortical afferents to caudate nucleus and putamen in primate: A fluorescence retrograde double labeling study. *Neuroscience, 10*, 1137–1150.

Payne, C., Machado, C. J., Bliwise, N. G., & Bachevalier, J. (2010). Maturation of the hippocampal formation and amygdala in *Macaca mulatta*: A volumetric magnetic resonance imaging study. *Hippocampus, 20*, 922–935.

Pitkänen, A., & Amaral, D. G. (1991). Demonstration of projections from the lateral nucleus to the basal nucleus of the amygdala: A PHA-L study in the monkey. *Experimental Brain Research, 83*, 465–470.

Pitkänen, A., & Amaral, D. G. (1993). Distribution of parvalbumin-immunoreactive cells and fibers in the monkey temporal lobe: The amygdaloid complex. *Journal of Comparative Neurology, 331*, 14–36.

Pitkänen, A., & Amaral, D. G. (1998). Organization of the intrinsic connections of the monkey amygdaloid complex: Projections originating in the lateral nucleus. *Journal of Comparative Neurology, 398*, 431–458.

Pitkänen, A., Kelly, J. L., & Amaral, D. G. (2002). Projections from the lateral, basal, and accessory basal nuclei of the amygdala to the entorhinal cortex in the macaque monkey. *Hippocampus, 12*(2), 186–205.

Pitkänen, A., & Kemppainen, S. (2002). Comparison of the distribution of calcium-binding proteins and intrinsic connectivity in the lateral nucleus of the rat, monkey, and human amygdala. *Pharmacology Biochemistry and Behavior, 71*, 369–377.

Porrino, L. J., Crane, A. M., & Goldman-Rakic, P. S. (1981). Direct and indirect pathways from the amygdala to the frontal lobe in rhesus monkeys. *Journal of Comparative Neurology, 198*, 121–136.

Price, J. L. (1986). Subcortical projections from the amygdaloid complex. *Advances in Experimental Medicine and Biology, 203*, 19–33.

Price, J. L., & Amaral, D. G. (1981). An autoradiographic study of the projections of the central nucleus of the monkey amygdala. *Journal of Neuroscience, 1*, 1242–1259.

Price, J. L., Russchen, F. T., & Amaral, D. G. (1987). The limbic region: II. The amygdaloid complex. In A. Bjorklund, T. Hokfelt, & L. W. Swenson (Eds.), *Handbook of chemical neuoroanatomy: Vol. 5. Integrated systems of the CNS* (Part I, pp. 279–388). Amsterdam: Elsevier.

Rosene, D. L., & Van Hoesen, G. W. (1977). Hippocampal efferents reach widespread areas of cerebral cortex and amygdala in the rhesus monkey. *Science, 198*, 315–317.

Russchen, F. T., Amaral, D. G., & Price, J. L. (1985a). The afferent connections of the substantia innominata in the monkey, *Macaca fascicularis. Journal of Comparative Neurology, 242,* 1–27.

Russchen, F. T., Bakst, I., Amaral, D. G., & Price, J. L. (1985b). The amygdalostriatal projections in the monkey. An anterograde tracing study. *Brain Research, 329,* 241–257.

Saunders, R. C., & Rosene, D. L. (1988). A comparison of the efferents of the amygdala and the hippocampal formation in the rhesus monkey: I. Convergence in the entorhinal, prorhinal, and perirhinal cortices. *Journal of Comparative Neurology, 271*(2),153–184.

Saunders, R. C., Rosene, D. L., & Van Hoesen, G. W. (1988). Comparison of the efferents of the amygdala and the hippocampal formation in the rhesus monkey: II. Reciprocal and non-reciprocal connections. *Journal of Comparative Neurology, 271,* 185–207.

Saygin, Z. M., Osher, D. E., Augustinack, J., Fischl, B., & Gabrieli, J. D. E. (2011). Connectivity-based segmentation of human amygdala nuclei using probabilistic tractography. *NeuroImage, 56,* 1353–1361.

Schumann, C. M., & Amaral, D. G. (2005). Stereological estimation of the number of neurons in the human amygdaloid complex. *Journal of Comparative Neurology, 491,* 320–329.

Schumann, C. M., Bauman, M. D., & Amaral, D. G. (2011). Abnormal structure or function of the amygdala is a common component of neurodevelopmental disorders. *Neuropsychologia, 49,* 745–759.

Schumann, C. M., Hamstra, J., Goodlin-Jones, B. L., Lotspeich, L. J., Kwon, H., Buonocore, M. H., et al. (2004). The amygdala is enlarged in children but not adolescents with autism; the hippocampus is enlarged at all ages. *Journal of Neuroscience, 24,* 6392–6401.

Schumann, C. M., Scott, J. A., Lee, A., Fletcher, A., Buoncore, M., Bauman, M. D., et al. (in preparation). *Amygdala growth from youth to adulthood in the macaque monkey.* Unpublished manuscript.

Setzer, M., & Ulfig, N. (1999). Differential expression of calbindin and calretinin in the human fetal amygdala. *Microscopy Research and Technique, 46,* 1–17.

Solano-Castiella, E., Anwander, A., Lohmann, G., Weiss, M., Docherty, C., Geyer, S., et al. (2010). Diffusion tensor imaging segments the human amygdala *in vivo. NeuroImage, 49,* 2958–2965.

Sorvari, H., Soininen, H., Paljärvi, L., Karkola, K., & Pitkänen, A. (1995). Distribution of parvalbumin-immunoreactive cells and fibers in the human amygdaloid complex. *Journal of Comparative Neurology, 360,* 185–212.

Sorvari, H., Soininen, H., & Pitkänen, A. (1996a). Calbindin-D28K-immunoreactive cells and fibres in the human amygdaloid complex. *Neuroscience, 75,* 421–443.

Sorvari, H., Soininen, H., & Pitkänen, A. (1996b). Calretinin-immunoreactive cells and fibers in the human amygdaloid complex. *Journal of Comparative Neurology, 369,* 188–208.

Stefanacci, L., & Amaral, D. G. (2000). Topographic organization of cortical inputs to the lateral nucleus of the macaque monkey amygdala: A retrograde tracing study. *Journal of Comparative Neurology, 421,* 52–79.

Stefanacci, L., & Amaral, D. G. (2002). Some observations on cortical inputs to the macaque monkey amygdala: An anterograde tracing study. *Journal of Comparative Neurology, 451,* 301–323.

Stefanacci, L., Suzuki, W. A., & Amaral, D. G. (1996). Organization of connections between the amygdaloid complex and the perirhinal and parahippocampal cortices in macaque monkeys. *Journal of Comparative Neurology, 375*, 552–582.

Tigges, J., Tigges, M., Cross, N. A., McBride, R. L., Letbetter, W. D., & Anschel, S. (1982). Subcortical structures projecting to visual cortical areas in squirrel monkey. *Journal of Comparative Neurology, 209*, 29–40.

Tigges, J., Walker, L. C., & Tigges, M. (1983). Subcortical projections to the occipital and parietal lobes of the chimpanzee brain. *Journal of Comparative Neurology, 220*, 106–115.

Turner, B. H., Gupta, K. C., & Mishkin, M. (1978). The locus and cytoarchitecture of the projection areas of the olfactory bulb in Macaca mulatta. *Journal of Comparative Neurology, 177*(3), 381–396.

Turner, B. H., Mishkin, M., & Knapp, M. (1980). Organization of the amygdalopetal projections from modality-specific cortical association areas in the monkey. *Journal of Comparative Neurology, 191*, 515–543.

Uematsu, A., Matsui, M., Tanaka, C., Takahashi, T., Noguchi, K., Suzuki, M., et al. (2012). Developmental trajectories of amygdala and hippocampus from infancy to early adulthood in healthy individuals. *PLoS One, 7*, e46970.

Ulfig, N., Setzer, M., & Bohl, J. (1998). Transient architectonic features in the basolateral amygdala of the human fetal brain. *Acta Anatomica (Basel), 163*, 99–112.

Ulfig, N., Setzer, M., & Bohl, J. (1999). Distribution of GAP-43-immunoreactive structures in the human fetal amygdala. *European Journal of Histochemistry, 43*, 19–28.

Ulfig, N., Setzer, M., & Bohl, J. (2003). Ontogeny of the human amygdala. *Annals of the New York Academy of Sciences, 985*, 22–33.

Van Hoesen, G. (1981). The differential distribution, diversity and sprouting of cortical projections to the amygdala in the rhesus monkey. In Y. Ben-Ari (Ed.), *The amygdaloid complex* (pp. 77–90). Amsterdam: Elsevier/North Holland.

Van Hoesen, G., & Pandya, D. N. (1975). Some connections of the entorhinal (area 28) and perirhinal (area 35) cortices of the rhesus monkey: I. Temporal lobe afferents. *Brain Research, 95*, 1–24.

Vogt, B. A., & Pandya, D. N. (1987). Cingulate cortex of the rhesus monkey: II. Cortical afferents. *Journal of Comparative Neurology, 262*, 271–289.

Webster, M. J., Ungerleider, L. G., & Bachevalier, J. (1991). Connections of inferior temporal areas TE and TEO with medial temporal-lobe structures in infant and adult monkeys. *Journal of Neuroscience, 11*, 1095–1116.

Weller, R. E., Steele, G. E., & Kaas, J. H. (2002). Pulvinar and other subcortical connections of dorsolateral visual cortex in monkeys. *Journal of Comparative Neurology, 450*, 215–240.

Witter, M. P., & Amaral, D. G. (1991). Entorhinal cortex of the monkey: V. Projections to the dentate gyrus, hippocampus, and subicular complex. *Journal of Comparative Neurology, 307*, 437–459.

Yukie, M. (2002). Connections between the amygdala and auditory cortical areas in the macaque monkey. *Neuroscience Research, 42*, 219–229.

CHAPTER 3

A Short History of the Lesion Technique for Probing Amygdala Function

DAVID G. AMARAL

Much of the research reviewed in this book is based on the behavioral conse-quences of various forms of lesions in experimental animals and human sub-jects. A consistent theme in this research is that alterations in emotional behav-ior that are characteristic of selective amygdala lesions are far different from the behavioral outcomes of damage to the temporal neocortex in which it is embedded or to the hippocampal formation that is its neighbor. The history of how this appreciation was gained parallels the efforts of neuroscience to local-ize specific functions to anatomically defined regions of the brain. It is a story of missed opportunities, of capitalizing on unexpected findings, and of incre-mental specification of the critical locus of brain damage leading to dramatic behavioral alterations. This chapter provides a selective review of research that extends back into the late 1880s dealing with lesions and amygdala function. It also highlights the era of psychosurgery in which the results from animal lesion studies were applied to the treatment of human epileptic and psychiatric patients. While much of the history of lesions and the amygdala is based on nonprimate animal studies, this chapter deals almost entirely with studies in nonhuman primates and human subjects.

Animal Studies

The practice of producing lesions of the brain and observing alterations of behavior in animal models dates back to the pioneering research of the French physiologist Pierre Flourens. In studies initiated in the early 1800s, Flourens (1842) produced lesions in the brains of pigeons and rab-bits, and concluded that the cerebral cortex is responsible for sensory perception, the cerebellum for motor coordination, and the medulla for heart rate, respiration and other vital bodily functions (Tizard, 1959). Shortly after these initial studies, a number of prominent names in the early era of neuroscience engaged in complementary electrical stimulation and lesion studies to define the functions of the cerebral cortex; many of these studies were carried out in nonhuman primates. It is important to appreciate the relative poverty of understanding related to the structure and function of the brain at the time of these early studies. It was not until 1870, when Gustav Fritsch and Eduard Hitzig, at the University of Berlin, published the remarkable finding that passing a weak electrical current through the cerebral cortex could lead to contractions of the limbs! This was the dawn of understanding that the brain and, more specifically, the cerebral cortex was made up of excitable tissue. David Ferrier, a London physician driven by an interest in understanding the cerebral basis of epilepsy, wanted to replicated these findings and carried out a series of studies at the West Riding Lunatic Asylum on animals ranging from frogs to monkeys. These studies identified motor regions of the cerebral cortex, and Ferrier's publication of his primate studies (1874, 1875) began to put the idea of cerebral localization on firm experimental ground. This early period of cerebral stimulation and ablation is portrayed in an interesting review by Millet (1998), who highlighted the use of neuroanatomical illustrations as a means of conveying these newly emerging data. There was considerable uncertainty about the function of much of the cerebral cortex and some clearly incorrect conclusions based, presumably, on the limitations of experimental techniques and behavioral observation. Ferrier reported, for example, that removal of the occipital lobes in monkeys did not result in visual impairments, and he thought that the angular gyrus was the primary visual cortex. This conclusion undoubtedly resulted from the relative sparing of much of the occipital lobes in his experimental animals. Nonetheless, many researchers of this era contributed to a substantial body of evidence that different functions were mediated by specific territories of the cerebral cortex. As reasonable as this perspective now seems, it did not go unchallenged. There was something of a countercurrent to the localizationalist perspective that was championed by several scientists, including the American psychologist Karl Lashley, who had a lifelong fascination with the organization of the visual system and also intensively studied the brain basis of learning and memory. He was perennially in search of the biological locus of memory, which he called the "engram." When these efforts were unsuccessful he quipped, "I sometimes feel, in reviewing the evidence on the localization of the memory trace, that the necessary conclusion is that learning just is not possible" (Lashley, 1950, pp. 477–478). His learning studies involved making lesions of various portions of the cortex and attempting to establish which led to a loss of memory function. These studies led to the proposal of mass action, which suggested that loss of memory performance was directly proportional to the amount of cortical tissue that was removed. His research on the visual system also suggested a lack of localization, since he believed that visual function was largely spared as long as some minimal amount of visual cortex was spared by a lesion. This led to the notion of equipotentiality or the idea that any portion of the cerebral cortex could perform any function. Lashley was a brilliant scientist and experimentalist, and I cite his work only to emphasize how little was really known about the location of function in the neocortex in the late 1800s and early 1900s. This short introduction leads to the first study germane to lesions and the function of the amygdala.

Sanger Brown, an American neurologist, was the student of Edward Albert Sharpey-Schafer, the Jodrell Professor of Physiology at University College London. In 1887, they collaborated on a series of studies aimed at identifying the visual cortex of the monkey brain (Brown & Schafer, 1888). They carried out unilateral or two-stage bilateral extirpations of portions of the occipital or temporal lobes and carefully studied the effects of these lesions on the behavior of the animals. One of these experiments (VI) was carried out on a large, male rhesus monkey. In a first surgery, the right temporal lobe was removed. This resulted in very little observable change in the animal's behavior. Five days after the first operation, the left temporal lobe was also removed. Rather than summarize the findings, I have reproduced this section of their paper so that the results are presented in the authors' own words:

> Results.—These severe operations were recovered from with marvellous rapidity, the animal appearing perfectly well even so early as the day after the establishment of the second lesion. A remarkable change is, however, manifested in the disposition of the Monkey. Prior to the operations he was very wild and even fierce, assaulting any person who teased or tried to handle him. Now he voluntarily approaches all persons indifferently, allows himself to be handled, or even to be teased or slapped, without making any attempt at retaliation or endeavouring to escape. His memory and intelligence seem deficient. He gives evidence of hearing, seeing, and of the possession of his senses generally, but it is clear that he no longer clearly understands the meaning of the sounds, sights, and other impressions that reach him. Every object with which he comes in contact, even those with which he was previously most familiar, appears strange and is investigated with curiosity. Everything he endeavours to feel, taste, and smell, and to carefully examine from every point of view. This is the case not only with inanimate objects, but also with persons and with his fellow Monkeys. And even after having examined an object in this way with the utmost care and deliberation, he will, on again coming across the same object accidentally even a few minutes afterwards, go through exactly the same process, as if he had entirely forgotten his previous experiments. His food is devoured

greedily, the head being dipped into the dish, instead of the food being conveyed to the mouth by the hands in the way usual with Monkeys. He appears no longer to discriminate between the different kinds of food; e.g., he no longer picks out the currants from a dish of food, but devours everything just as it happens to come. He still, however, possesses the sense of taste, for when given a raisin which has been partly filled with quinine he shows evident signs of distaste, and refuses to eat the fruit.

It is also clear that he still both sees and hears. The field of vision appeared at first somewhat limited, and he also seemed to see somewhat indistinctly, making, for example, one or two unsuccessful attempts to pick up a currant from the floor before finally succeeding. This condition, however, soon passed off. He reacts to all kinds of noises, even slight ones, such as the rustling of a piece of paper, but shows no consequent evidence of alarm or agitation, although his attention is evidently attracted by sounds. Thus he was observed to follow with his head the sound of footsteps passing along the corridor just outside his room, directing his attention to them as long as one could oneself distinctly hear them.

This peculiar mental condition was observed for some weeks, becoming gradually less noticeable. A week after the second operation it is noted that he appears brighter in disposition, and is again commencing to display signs of tyrannising proclivities towards his mate, for which he had been remarkable previously. About this time a strange Monkey, wild and savage, was put into the common cage. Our Monkey immediately began to investigate the new comer in the way described, but his attentions were repulsed, and a fight resulted, in which he was being considerably worsted. The animals were, however, separated and tied up away from one another, but our Monkey soon managed to free himself, and at once proceeded, without any signs of fear or suspicion, again to investigate the stranger, having apparently already entirely forgotten the result of his former investigation.

Two weeks after the second operation it is noted that this Monkey continues to "investigate" objects, but with diminishing frequency and thoroughness. He is either rapidly regaining some of his former experience and memory, or forming altogether new ones. He now takes his food up with his hands, and also pays a more natural attention to his fellows than before. All his senses are acute.

Five weeks after the operation his curiosity has sensibly diminished, and he is slowly regaining his former mercurial temperament, continuing, however, tame.

This Monkey was kept for nearly eight months after the operation. Long before the expiration of that time he had regained full possession of his mental faculties, and became one of the brightest and most intelligent animals that we had experience of, domineering over all the other Monkeys which were kept in the same cage with him. He was shown to and tested before the Physiological and Neurological Societies, and was also seen privately by several eminent neurologists. With regard to this Monkey there was no difference of opinion expressed, but it was universally admitted that all his senses, including that of hearing, were perfectly acute. Indeed, it was eventually impossible to detect any abnormality of the cerebral functions.

The animal eventually died of dysentery, after a short illness.

Autopsy.—With the exception of the large intestine, which is ulcerated and inflamed, all the organs appear healthy. In the brain the whole of the temporal lobe is completely removed upon both sides; the lesion extending quite up to the Sylvian fissure on the outer surface, and reaching to the inner edge of the hemisphere on the under surface. On the right side the lesion does not quite reach the parietooccipital fissure on the external surface, but on the left side the removal extends quite up to this fissure. A very small piece of the antero-inferior edge of the lobe remains on the left side, but this is undermined and cut off from the medullary centre. No trace of the superior temporal gyrus is left on either side, except a part of the grey matter bounding the Sylvian fissure below, and this grey matter is devoid of its corresponding medullary centre.

Remarks.—This is the most extensive bilateral lesion of the whole temporal region which we have performed. What is most remarkable about it is the immediate loss and ultimate recovery of the intellectual faculty. On localisation of functions the experiment throws no direct light; what evidence there is being entirely negative. (pp. 310–312)

The illustration that represents the extent of this lesion is reproduced here as Figure 3.1. It is clear that this massive, bilateral lesion not only removes nearly the entirety of temporal neocortex but also the bulk of the medial temporal lobe, including both the amygdala and the hippocampal formation.

Many of the other experiments reported in this paper had lesions confined to the lateral temporal neocortex. And none of these led to the unusual changes in personality and behavior that were seen in experiment VI. What is so remarkable about the observations in this paper is that they so accurately presaged the observations by Klüver and Bucy (1939) on their experimental monkey Aurora, to which we turn next, and that they were so completely ignored.

Fifty years after the publication of Brown and Schafer (1888), Heinrich Klüver, a University of Chicago psychologist, and Paul Bucy, a Chicago-area neurosurgeon, teamed up to carry out studies that were similar in style. Klüver had earlier carried out studies of the visual system with Lashley, which involved lesions of the occipital lobe. But, the studies with Bucy were aimed at understanding which areas of the brain mediated the hallucinatory images induced by mescaline. Klüver was fascinated with the psychotropic effects of mescaline and had personally experienced the effects of sampling peyote buttons. While Klüver was primarily interested in determining the brain regions involved in producing

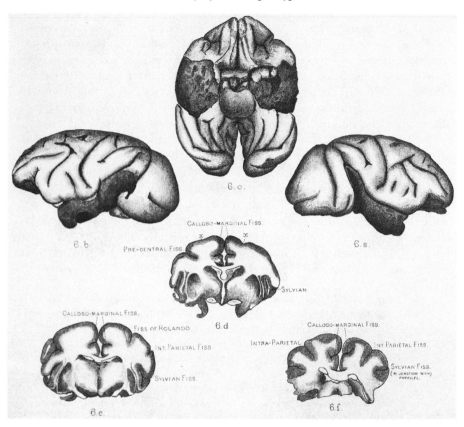

FIGURE 3.1. A reproduction of a figure from the paper by Brown and Schaffer (1888) that illustrates the extent of the bilateral lesion in the rhesus monkey, described in the quoted material in the text. Virtually the entire temporal lobe is resected bilaterally.

the visual impressions induced by mescaline, he understood that this would be impossible to determine in nonhuman primate experiments. But, Klüver also knew that mescaline induced jaw movements in monkeys that resembled the facial motor responses in humans with temporal lobe epilepsy. These were thought to be mediated by medial portions of the temporal lobe. He thought that if temporal lobe lesions halted the mescaline-induced jaw movements, that this would be a first step towards establishing the locus of the visual hallucinations to the temporal lobe. Since Klüver had never carried out temporal lobectomies, he enlisted the aid of Bucy to handle the complex surgery. Bucy argued that prior to doing the technically more difficult selective medial temporal lobectomy, they should try a complete temporal lobectomy first.

Their first experiment was carried out on an adult, female rhesus monkey (Aurora) in December 1936. This was a highly vicious monkey that was offered to Klüver because of his expertise in working with adult rhesus monkeys. Bucy (1985) recounted that he first removed the left temporal lobe. On the morning after the surgery, Klüver called him to ask, "What did you do to my monkey?" When Bucy arrived to evaluate the monkey, he found that the previously aggressive animal had become tame. This is somewhat odd, since unilateral temporal lobectomy is usually without major effect on emotionality and suggests that there may have been some preexisting damage to the right medial temporal lobe. Anyway, in the second surgery, carried out about a month and a half later, the right temporal lobe was removed. Thereafter, Klüver carried out detailed behavioral observations of Aurora for the next 4 months. He chronicled a series of behavioral changes he initially called the "temporal lobe syndrome" but which later came to be known as the Klüver–Bucy syndrome. Here are some of the findings reported in the 1938 paper:

> Sensory and Motor Factors—From the very beginning the monkey had no difficulty picking up objects. . . . The ability to localize position in space and to recognize the shape of objects did not seem to be impaired even if the objects were placed on surfaces exhibiting complex visual patterns. . . . Although quantitative data are lacking, it may be inferred from the various observations and tests that the ability of the monkey to appreciate differences in brightness, size, shape, distance or position was not seriously, if at all disturbed . . . she showed no visual defect when climbing, running or jumping around. . . . We also failed to find changes in cutaneous sensitivity. . . . it is difficult to say whether her sense of smell is impaired. On the one hand, she did not appear to utilize olfactory cues or respond differentially to various olfactory stimuli, whereas on the other hand, she went through the motion of "smelling" by holding objects repeatedly before her nostrils. . . . From general observation it appeared that there was no motor deficit.
>
> Psychic Blindness—Following the second operation, it was incidentally observed that while the monkey showed no gross defect in the ability to discriminate visually, she seemed to have lost entirely the ability to recognize and detect the meaning of objects on the basis of optical criteria alone. . . . Subsequently, the reactions of the monkey to various objects were studied more systematically [and] may be briefly summarized as follows:
>
> 1. The hungry animal picks up all objects within reach. . . . She finally discards those which are not edible. She approaches any animate or inanimate object without hesitation and even picks up and examines, or tried to examine, objects which represent strong emotional stimuli for normal monkeys.
> 4. She examines all available objects. If the first object she picks up is the only piece of food . . . she eats it and then continues to examine the remaining objects.

5. Even though some of the objects have been presented previously, the monkey nevertheless, examines such objects as if they were being presented for the first time.

Emotional Changes—The rather startling changes in her emotional reactions remain to be considered. The picture she presented after the second operation was one of complete loss of all emotional reactions. In spite of being active and exhibiting great interest and curiosity in her surroundings at all times, she appeared never to discover anything causing resentment, anger, fear or pleasure. . . . The tendency to approach and contact every object in sight was so strong that she never wavered or hesitated even when approaching a strange person, a cat, a dog or a snake. . . . During the first few months all modes of affective expression as evidences by vocalization and rhythmical lip, tongue and jaw movements accompanying various sounds had completely disappeared.

The description of the behavioral alterations provided in the paper by Klüver and Bucy (1938) is remarkable both for the level of detail and for the similarity to the findings for monkey VI in Brown and Schafer. Remarkably, the paper by Brown and Schafer (1888) was not cited in Klüver and Bucy (1938). A comprehensive biographical sketch of Klüver has been produced by Nahm (1997), who indicates that Klüver carried out a literature search only after he made the observations of Aurora and came across the paper by Brown and Schafer (1888). Nahm (1997) also advanced a set of interesting suggestions as to why the findings reported by Brown and Schafer (1888) were largely ignored but caused intense interest when presented by Klüver and Bucy (1938). Nahm (1997) pointed out that Klüver was not particularly interested in the localization of the functions that were lost after these lesions. And, in fact, for the purposes of this chapter, the amygdala is never mentioned in the 1938 paper. Moreover, the extent of the lesion was not fully documented until later, in a very detailed paper by Bucy and Klüver (1955). As illustrated in Figure 3.2, which is taken from that paper, the lesion is as extensive and very similar to the one produced in experiment VI by Brown and Schafer (1888).

The establishment of the temporal lobe syndrome, and particularly the emotional changes that these lesions produced, did set off a chain reaction of studies that ultimately attributed the emotional changes that Klüver and Bucy reported to damage of the amygdala.

Two papers published in 1953 attempted to refine the understanding of which brain damage led to the Klüver–Bucy syndrome. Pribram and Bagsaw (1953) based their placement of lesions on findings from strychnine neuronography that suggested prominent medial temporal lobe connections with the orbitofrontal cortex. They produced lesions is a variety of primates that involved posterior orbital cortex, temporal pole, periamygdaloid cortex, and amygdala. While they confirmed many

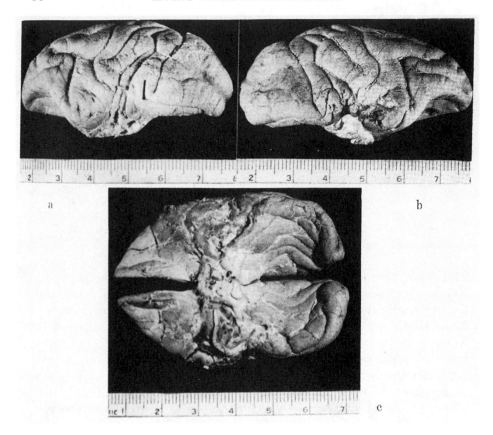

FIGURE 3.2. A reproduction of an illustration in Bucy and Klüver (1955, Plate 1), showing the appearance of the lateral (Panels A and B) and ventral (Panel C) surfaces of the animal (Aurora) described in their 1938 paper. The lesion is as extensive as the one reported by Brown and Schaffer (1888, Experiment VI).

of the emotional changes reported by Klüver and Bucy, this paper did not provide evidence that the amygdala was specifically involved.

The other paper that appeared in 1953 was by Walker, Thomson, and McQueen. Working at the Johns Hopkins University Medical School, these investigators carried out 11 experiments on young rhesus monkeys in which the anterior medial temporal lobe, including the amygdala, was damaged by suction ablation. The behavioral consequences of these lesions were studied in a number of contexts following the lesions. One unique aspect to this paper is that one of the investigators carried out preoperative behavioral assessments for 1 week up to 2 months in order to get a sense of the prelesion personality of the subject monkeys. These investigators not only chronicled the behavioral changes that resulted from the lesions, but they also described the amount of damage to the amygdala in each case. They observed dramatic emotional changes in some of their animals but not in others. For cases in which only superficial cortex was damaged, they saw little behavioral change. Hippocampal damage was also not associated with behavioral changes. The authors concluded,

> At first glance the damage to the amygdaloid complex seems to correlate with the degree of behavioral change but on a second look it is apparent that Monkey 65 challenges this conclusion. In this animal the left amygdaloid complex was practically entirely removed and on the right side the anterior and inferior portions of that mass were ablated. The monkey, however, exhibited no behavioral changes. Except for this experiment the thesis might be defended that damage to the amygdala was responsible for the alterations in conduct. . . . Thus we may only conclude that the amount of damage to the amygdaloid complex in general correlates fairly well with the degree of social and environmental (tameness) change of conduct. (pp. 89–91)

Thus, the conclusion from this paper is that the taming and other changes in emotional behavior were likely due to damage to the amygdala, but the behavioral changes may be related to either how much or what part of the amygdala was damaged. The idea that the size of the lesion matters will reemerge when we discuss the more recent paper by Aggleton and Passingham (1981b).

Lawrence Weiskrantz, a graduate student with Karl Pribram, undertook an analysis of monkeys with anteromedial temporal lobe lesions for his dissertation research. This work, published by Weiskrantz in 1956, was an extension of the paper by Pribram and Bagshaw (1953) discussed previously. Not only did Weiskrantz want to further specify the regions of the temporal lobe that led to reduction of fear and tameness, but he also wanted to evaluate further the behavioral ramifications of a lesion that decreased fear. "Are changes found in more than one 'emotional' situation? Are the 'emotional' changes artifactually produced, or at least influenced by other behavioral changes such as altered activity level, paralysis, stupor, blindness, etc.?" (Weiskrantz, 1956, p. 381). In addition to direct observations, the animals were formally tested on a conditioned avoidance and conditioned depression task. Efforts were also made to provide a quantitative measure of tameness. Weiskrantz produced one-stage bilateral lesions that involved either the temporal pole and amygdaloid (AM) complex or the inferotemporal (IT) cortex. Figure 3.3 summarizes some of the AM lesions that were produced.

Clearly, these lesions were much more discrete than others that had been produced in the past. Weiskrantz (1956) provided the following summary of the general behavioral changes observed following surgery:

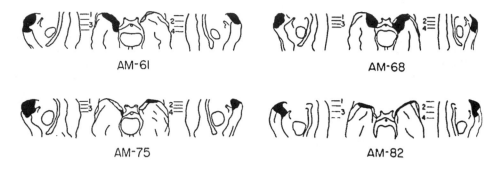

AM-61

AM-68

AM-75

AM-82

FIGURE 3.3. Illustrations adapted from the paper by Weiskrantz (1956). These more discrete lesions involved the temporal polar cortex, as well as the amygdala, and produced many of the changes in emotional behavior that were observed by Brown and Schaffer (1888) and Klüver and Bucy (1938).

> Postoperatively there was an immediate and unmistakable difference in appearance and behavior between AM operates and controls. The AM animals permitted petting and handling without visible excitement, or even approached and reached for observers. On the other hand, control operates continued to display their fear of and hostility toward humans by running to the farthest corner of the cage, frequently urinating and defecating, grimacing, and screeching. The AM operates were also altered in their reactions to sticks and gloves, handling and chewing them without hesitation. Controls showed the same violent behavior toward these objects as they had preoperatively. The excessive oral examination of objects reported by Klüver and Bucy (for temporal lobectomized animals) was also observed in the present group of AM operates, but diminished after a week to ten days. In some cases, food ingestion was quite indiscriminate, and included feces and horse meat. Hypersexuality, reported by other investigators . . . was never observed, but this may have been because of the sexual immaturity of all experimental animals and their isolation in single cages during the course of experimentation. (p. 385)

The major results of this paper are summarized in the paper's Discussion section.

> In both the avoidance and the depression situations: (a) man was less of a disturbing or aversive factor to the AM operates than to controls; (b) the AM operates had a slower rate of acquisition than sham operates, but in both situations one IT operate deviated from the sham operate level; and (c) the AM operates had a faster rate of extinction for conditioned avoidance and depressive behavior established preoperatively. (pp. 387–388)

This paper thus went some way toward a confirmation that damage to the amygdala and immediately surrounding tissue was sufficient to produce tameness in monkeys and was the first to propose a possible mechanism (i.e., that the monkeys extinguished a preoperatively acquired fear of humans). Weiskrantz does not conclude that damage to the amygdala is the only lesion that results in these emotional changes but provides evidence that inferotemporal cortex lesions, which were studied as controls, certainly do not. Weiskrantz also suggests that the total syndrome of altered behaviors produced by lesions of the amygdala can not be subsumed under the general notion of reduction of fear. The indiscriminate eating of foods such as meat or even feces, he argued, is difficult to align with a reduction of fear. Rather, "the effect of amygdalectomy, it is suggested, is to make it difficult for reinforcing stimuli, whether positive or negative, to become established or to be recognized as such" This hypothesis has been tested in much of the work of Betsy Murray, some of which is summarized in Murray and Rhodes (Chapter 9, this volume). Despite the caveats that Weiskrantz raises in the Discussion section of this paper, it is generally acknowledged that this was the first paper to establish firmly that lesions of the amygdala could result in the tameness and other emotional changes first observed by Brown and Sanger (1888).

There were a number of technical breakthroughs in the post–World War II era that enabled much more sophisticated neuroscientific research, as well as more selective neurosurgery. One of these was the widespread development and use of the stereotaxic apparatus. Robert Henry Clarke, a British surgeon and anatomist, conceived of the idea of developing a rigid frame in which the head of an experimental animal or human patient could be placed to enable the precise lesion of a brain region based on predetermined three-dimensional coordinates. The first stereotaxic apparatus was built in London in 1905, at a cost of £300 and patented by Clarke 9 years later. In the interim, it was used for a series of collaborative studies of the cerebellum between Clarke and neurosurgeon Victor Horsely (reviewed in Fodstad, Hariz, & Ljunggren, 1991). While the stereotaxic apparatus was sporadically used, it was widely adopted and commercialized for experimental and human neurosurgical use in the 1950s and 1960s. The first experimental instrument, for example, was built in the early 1930s at Northwestern University. By 1947, there were only 50 stereotaxic apparatuses in use in the United States, and these were mainly built in university fabrication laboratories. It was not until 1956 that David Kopf started a factory in his garage in California producing Kopf stereotaxics.

I mention this history of the stereotaxic apparatus because the next step in determining that lesions of the amygdala were responsible for the emotional changes of the temporal lobe syndrome came from the use of stereotaxic placement of radiofrequency lesions in the monkey by

Aggleton and Passingham (1981b). Using a David Kopf stereotaxic apparatus, the lesions were produced by lowering a radiofrequency probe into the amygdaloid complex. These investigators had previously established an X-ray-based atlas of the rhesus monkey's temporal fossa (Aggleton & Passingham, 1981a), and this strategy was used to guide the probe to an appropriate region within the amygdaloid complex. Perhaps the major contribution of this paper was to establish that a total bilateral lesion of the amygdaloid complex with minimal damage to surrounding tissue can lead to the full Klüver–Bucy syndrome. Interestingly, when the lesion of the amygdala was subtotal, the resulting behavioral modification was much more subtle.

If we fast-forward to the 1990s, there was one remaining issue that needed to be resolved. We and others had demonstrated that fibers arising from regions other than the amygdala, such as the perirhinal cortex, traveled immediately adjacent to or even within the substance of the amygdala en route to the orbitofrontal cortex or other brain destinations (Lavenex, Suzuki, & Amaral, 2002) and ablative lesions of the amygdala were shown to disrupt some of these projections (Goulet, Dore, & Murray, 1998). The question arose, therefore, of whether the behavioral alterations resulting from lesions confined to the amygdaloid complex were due to damage of amygdala neurons and their connections or, at least in part, to some of the fibers of passage that traverse the amygdala but arise and terminate in different brain regions. This issue was first investigated directly by Meunier, Bachevalier, Murray, Malkova, and Mishkin (1999). They were able to do this due to the development of a new drug-induced "neurotoxic" form of lesion using ibotenic acid. This toxin, which killed neuronal cell bodies but did not damage axons of passage, could be injected into the amygdala at several locations to produce a really selective amygdala lesion (Jarrard, 1989). These authors concluded that

> relative to controls, monkeys with neurotoxic lesions showed the same array of behavioural changes as those with aspiration lesions, i.e. reduced fear and aggression, increased submission, and excessive manual and oral exploration. Even partial neurotoxic lesions involving less than two-thirds of the amygdala significantly altered fear and manual exploration. These findings convincingly demonstrate that the amygdala is crucial for the normal regulation of emotions in monkeys. Nevertheless, because some of the symptoms observed after neurotoxic lesions were less marked than those seen after aspiration lesions, the emotional disorders described earlier after amygdalectormy in monkeys were likely exacerbated by the attendant fibre damage. (Meunier et al., 1999, p. 4403)

Subsequently, we (Emery et al., 2001) have replicated the finding that selective ibotenic acid lesions produce profound changes in emotional behavior in adult rhesus monkeys. We have also used this technique to carry out selective lesions in neonatal rhesus monkeys, and the results of those studies are reported by Bliss-Moreau, Moadab, and Amaral (Chapter 6, this volume). Thus, in studies spanning the time period of 1880–2000, it has now been convincingly demonstrated that selective damage to the neurons of the amygdala produces a syndrome of behavioral changes that resembles in many respects the overt behavioral changes first observed by Brown and Schafer (1888). There are still many questions to resolve. For example, it is not clear what part each of the 13 nuclei and cortical regions of the amygdaloid complex plays in the evocation of normal fear and species-typical emotional responses. Given the known neurocircuitry of the amygdala, it remains somewhat mysterious why lesions of key regions do not lead to the same behavioral sequelae. The lateral nucleus, for example, receives much of the sensory information that enters the amygdala. One would expect that selective lesions of this nucleus bilaterally should results in a profound change in the animal's behavior. But there is little evidence to support that hypothesis at the moment.

Human Studies

The 1950s, '60s, and '70s ushered in a steady increase of neurosurgical procedures for the treatment of brain disorders, ranging from Parkinson's disease to epilepsy to behavioral problems. Based on the findings of decreased aggression in monkeys published by Klüver and Bucy (1955), many neurosurgeons attempted lesions of the amygdaloid complex to alleviate aggressive outbursts and other destructive emotional behaviors. These tended to be done in greater numbers in countries such as Japan and India, in which proper behavior, particularly of children, has very narrow social norms.

Probably the paper by Hrayr Terzian and Giuseppe Ore (1955), based on work carried out in Italy, was the first to report a surgery motivated by Klüver and Bucy's findings. The Introduction to this paper states, "More or less complete bilateral removal of the temporal lobes has been recently practiced in man also, both for the purpose of removing bilateral epileptogenic foci and, directly inspired in this by the experimental work of Klüver and Bucy, for the purpose of modifying aggressive behavior and agitation in schizophrenic subjects" (p. 374).

The authors describe a single patient in the following way:

> A 19 year old boy was admitted to the hospital on August 26, 1952 with a history of seizures. When three years old he was afflicted by an attack of fever lasting seven days. Some months later he began to suffer from epileptic attacks of psychomotor and grand mal type, with rotation of the head and eyes to the right, and they were followed by paresis of the right extremities. Almost all these attacks were preceded by terrifying

visual hallucinations, rarely by auditory hallucinations. Fits of minor scale were followed by long states of confusion with various automatisms from the most simple to the most complex. In addition to this the patient presented considerable changes of character, which became more accentuated in the following years and were accompanied by paroxysms of aggressive and violent behavior. Several times during these attacks, he attempted to strangle his mother or to crush his younger brother under his feet. (p. 374)

They then described how this patient was subjected to a two-stage bilateral resection of the anterior medial temporal lobe. The main point of the paper was that the surgery resulted in a dramatic reduction in aggression, with a concomitant increase in sexual behavior—changes likened to the Klüver–Bucy syndrome. Unfortunately, for this patient, the seizures returned two months after the surgeries. However, they were never of the psychomotor type.

Perhaps the most famous patient who received bilateral amygdala removal is H. M. His life and contributions to science are chronicled in a book by Suzanne Corkin (2013). And a delightful account of H. M.'s personality can be found in Ogden and Corkin (1991). H. M. suffered from serious epileptic seizures that were not treatable by standard medications. Although his seizures were life threatening, he did not have any of the aggressive behavioral abnormalities that would make him a candidate for bilateral amygdalectomy. Rather, the neurosurgeon William Scoville decided to attempt the "frankly experimental operation" of bilateral hippocampectomy for the alleviation of H. M.'s seizure. However, the approach of resecting the medial temporal lobe through 1½ inch trephine holes in H. M.'s forehead necessitated the removal of the temporal pole and the amygdala, which obscure the view of the rostral hippocampal formation (Scoville & Milner, 1957). The first magnetic resonance imaging (MRI) study of H. M. (Corkin, Amaral, Gonzalez, Johnson, & Hyman, 1997) confirmed that his amygdala on both sides of his brain were entirely removed. In all of the published accounts of H. M., there is virtually no information related to how the loss of his amygdala changed his behavior; the focus has been almost entirely on his memory and cognitive changes.

According to Corkin (2013), H. M. was always an easygoing person, and this did not change following his surgery. After his surgery, he was said to be a very affable person with a good sense of humor (Ogden & Corkin, 1991). Certainly there was no report of H. M. demonstrating components of the Klüver–Bucy syndrome. Howard Eichenbaum did carry out a few studies that addressed the issue of amygdala function. For example, Eichenbaum, Morton, Potter, and Corkin (1983) demonstrated that H. M. had normal ability to detect odors but failed to discriminate between odors—presumably due to damage of the piriform cortex and regions of the periamygdaloid cortex. Similarly, Hebben, Corkin, Eichenbaum, and Shedlack (1985) reported that H. M. was deficient in his ability to report internal states such as hunger and was less sensitive to pain than other amnesic patients without amygdala damage. Again, these alterations were attributed to the loss of amygdala function. But there was apparently no direct evaluation of H. M.'s ability to detect and to have an emotional response to fearful stimuli or facial expressions. So, as much as H. M. taught the world about the hippocampal formation and memory function, the behavioral consequences of the loss of his amygdala were never adequately evaluated.

Some psychotic patients received amygdalectomies in the early 1950s through a direct surgical approach. Freeman and Williams (1952), for example, bilaterally lesioned the amygdala through a middle temporal gyrus approach in five patients suffering from auditory hallucinations. The claim is made that these hallucinations were eliminated in four of the five patients, although "the abnormal behavior associated with psychosis has been less influenced" (p. 461). As with neuroscience research in general, the advent of the stereotaxic apparatus provided an enabling tool for surgical manipulation of the human brain (Spiegel, Wycis, Marks, & Lee, 1947). Between 1960 and 1970, over 40,000 stereotaxic procedures were carried out worldwide (al-Rodhan & Kelly, 1992). The vast majority of these were for movement disorders or for the alleviation of chronic pain. But, something on the order of 1,000 patients worldwide received unilateral or, more often, bilateral amygdalectomy for the treatment of epilepsy, behavioral problems, or both. This was the era of psychosurgery that began with the introduction of the prefrontal lobotomy. Without more effective drugs for treating psychosis or aggressive behaviors, neurosurgeons in many countries resorted to lesions of brain regions, including the amygdala.

Human stereotaxic surgeries of the amygdala began in Japan by the neurosurgeon Hirotaro Narabayashi. Narabayashi designed his own stereotaxic apparatus and used this for carrying out bilateral amygdalectomies in a large number of patients (Fountas & Smith, 2007). One of his earliest reports appeared in 1963 (Narabayashi, Ngao, Saito, Yoshida, & Nagahata, 1963). The title of this paper, "Stereotaxic Amygdalotomy for Behavior Disorders" is telling. The goal of the authors is expressed in the following way:

> It was originally our intention to investigate the value of amygdalotomy upon patients with temporal lobe epilepsy characterized by psychomotor seizures and focal spike discharges on the electroencephalogram as well as marked behavior disturbances such as hyperexcitability, assaultive behavior, or violent aggressiveness. The indications for amygdalotomy were then extended to include patients without clinical

manifestations of temporal lobe epilepsy but with EEG [electroence-phalic] abnormalities and marked behavior disturbances. Finally, cases of behavior disorders without epileptic manifestations, clinically and electrically, but associated with various degrees of feeblemindedness or with subnormal intelligence were also included in the series. It has been our intention to improve the emotional state of the patient with behavior disorders and not primarily to utilize this technique in order to achieve control of epileptic seizures. (p. 1)

They go on to describe the initial group of patients and the operative procedures:

> Sixty patients were subjected to stereotaxic amygdalotomy. There were 38 male and 22 female patients who ranged in age from 5 to 35 years. Forty-six of the cases were diagnosed as having epilepsy of various eti-ologies and had both clinical seizures as well as EEG abnormalities. The other 14 patients had no history of seizures, although six of them showed either unilateral or bilateral fronto-temporal spike abnormali-ties on the EEG. The period of postoperative observation ranged from 3 to 48 months in duration.
>
> Blocking or destruction of the nucleus was obtained by means of an injection of 0.6 to 0.8 ml of a mixture of oil and wax to which lipi-odol had been added. (p. 2)

Lipiodol, also known as ethiodized oil, is a poppyseed oil that when mixed with the wax produces a space occupying lesion.

The postoperative evaluations of these patients were generally very subjective. Here is the way the outcome of one of these patients was described:

> Case 6.–This 7-year-old boy had been diagnosed as having symptom-atic epilepsy with right spastic hemiplegia and imbecility. The child manifested a severe behavior disturbance with erethic tendencies, explosiveness, and uncontrollable hyperactivity. The EEG revealed a general dysrhythmia with spike discharges bilaterally and a right-sided predominance. The clinical improvement following the first operation although notable was not felt to have sufficiently affected the boy's emotional problems. Following the second operation, however, the change in behavior was so complete, the patient had become so obedi-ent and cooperative that it was almost impossible to imagine that it was the same child who had been so wild and uncontrollable preopera-tively. The electroencephalogram no longer revealed spike discharges on either side. This was our first case of bilateral amygdalotomy and clinically no manifestations of the Klüver–Bucy syndrome could be observed. This lack of undesirable side-effects of bilateral amygdalot-omy must be taken into account in trying to understand the neuro-physiologic role of the amygdaloid nucleus. (pp. 6–7)

It appears that on the order of 100 patients received amygdalectomy by Narabayashi and colleagues—at least that is the number that is reported in the literature. Although there are papers that report long-term follow-up (Narabayashi, 1980; Narabayashi & Uno, 1966) of these patients, they are scientifically unsatisfying for reasons to which we return later. Narabayashi was primarily interested in extrapyramidal disorders, including Parkinson's disease, and the "limbic surgeries" were only of incidental interest.

The largest number of stereotaxic amygdalectomies was carried out in India. These were carried out at the Institute of Neurology of Madras (now Chennai) under the leadership of B. Ramammurthi, who received his medical degree from the Madras Medical College, where he also obtained the Master of Surgery degree. He then did a Fellowship at the Royal College of Surgeons of Edinburgh and traveled to Newcastle to obtain specialized training in neurosurgery. On returning to India, he was appointed as a Lecturer at the Madras Medical College. Amid doubts from the senior faculty that he had the requisite skills in neurosurgery, he endeavored to build a neurosurgical department from the ground up. By 1956, he had established his reputation as the top neurosurgeon in the country and recruited a number of bright young trainees, such as V. Balasubramaniam, T. S. Kanaka, and others. The stereotaxic neurosurgery unit was established in the early 1960s; thereafter, 481 patients underwent stereotaxic ablations of portions of the amygdala (Ramamurthi, 1988). A variety of techniques were used to lesion the amygdala, including radiofrequency lesions, physical disruption with a Bertrand loop, or injection of the same wax mixture used by Narabayashi et al. (1963).

In summarizing the opus of his stereotaxic neurosurgery practice, Ramamurthi recounts that of the 1,774 stereotaxic operations he performed over a 28-year career, 603 operations were done for the control of aggressive behavior. Of these, 481 were bilateral amygdalectomies and 122 were posterior hypothalamotomies (Ramamurthi, 1988). In describing the patient population, he states:

> Most of the patients were children below the age of 15 who had developed aggressive behaviour disorder of restlessness as a result of some insult to the brain. The types of behaviour problems included physical aggression, hyperkinesis, wandering tendency, destructive and self destructive tendencies. In some instances, the behaviour disorder was associated with epilepsy. . . . (p. 152)

Ramamurthi (1988) indicated that 39% of the patients showed good to excellent improvement, whereas 37% showed moderate improvement. Exactly how these evaluations were carried out, though, is not clear. Again, we return to this topic later. Ramamurthi and colleagues were major contributors to the literature on stereotaxic surgery and provided substantial detail on the methodologies that were employed. Balasubramaniam, in particular, provided a number of papers on various facets of amygdalotomy and hypothalamotomy (see, e.g., Balasubramaniam, Kanaka, Temanujam, & Ramamurthi, 1969; Balasubramaniam & Ramamurthi, 1970; Balasubramaniam, Ramamurthi, Jagannathan, & Kalyanaraman, 1967).

Stereotaxic surgeries of the amygdala were done in many centers around the world. A small number were carried out in Thailand (Chitanondh, 1966) and Australia (White & Williams, 2009), and a somewhat larger number in Scotland (Hitchcock & Cairns, 1973). Robert Heimburger and colleagues (Heimburger, 1975; Heimburger, Whitlock, & Kalsbeck, 1966) carried out unilateral or bilateral amygdalectomies in 58 patients at the Indiana University Medical Center in the United States. Fourteen of the patients had intractable seizures, 12 had unmanageable behavior, and the remainder had both conditions (Heimburger, Small, Small, Milstein, & Moore, 1978). The series of reports from this group was distinctive in several respects. First, there was substantial detail related to the part of the amygdala that needed to be lesioned for optimal result. And substantial information related to the establishment of appropriate coordinates was also provided. Second, 1 to 11 years after the initial stereotaxic surgeries, long-term follow-up of the patients was carried out by research staff members of the Department of Psychiatry who were not involved in the initial care of the patients. Third, standardized assessment measures were employed. Patients were tested with the Spitzer Status Schedule, a structured psychiatric interview, and the Halstead–Reitan–Wepman Neuropsychological Test Battery. The postsurgical assessments were compared with similar testing done presurgically. The results of this testing were discussed by the research team and a consensus was reached on whether the patient had improved. The conclusion was that 43% of the patients with seizures improved due to the surgery, whereas only 38% of those with behavioral problems showed significant improvement. Seventeen of the 44 patients with behavioral problems had improved, whereas 25 showed no improvement and two seemed worse. This program can be considered a model for how translational research should be conducted, since reliable objective methods of assessment were used, including structured psychiatric interviews, along with physical and neurological examinations. Unfortunately, this level of scientific rigor was more the exception that the rule.

Another example in which scientific benefit was linked to bilateral amygdalectomy in human patients is a paper that is probably the most recent and last report of this procedure being carried out. Lee et al. (1998) reported on two young adult patients who received bilateral amygdalectomy for intractable aggression in the late 1980s. This paper was distinctive in many ways. First, postoperative MRIs of the lesions were shown for both patients. Second, psychophysiological measures including electromyography of facial muscles and skin conductance responses measured from the hands were carried out. Autonomic alterations were observed in both patients following surgery. Although both patients had declines in aggression, they continued to have difficulty controlling aggressive outbursts. Surgery on one patient was considered to be a moderate success, while the other was considered a failure.

It is interesting how the follow-up paper by Heimburger et al. (1978) begins. The first lines of the Introduction are as follows:

> The controversy regarding surgery to improve abnormal behavior has become so intense that legislation has been passed in many parts of the world to ban its use. Those who advocate this method of therapy find it safe and effective in relieving a significant percentage of patients who have been resistant to other forms of therapy. Those who oppose it fear that it will be used indiscriminately and punitively. . . . (p. 43)

Clearly, the unbridled enthusiasm for psychosurgery that emanated from the medical community in the early 1950s (Freeman, 1953), gave way to very substantial societal concern by the mid-1970s. State courts were banning the use of psychosurgery on prisoners (Future of psychosurgery in doubt, 1973). This increased level of concern was due in part to the increasingly more publicized failures of prefrontal lobotomy. The appearance of the Milos Forman film, *One Flew over the Cuckoo's Nest,* probably contributed to the public's concern with brain surgery for behavior control. The widespread public concern with these procedures led the U.S. Congress to establish the National Commission for the Protection of Human Subjects of Biomedical and Behavioral Research (1977), which carried out a comprehensive investigation of psychosurgery. One of the activities of the Commission was to sponsor a literature review of post-operative evaluation procedures for patients undergoing psychosurgery (Valenstein, 1980). Among many findings in this review was that 58.8% of all articles on psychosurgery had no objective outcome measures; 11.8% had objective psychiatric evaluations, and 8.8% had objective personality tests. Taken together, amygdalectomies for aggressive patients resulted in only 28% of the cases in which the patients were judged to have improved significantly. It is beyond the scope of this article to delve deeply into the ethics of psychosurgery and, more specifically, the ethics of bilateral amygdala lesions for the control of unmanageable behavior. But given that on the order of 1,000 human patients received lesions of the amygdala, the question naturally arises, what did we learn from this era of human amygdala lesions? The answer, regrettably, is very little. The following is a series of points that summarize findings across many papers dealing with this topic:

- It was extremely rare to observe anything approaching the characteristics of the Klüver–Bucy syndrome in human patients with bilateral amygdala lesions. While it is difficult to draw a direct comparison, it would appear that the loss of the amygdala in the human may lead to a less marked reduction in emotional behavior than in the nonhuman primate.
- There was rarely adequate objective preoperative and postoperative evaluation of the cognitive and emotional status of the amygdalectomy patients.
- There was very little control over the size and position of the lesions produced in these patients. What is most astonishing is that there is not a single postmortem neuropathological evaluation of these lesions presented in the literature! There was therefore no attempt to correlate the size and location of the lesion with the clinical and behavioral outcome. Thus, there was no way to correct and improve the procedure.
- The procedures that were used to induce the lesion of the amygdala varied widely, but the literature does not progress to a strategy that was most effective, since there was very little objective comparison.

A comparison of the literatures on monkey and human amygdalectomies was previously reviewed by John Aggleton (1992). He came to very much the same conclusion that the era of amygdala lesions in human patients provided both modest therapeutic benefits and limited new scientific information. This era is in stark contrast to the elegant studies of patients with Urbach–Wiethe syndrome chronicled in this volume by neuroscientists such as Ralph Adolphs, Jack van Honk and René Hurlemann. These investigations give us faith that we have indeed come a long way in the sophistication with which translational research is carried out.

The India Project

The topic of human amygdalectomies has been discussed in our laboratory for many years. In 2000, a young MD, PhD student, Noah Merin, was rotating through our laboratory and became fascinated with the patients who underwent surgery in India. Since the period of bilateral amygdalectomy surgery extended from 1964 through 1988, and since the majority of the surgeries were performed on children between 4 and 12 years of age, we wondered whether it might be possible to identify some of these patients who would be middle-aged and carry out cognitive testing, along with detailed MRI studies of both the lesion locations and any potential brain reorganization. These ideas were prompted by the knowledge that there were actually very few human subjects who had undergone this type of testing anywhere in the world.

With funding from the Early Experience and Brain Development Network of the MacArthur Foundation, we carried out an exploratory feasibility study by having Mr. Merin journey to Chennai, India, during the summer of 2000. The first question we asked was whether there was a physician associated with the patients who was willing to collaborate on the project. As reviewed earlier, many of the surgeries were carried out by Dr. B. Ramamaurthi and Dr. C. Balasubramaniam, both of whom were retired. However, they were interested in the project and endorsed it. They recommended that we consult with Dr. Mohan Sampath Kumar, who was Head of Neurology and Neurosurgery at the Government General Hospital in Chennai (Madras Medical College). He agreed to coordinate the work in Chennai and to collaborate on all facets of the project. We were also able to determine that medical records for the neurosurgery patients did exist, that a 1.5 T (tesla) Siemens MRI scanner was available for scanning the patients, and that a neuropsychologist, Dr. Virudhagirinathan, worked at the Government Hospital and had personally translated from English to Tamil many of the cognitive measures we were interested in employing and would be willing to provide office space, testing rooms, and time to carry out neuropsychological testing of the patients. Mr. Merin determined which authorizations would need to be obtained from the Indian Government to pursue the collaboration. He was accompanied by Dr. Vinod Menon, a South Indian native (now Professor at Stanford University), who not only facilitated some of the meetings but provided consultation on study design and budget.

Based on these preliminary findings, additional funding was provided by the MacArthur Foundation to carry out an extended pilot study. The goal was to recruit five bilateral amygdalectomy patients and carry out neuropsychological and MRI analyses. Having received authorization from the Indian government, as well as institutional review board (IRB) approval from the University of California, Davis (UC Davis), Mr. Merin returned to Chennai the following summer to oversee this pilot study.

We were very appreciative that all of the physicians associated with this program of neurosurgery, including doctors Ramamurthi, Balasubramaniam, and Kaliyaliraman (all retired), and the doctors they trained in stereotaxic neurosurgery (doctors Kanaka, Chendilnathan, and Mohendran) provided advice and support for this project. A first goal was to look for the medical records of the surgery patients.

Unfortunately, the condition of the records of patients who underwent bilateral amygdalectomy was poor. All of the senior doctors told us that pre-1995 records at the Government Hospital were destroyed at the insistence of the government in 1998. During the course of an investigation in the Records Department of the Government Hospital, we discovered that this was not strictly true. To make room for more recent records, pre-1995 records were stacked in several large rooms and alcoves in an unused wing of the hospital (Figure 3.4). Mr. Merin and two Indian technicians, hired as a research assistant and medical social worker (for patient recruitment), respectively, attempted sorting through the very large piles of uncatalogued paper bundles. They found records dating back to 1972, suggesting that the piles of millions of records might contain files pertaining to the 481 patients who underwent bilateral amygdalectomy between 1964 and 1986. The task of sorting through these records to find those related to the patients of interest, however, would be daunting and was ultimately abandoned.

In order to continue the pilot project, we resorted to an appeal to the neurosurgeons and neurologists who continued to provide medical care to some of the patients who had undergone bilateral amygdalectomy. During the course of the summer, Mr. Merin and colleagues recruited three patients with purported bilateral amygdalectomies. All three consented to MRI scanning and expressed interest in participating in a study of social cognition. All three patients were supplied to us directly by the doctors who performed the surgeries, who continued to see the patients to treat persistent epilepsy and monitor the patient's regimens of antiepileptic medication. The collaborating physicians estimated that additional patients could be solicited through other doctors in the Department of Neurology.

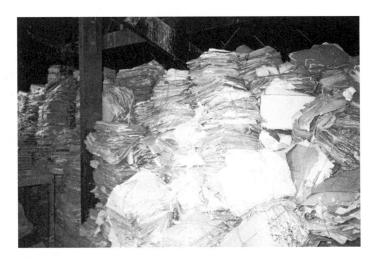

FIGURE 3.4. A photograph taken by Noah Merin, MD, of pre-1995 records of patients who had undergone bilateral lesions of the amygdala at Government General Hospital in Chennai.

Of the three patients that were scanned during the summer of 2001, one (patient V. K.) was found to have bilateral lesions affecting much of the anterior amygdala, with minimal damage to other brain structures (Figure 3.5). Some hippocampal atrophy was present in this patient, due, most likely, to his history of epilepsy and its treatment by antiepileptic medication. V. K. was 57 years old in 2001. He received bilateral amygdalectomy at age 27 in an attempt to control violent and aggressive behavior. Presurgically, he was said to be extremely violent and aggressive without provocation. He was highly excitable, and his behavior caused a great deal of problems for his family members. He was epileptic and prior to surgery experienced seven to eight episodes per day. Postsurgically, his violent behavior was said to be greatly reduced and his behavior overall was manageable. Episodes of seizures had been reduced to one every 4 or 5 months. His social behavior had improved. He is now functionally

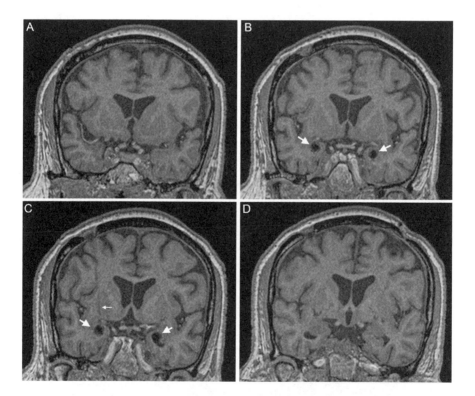

FIGURE 3.5. Magnetic resonance coronal images of the brain of patient V. K., who received a bilateral stereotaxic lesion of the amygdala when he was 27. Images are arranged from rostral (A) to caudal (D). The lesion within the substance of the amygdala is indicated by large white arrows in panels B and C. The electrode track is indicated by a small arrow in panel C.

independent, though under the supervision of his elder brother. He is socially remote and does not watch TV or read.

During the course of interviews with the senior physicians who performed the surgeries, we learned that the majority of the children who received bilateral amygdalectomies had intellectual disability. This fact was not clear from the follow-up reports published by this group of surgeons. It was not clear, therefore, what percentage of patients who were operated on as children would have cognitive abilities that would permit neuropsychological and experimental social testing. Therefore, we decided that any potential subject would need to be administered an abbreviated IQ test (e.g., the Tamil translation of the Wechsler Abbreviated Scale of Intelligence [WASI]) prior to MRI scanning.

As a follow-up to this visit, our collaborators, doctors Sampath Kumar and Virudhagirinathan, visited UC Davis, and the first three patients were discussed in detail. During these meetings, we established inclusion–exclusion criteria based on lesion quality, planned the neuropsychological screening protocol, and discussed the outlook for the project. After this, we were sent records from two additional patients who had been selected and had undergone MRI analysis. As a result of this analysis, we found that only a single patient of the five (V. K.) had bilateral lesions that were restricted to the amygdaloid complex. The other patients had either unilateral amygdala damage or significant damage to other brain structures, including the insular cortex, ventrolateral prefrontal cortex, white matter dorsolateral to the amygdala, and entorhinal cortex. While these findings were disappointing, given the relatively modest guidance procedures that were in place at the time of the surgeries, they perhaps should not have been unanticipated.

In the end, we decided not to pursue a larger study of this patient population, and our preliminary results were not published due, in part, to the poor quality of the medical records related to these patients. We were also concerned about the substantial premorbid intellectual and medical conditions that affected the patients, and the realization that a large number of subjects would need to be evaluated in order to attain a reasonably sized cohort of subjects with bilateral lesions largely confined to the amygdaloid complex.

The clinicians who treated these patients were primarily interested in benefiting the patients and their families. Contributing to a deeper understanding of the function of the human amygdala was not their major interest. Conducting informative translational neuroscience is difficult in the best of conditions and requires adequate planning and partnership with the patients. It is always easier to carry out these complex studies prospectively rather than retrospectively.

Conclusion

Aggleton (1992) concludes his chapter in *The Amygdala* by stating:

> While there is reason to believe that there are differences in the extent of the emotional changes that follow amygdala damage in man and other primates, there are no grounds to suggest that these effects are qualitatively different. It would appear, therefore, that detailed studies of the monkey amygdala will continue to help us determine how the functions of the human amygdala are realized. (p. 494)

Given that it is likely that no human patients will undergo bilateral neurosurgical lesions of the amygdala in the future, we need to rely on studies of the nonhuman primate to understand both the normal functions of the amygdala and how its pathology leads to epilepsy, aggression, and anxiety. The patients with Urbach–Wiethe syndrome described in this book will certainly contribute to our understanding. But fundamental questions of plasticity and compensation that are raised about these patients need to be answered experimentally using the nonhuman primate model. I hope that this review of the parallels between humans and monkeys living without an amygdala will provide justification for the validity of the model and the value of the experimental approach.

ACKNOWLEDGMENTS

The primary research is supported by grants from the National Institutes of Health (Nos. R37 MH 57502, 5 R01 MH41479, and 5 R01 NS16980). The India Project was supported by the Early Experience and Brain Development Network of the MacArthur Foundation. I thank Noah Merin, MD, for his substantial efforts on the India Project and our gracious Indian colleagues.

REFERENCES

Aggleton, J. P. (1992). The functional effects of amygdala lesions in humans: A comparison with findings from monkeys. In J. P. Aggleton (Ed.), *The amygdala: Neurobiological aspects of emotion, memory and mental dysfunction* (pp. 485–503). New York: Wiley-Liss.

Aggleton, J. P., & Passingham, R. E. (1981a). Stereotaxic surgery under X-ray guidance in the rhesus monkey, with special reference to the amygdala. *Experimental Brain Research, 44*(3), 271–276.

Aggleton, J. P., & Passingham, R. E. (1981b). Syndrome produced by lesions of the amygdala in monkeys (*Macaca mulatta*). *Journal of Comparative and Physiological Psychology, 95*(6), 961–977.

al-Rodhan, N. R., & Kelly, P. J. (1992). Pioneers of stereotactic neurosurgery. *Stereotactic and Functional Neurosurgery, 58*(1–4), 60–66.

Balasubramaniam, V., Kanaka, T. S., Ramanujam, P. V., & Ramamurthi, B. (1969). Sedative neurosurgery. A contribution to the behavioural sciences. *Journal of the Indian Medical Association, 53*(8), 377–381.

Balasubramaniam, V., & Ramamurthi, B. (1970). Stereotaxic amygdalotomy in behavior disorders. *Confinia Neurologica, 32*(2), 367–373.

Balasubramaniam, V., Ramamurthi, B., Jagannathan, K., & Kalyanaraman, S. (1967). Stereotaxic amygdalotomy. *Neurology India, 15*(3), 119–122.

Brown, S., & Schafer, E. A. (1888). An investigation into the functions of the occipital and temporal lobes of the monkety's brain. *Philosophical Transactions of the Royal Society B: Biological Sciences, 179*, 303–327.

Bucy, P. C. (1985). Heinrich Klüver. In P. C. Bucy (Ed.), *Neurosurgical giants: Feet of clay and iron* (pp. 349–353). New York: Elsevier Science.

Bucy, P. C., & Klüver, H. (1955). An anatomical investigation of the temporal lobe in the monkey (*Macaca mulatta*). *Journal of Comparative Neurology, 103*(2), 151–251.

Chitanondh, H. (1966). Stereotaxic amygdalotomy in the treatment of olfactory seizures and psychiatric disorders with olfactory hallucination. *Confinia Neurologica, 27*(1), 181–196.

Corkin, S. (2013). *Permanent present tense.* New York: Basic Books.

Corkin, S., Amaral, D. G., Gonzalez, R. G., Johnson, K. A., & Hyman, B. T. (1997). H. M.'s medial temporal lobe lesion: Findings from magnetic resonance imaging. *Journal of Neuroscience, 17*(10), 3964–3979.

Eichenbaum, H., Morton, T. H., Potter, H., & Corkin, S. (1983). Selective olfactory deficits in case H. M. *Brain, 106*(2), 459–472.

Emery, N. J., Capitanio, J. P., Mason, W. A., Machado, C. J., Mendoza, S. P., & Amaral, D. G. (2001). The effects of bilateral lesions of the amygdala on dyadic social interactions in rhesus monkeys (*Macaca mulatta*). *Behavioral Neuroscience, 115*(3), 515–544.

Ferrier, D. (1874). Experiments on the brain of monkeys—No. 1. *Proceedings of the Royal Society of London, 23*, 409–432.

Ferrier, D. (1875). The Croonian Lecture: Experiments on the brain of monkeys (second series). *Transactions of the Royal Society of London, 165*, 433–488.

Flourens, M. J. P. (1842). *Experimental research on the properties and functions of the nervous system in vertebrate animals.* Paris: J. B. Ballière.

Fodstad, H., Hariz, M., & Ljunggren, B. (1991). History of Clarke's stereotactic instrument. *Stereotactic and Functional Neurosurgery, 57*(3), 130–140.

Fountas, K. N., & Smith, J. R. (2007). Historical evolution of stereotactic amygdalotomy for the management of severe aggression. *Journal of Neurosurgery, 106*(4), 710–713.

Freeman, W. (1953). Ethics of psychosurgery. *New England Journal of Medicine, 249*(20), 798–801.

Freeman, W., & Williams, J. M. (1952). Human sonar: The amygdaloid nucleus in relation to auditory hallucinations. *Journal of Nervous and Mental Disease, 116*(5), 456–462.

Fritsch, G., & Hitzig, E. (1870). Uuber die elektrische Erregbarkeit des Grosshirns

[Electric excitability of the cerebrum]. *Archiv für Anatomie, Physiologie und Wissenschaftliche Medicin, 3,* 300–332.

Future of psychosurgery in doubt. (1973). *Nature, 244*(5412), 128–129.

Goulet, S., Dore, F. Y., & Murray, E. A. (1998). Aspiration lesions of the amygdala disrupt the rhinal corticothalamic projection system in rhesus monkeys. *Experimental Brain Research, 119*(2), 131–140.

Hebben, N., Corkin, S., Eichenbaum, H., & Shedlack, K. (1985). Diminished ability to interpret and report internal states after bilateral medial temporal resection: Case H. M. *Behavioral Neuroscience, 99*(6), 1031–1039.

Heimburger, R. F. (1975). Stereotaxic coordinates for amygdalotomy. *Confinia Neurologica, 37*(1–3), 202–206.

Heimburger, R. F., Small, I. F., Small, J. G., Milstein, V., & Moore, D. (1978). Stereotactic amygdalotomy for convulsive and behavioral disorders: Long-term follow-up study. *Applied Neurophysiology, 41*(1–4), 43–51.

Heimburger, R. F., Whitlock, C. C., & Kalsbeck, J. E. (1966). Stereotaxic amygdalotomy for epilepsy with aggressive behavior. *Journal of the American Medical Association, 198*(7), 741–745.

Hitchcock, E., & Cairns, V. (1973). Amygdalotomy. *Postgraduate Medical Journal, 49*(578), 894–904.

Jarrard, L. E. (1989). On the use of ibotenic acid to lesion selectively different components of the hippocampal formation. *Journal of Neuroscience Methods, 29*(3), 251–259.

Klüver, H., & Bucy, P. C. (1938). An analysis of certain effections of bilateral temporal lobectomy in the rhesus monkey with special reference to "psychic blindness." *Journal of Psychology, 5,* 33–54.

Klüver, H., & Bucy, P. C. (1939). Preliminary analysis of functions of the temporal lobes in monkeys. *Archives of Neurology and Psychiatry, 42,* 979–1000.

Lashley, K. (1950). In search of the engram. In Society's Symposium IV, Physiological *Mechanisms in animal behavior* (pp. 454–482). Oxford, UK: Academic Press.

Lavenex, P., Suzuki, W. A., & Amaral, D. G. (2002). Perirhinal and parahippocampal cortices of the macaque monkey: Projections to the neocortex. *Journal of Comparative Neurology, 447*(4), 394–420.

Lee, G. P., Bechara, A., Adolphs, R., Arena, J., Meador, K. J., Loring, D. W, et al. (1998). Clinical and physiological effects of stereotaxic bilateral amygdalotomy for intractable aggression. *Journal of Neuropsychiatry and Clinical Neurosciences, 10*(4), 413–420.

Meunier, M., Bachevalier, J., Murray, E. A., Malkova, L., & Mishkin, M. (1999). Effects of aspiration versus neurotoxic lesions of the amygdala on emotional responses in monkeys. *European Journal of Neuroscience, 11*(12), 4403–4418.

Millett, D. (1998). Illustrating a revolution: an unrecognized contribution to the golden era of cerebral localization. *Notes and Records of the Royal Society of London, 52*(2), 283–305.

Nahm, F. K. (1997). Heinrich Klüver and the temporal lobe syndrome. *Journal of the History of the Neurosciences, 6*(2), 193–208.

Narabayashi, H. (1980). From experiences of medial amygdalotomy on epileptics. *Acta Neurochirurgica Supplementum, 30,* 75–81.

Narabayashi, H., Nagao, T., Saito, Y., Yoshida, M., & Nagahata, M. (1963). Stereotaxic amygdalotomy for behavior disorders. *Archives of Neurology, 9*, 1–16.

Narabayashi, H., & Uno, M. (1966). Long range results of stereotaxic amygdalotomy for behavior disorders. *Confinia Neurologica, 27*(1), 168–171.

National Commission for the Protection of Human Subjects of Biomedical and Behavioral Research. (1977). Use of psychosurgery in practice and research: Report and recommendations of the National Commission for the Protection of Human Subjects of Biomedical and Behavioral Research. *Federal Register, 42*(99), 26318–26332.

Ogden, J. A., & Corkin, S. (1991). Memories of H. M. In C. Wickliffe, M. Abraham, C. Corballis, & K. G. White (Eds.), *Memory mechanisms: A tribute to G. V. Goddard* (pp. 195–215). Mahway, NJ: Erlbaum

Pribram, K. H., & Bagshaw, M. (1953). Further analysis of the temporal lobe syndrome utilizing fronto-temporal ablations. *Journal of Comparative Neurology, 99*(2), 347–375.

Ramamurthi, B. (1988). Stereotactic operation in behaviour disorders: Amygdalotomy and hypothalamotomy. *Acta Neurochirurgica Supplementum, 44*, 152–157.

Scoville, W. B., & Milner, B. (1957). Loss of recent memory after bilateral hippocampal lesions. *Journal of Neurology, Neurosurgery and Psychiatry, 20*(1), 11–21.

Spiegel, E. A., Wycis, H. T., Marks, M., & Lee, A. J. (1947). Stereotaxic apparatus for operations on the human brain. *Science, 106*(2754), 349–350.

Terzian, H., & Ore, G. D. (1955). Syndrome of Klüver and Bucy: Reproduced in man by bilateral removal of the temporal lobes. *Neurology, 5*(6), 373–380.

Tizard, B. (1959). Theories of brain localization from Flourens to Lashley. *Medical History, 3*(2), 132–145.

Valenstein, E. S. (1980). Review of the literature on postoperative evaluation. In E. S. Valenstein (Ed.), *The psychosurgery debate* (pp. 141–163). New York: Freeman.

Walker, A. E., Thomson, A. F., McQueen, J. D. (1953). Behavior and the temporal rhinencephalon in the monkey. *Bulletin of the Johns Hopkins Hospital, 93*(2), 65–93.

Weiskrantz, L. (1956). Behavioral changes associated with ablation of the amygdaloid complex in monkeys. *Journal of Comparative and Physiological Psychology, 49*(4), 381–391.

White, R., & Williams, S. (2009). Amygdaloid neurosurgery for aggressive behaviour, Sydney, 1967–1977: Societal, scientific, ethical and other factors. *Australasian Psychiatry, 17*(5), 410–416.

CHAPTER 4

The Role of the Rodent Amygdala in Early Development

EMMA SARRO

REGINA M. SULLIVAN

The amygdala is highly involved in both social and emotional behaviors in adults. This chapter reviews the literature on the changing role of the amygdala during development and specifically outlines the neurobiology of infant attachment learning and underlying neural circuitry in both human and animal models. This circuitry serves to keep the infant close to the caregiver, as well as to shape the emotional behavior of the pup to match and respond to the ever-changing environment. Moreover, the quality of care from the mother can alter the amygdala's developmental trajectory to produce enduring effects on social behavior and depressive-like symptoms throughout the lifespan. This literature suggests that while the amygdala is rarely engaged in cognitive, social, and emotional behaviors during early life, poor-quality caregiving appears to program the amygdala to cause profound differences in later-life amygdala function, altering cognitive, social, and emotional learning and expression.

The amygdala is a brain area often implicated in adult behaviors, including cognitive, social, and emotion-related behaviors. Here we review the literature on the changing role of the amygdala during development and suggest that, in fact, during early life, the amygdala is rarely engaged in behaviors that involve social and emotional aspects of cognition in early life. Despite this, early-life environment and attachment quality can alter amygdala development and produce profound differences in adult amygdala function, altering cognitive, social, and emotional learning and expression.

The early-life environment of the infant is primarily encompassed by the caregiver, with emotional and social behavior of the infant channeled within the attachment system that bonds infant and mother. This mutual attachment, which is typically formed rapidly and has wide phylogenetic representation, includes chicks, rodents, nonhuman primates, and humans. Attachment can occur throughout the lifespan and includes the mother attaching to her offspring, the offspring attaching to the caregiver, and mates attaching to one another. While an attachment neural circuit has not yet been identified in humans at any stage of development, based on our behavior and our strong need to form social bonds, it is safe to assume that it exists. Indeed, our ability to develop attachments goes beyond bonds with other humans; it can include other species in the form of pets. The existence of a neural circuitry for attachment and its importance in healthy development was first hypothesized by Bowlby (1965).

Human infants exhibit attachment behaviors in response to their caregiver within minutes of birth, with the mother's voice evoking attachment-related behaviors (DeCasper & Fifer, 1980; Mennella, 1995; Schaal, Marlier, & Soussignan, 1995; Lecanuet & Schaal, 1996; Varendi, Porter, & Winberg, 1996). Features of the mother, such as her odor or visual presence, can reduce crying and pain (Schaal et al., 1995; Sullivan & Toubas, 1998; Vervoort et al., 2008). New characteristics of the caregiver are rapidly learned, including facial features, and new sounds and odors, all of which involve the infant learning and remembering the caregiver, and continuously seeking closeness to the caregiver (DeCasper & Fifer, 1980; Schleidt & Genzel, 1990; Bolhuis & Honey, 1998; Sullivan & Toubas, 1998). This robust infant attachment learning, presumably shaped by evolution, ensures that the infant's display of social, emotional, and proximity-seeking behavior engages the caregiver to provide the food, protection, and warmth necessary for survival.

For ethical reasons, the neurobiology of infant attachment in humans is presently unavailable for exploration, although the adult literature on romantic attachment might provide clues (Bartels & Zeki, 2000, 2004). Thus, most of our understanding of early-life attachment learning is derived from the study of other mammals, including rodents and nonhuman primates. Indeed, due to the widespread of phylogenetic representation of robust attachment in altricial species, other species have provided considerable information about the attachment circuit, especially the involvement of the amygdala (in this volume, see Bliss-Moreau, Moadab, & Amaral, Chapter 6; Bachevalier, Sanchez, Raper, Stephens, & Wallen, Chapter 7). Attachment between the caregiver and offspring was first identified as "imprinting" and demonstrated the importance of learning within a biologically predisposed system present at birth (Hess, 1962; Salzen, 1970; Rajecki, Lamb, & Obmascher, 1978; Bolhuis & Honey, 1998). Attachment and its supporting neurobiology have now been demonstrated in several mammals (Polan & Hofer, 1998; Insel & Young, 2001; Hofer & Sullivan, 2008; Sullivan & Holman, 2010). Importantly, while this animal work provides understanding and insights into the neurobiology of human attachment and the role of the amygdala, human attachment shows far greater complexity (Rosen & Burke, 1999; Stovall & Dozier, 2000; Higley & Dozier, 2009).

Here, we review the literature on the neurobiology of infant attachment learning both in human and animal models. We focus on unique features of learning that narrow what is learned to enhance attachment and how this alters the infant's social behavior. Next, we review the literature on how the quality and experiences within attachment and infant social behavior alter the amygdala's developmental trajectory to produce enduring effects throughout the lifespan.

Infant Attachment Learning

Attachment learning, which underlies the infant's main objective to stay close to the caregiver to procure nutrition and protection, is usually guided by a specific sensory stimulus. For example, in the infant rat, the attachment behavior is controlled primarily by the maternal odor (Galef & Kaner, 1980; Leon, 1992), often combined with somatosensory stimuli when the animal is in direct contact with the mother (Hofer, Shair, & Singh, 1976; Teicher & Blass, 1977). In fact, removing the maternal odor has a negative impact on pups' survival (Singh & Tobach, 1975). Many experiments from our laboratory and others have shown that the maternal odor is a learned stimulus, and not a pheromone (Leon, 1975; Hofer et al., 1976; Rudy & Cheatle, 1977; Teicher & Blass, 1977; Brunjes & Alberts, 1979; Galef & Kaner, 1980; Pederson, Williams, & Blass, 1982; Campbell, 1984; Sullivan, Brake, Hofer, & Williams, 1986; Sullivan, Wilson, Wong, Correa, & Leon, 1990; Miller, Jagielo, & Spear, 1989; Leon, 1992; Terry & Johanson, 1996; Moriceau, Shionoya, Jakups, & Sullivan, 2009). This has been proven by showing that pups can learn and approach other novel odors that take on the characteristics of maternal odor (Galef & Sherry, 1973; Teicher, Flaum, Williams, Eckhert, & Lumia, 1978; Haroutunian & Campbell, 1979; Johanson & Hall, 1979; Galef & Kaner, 1980; Johanson & Teicher, 1980; Brake, 1981; Caza & Spear, 1984; Camp & Rudy, 1988; Duveau & Godinot, 1988; Sullivan et al., 1990; Sullivan, Landers, Yeaman, & Wilson, 2000a; Sullivan, Stackenwalt, Nasr, Lemon, & Wilson, 2000b; Roth & Sullivan, 2005; Moriceau et al., 2009; Sevelinges, Levy, Mouly, & Ferreira, 2009; Al Ain, Belin, Schaal, & Petris, 2012). Thus, approach toward the maternal odor is often used as a measure of attachment, and pairing a novel odor with a reward (e.g., milk, warmth, nursing, or tactile stimulation) can produce learned attachment (Galef & Sherry, 1973; Teicher et al., 1978; Johanson & Teicher, 1980; Pederson et al., 1982; Sullivan et al., 1986; Weldon, Travis, & Kennedy, 1991; McLean, Darby-King,

Sullivan, & King, 1993; Wilson & Sullivan, 1994; Cheslock, Varlinskaya, Petrov, & Spear, 2000; Moriceau et al., 2009; Sevelinges et al., 2009).

While odorants are hugely important for infant attachment learning, somatosensory information also plays a large role from the first day of life throughout development. Thus, manipulation of somatosensory input can have a dramatic impact on pup survival, as well as tactile learning and behavior in adulthood. For example, nipple attachment is disrupted when the infraorbital nerve, which innervates the whiskers, is severed (Hofer, Fisher, & Shair, 1981). In addition, removing whiskers during development delays nipple attachment and interferes with adult learning and whisker behavior (Carvell & Simons, 1996; Sullivan et al., 2003). Learning can also be measured in pups as young as 1 day old by manipulation of whiskers through whisker stimulation, or pairing this with reward, resulting in a marked increase of activity and head movements (Landers & Sullivan, 1999b). In slightly older pups (approximately postnatal day [PN] 12), when whiskers are able to move, dewhiskering manipulations result in abnormal head movements and exploration behaviors (Welker, 1964; Landers & Zeigler, 2006), which leads to impairments in the ability of pups to approach the mother and obtain milk.

Important to note here is that within the natural environment of the nest, a multitude of sensory information (including odor, somatosensory, and taste information) is constantly being used by the pup, and all play a role in the interactions between pup and mother.

Attachment Learning Neurobiology

The neurobiology of the attachment circuitry seems to have two primary roles during the early development of the infant: first, to keep the infant close to and preferring the presence of the caregiver, and second, to shape pups' emotional behavior to match and respond to the ever-changing environment during early life. The specialized neural circuitry involved in promoting the relationship between infant and caregiver has been uncovered with studies using animal models of infant attachment, (i.e., rat) and is the main focus of this section. One primary component of the resulting behavior is that infants learn a preference for the caregiver; a behavior acquired through hyperfunctioning of the locus coeruleus (LC) and release of norepinephrine (NE). Specifically, a unique developmental characteristic of the infant LC is that it produces larger than normal amounts of NE efflux to areas such as the olfactory bulb and anterior piriform cortex. A secondary, but equally important, component of this attachment circuitry is that infants display a reduced ability to learn an aversion to painful stimuli during this early period of development, such as an aversion to an abusive caregiver. This seems to be primarily related to a delayed functional maturation of the amygdala's experience-dependent plasticity. As the infant matures and begins to make brief excursions outside the nest, amygdala-dependent fear learning functionally emerges (Sullivan et al., 2000b) (see Figure 4.1). Finally, developmental experience, such as stress, can alter the normal development of the attachment circuitry (Adriani & Laviola, 2004; Hensch, 2004; Crews, He, & Hodge, 2007; Sullivan & Holman, 2010; Landers & Sullivan, 2012).

A critical site for neural plasticity underlying the rodent olfactory attachment learning circuitry is within the olfactory bulb, displaying both physiological and anatomical changes associated with the maternal odor. As introduced earlier, an overabundant release of NE from the LC is critical for learning related plasticity (Sullivan & Leon, 1986; Sullivan, Wilson, & Leon, 1989; Sullivan & Wilson, 1991; Wilson, Sullivan, & Leon, 1987; Woo, Coopersmith, & Leon, 1987; Johnson, Woo, Duong, Nguyen, & Leon, 1995; Fleming, O'Day, & Kraemer, 1999; Upton & Sullivan, 2010) (see Figure 4.1). This has been assessed in naturalistic settings both within the nest and outside the nest, and learning-induced plasticity has been demonstrated through an enhancement of the olfactory bulb response to learned odors (i.e., maternal or conditioned odors) and measured using a variety of techniques that include, 2-deoxyglucose uptake, c-Fos immunohistochemistry, electrophysiology, cyclic adenosine-3',5'-monophosphate (AMP) response element-binding protein (CREB) phosphorylation, and optical imaging (Coopersmith & Leon, 1986; Wilson et al., 1987; Woo et al., 1987; Johnson et al., 1995; Sullivan et al., 2000b; Yuan, Harley, Darby-King, Neve, & McLean, 2003; Yuan, Harley, McLean, & Knopfel, 2002; Zhang, Okutani, Inoue, & Kaba, 2003; Roth & Sullivan, 2005; Raineki, Moriceau, & Sullivan, 2010). In fact, NE has been found to be both necessary and sufficient for the learning-induced changes in the neural activity, as well as pup behavior (Shipley, Halloran, & de la Torre, 1985; Sullivan et al., 1989; McLean & Shipley, 1991; Sullivan, Zyzak, Skierkowski, & Wilson, 1992; Sullivan & Wilson, 1994; Rangel & Leon, 1995; Langdon, Harley, & McLean, 1997; Okutani, Kaba, Takahashi, & Seto, 1998; McLean, Harley, Darby-King, & Yuan, 1999; Sullivan et al., 2000a; Roth, Wilson, & Sullivan, 2004). NE release appears to work by preventing the primary output neurons of the olfactory bulb from habituating during a period of stimulation (a normal response to repeated stimulation) (Wilson & Sullivan, 1991). Mechanistically, NE's maintenance of mitral-tufted neurons' odor response seems to increase CREB phosphorylation and activity of immediate, early, and late response genes (McLean et al., 1999), a mechanism often found in adult learning and memory systems (Carew, 1996; Carew & Sutton, 2001; Tao, Finkbeiner, Arnold, Shaywitz, & Greenberg, 1998).

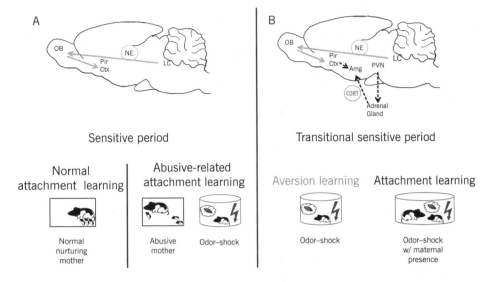

FIGURE 4.1. Active circuitry during the sensitive period (until PN 10) and transitional sensitive period (PN 10–PN 15) of attachment learning. Models of abusive–related attachment used in the laboratory during both periods are schematically depicted. (A) The circuitry active during the sensitive period (before PN 10) and models of abuse-related attachment. Normal attachment learning (left) and abusive-related attachment learning from an abusive mother (given minimal bedding) or odor–shock conditioning (pairing an odor with a hind limb shock to mimic pain associated with abuse) both activate the simple circuit highlighted in gray. This circuit involves hyperactive locus coeruleus (LC) release of norepinephrine (NE) into the olfactory bulb (OB). Changes can be measured in both the OB and piriform cortex (Pir Ctx). (B) During the transitional period (PN 10–PN 15), as pups begin to mature, more adult-like amygdala (Amg)-dependent learning can occur if the mother is not present. The shock induces a release of corticosterone (CORT) from the adrenal gland, leading to plasticity within the Amg. Aversion learning can occur during odor–shock conditioning without the mother, activating the circuitry highlighted by the black, dashed arrows. If the mother is present, only sensitive period circuitry is activated, since her presence can block the release of CORT and attachment learning occurs (circuitry within gray arrows only).

Interestingly, the amount of NE released into the olfactory bulb changes during the course of early development. Specifically, prior to PN 10 in rat pups, a significantly greater amount of NE is released into the olfactory bulb (Sullivan et al., 1989, 1992; Sullivan & Wilson, 1994; Rangel & Leon, 1995). This appears to result from a lack of recurrent collateral inhibition in the pups' LC. In adults (and older pups), inhibitory autoreceptors appear to decrease NE release from the LC projections (Nakamura, Kimura, & Sakaguchi, 1987; Nakamura & Sakaguchi, 1990; Marshall, Christie, Finlayson, & Williams, 1991; Winzer-Serhan, Raymon, Broide, Chen, & Leslie, 1997). This emergence of functional LC inhibitory autoreceptors has become one marker that signals the end of a specific sensitive period during which pups possess an enhanced ability to learn an attachment to new odors. Following this sensitive period, NE then acts as a modulator of learning, as has been shown repeatedly in adult models of learning (Ferry & McGaugh, 2000; McGaugh, 2006). A similar action of NE has been found in the developing somatosensory system (Levin, Craik, & Hand, 1988; Simpson, Wang, Kirifides, Lin, & Waterhouse, 1997; Landers & Sullivan, 1999a).

Another aspect of odor associations is the hedonic value or meaning to the odor. The piriform cortex plays a prominent role in processing hedonic value and receives direct projections from the olfactory bulb (Schwob & Price, 1984; Haberly, 2001). More specifically, the limbic structures and intracortical circuits are activated in older pups and adults to learned odors (Roth & Sullivan, 2005).

Infant Attachment Associated with Pain or Abuse

An important aspect of attachment learning is that regardless of the quality of care received, including pain from the caregiver, the infant learns an attachment to the caregiver (Roth & Sullivan, 2005; Raineki et al., 2010; Raineki, Rincon Cortes, Belnoue, & Sullivan, 2012). This occurs in myriad species, such as infant chicks, dogs, and nonhuman primates (Harlow & Harlow, 1965; Salzen, 1970; Suomi, 1997; Bolhuis & Honey, 1998; Maestripieri, Tomaszycki, & Carroll, 1999; Sanchez, Ladd, & Plotskey, 2001). Interestingly, infants are capable of detecting pain (King, Heath, Debs, Davis, Hen, & Barr, 2000; King & Barr, 2003; Fitzgerald, 2005), raising the question of why pain does not engage the amygdala-dependent fear-learning system. To address this, our laboratory has modeled this abuse-related attachment in rat pups using two distinct procedures: pain directly from the mother (abusive care) and odor–pain classical conditioning, inducing pain with either 0.5-mA electric shock or tail pinch (see Figure 4.1). Specifically, the first model is a naturalistic paradigm, in which the mother is provided with insufficient bedding for

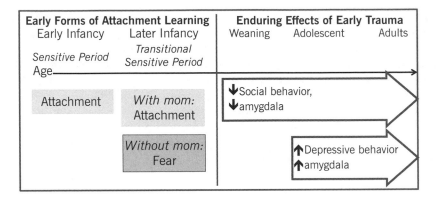

FIGURE 4.2. Timeline of attachment learning and the effects of early-life maltreatment on later-life social and emotional behavior in the rat model. Early on, infants learn attachment regardless of the quality of care, whereas slightly older infants (PN 10–PN 15) either learn to fear a traumatic associated stimulus when away from the mother or learn an attachment if acquisition takes place with the mother. Despite this, early-life trauma leads to lifelong amygdala-dependent behavioral deficits, such as poor social behavior, with onset prior to weaning and depressive-like behaviors, with onset postweaning (Sullivan & Leon, 1986; Sullivan et al., 2000b; Raineki et al., 2010; Sevelinges et al., 2011; Raineki et al., 2012).

nest building, leading to abusive maternal behavior in the home cage. The second model is an infant odor–shock conditioning paradigm, in which a novel stimulus (i.e., odor) is paired with a mild electric shock—mimicking pups' painful interactions with an abusive mother (Raineki et al., 2010, 2012). Both procedures lead to the behavioral approach toward the conditioned odor by the pup and support nipple attachment, not avoidance (see Figures 4.1 and 4.2, Early Infancy) (Rudy & Cheatle, 1977; Haroutunian & Campbell, 1979; Sullivan et al., 1986; Raineki et al., 2010; Sullivan et al., 2000a). However, as we address below, in order for this paradoxical odor preference–pain phenomenon to occur, there must be a suppression of the amygdala-dependent fear (Sullivan et al., 2000a), which normally occurs in adults in response to threatening stimuli (Fanselow & Gale, 2003; LeDoux, 2000, 2003, 2007).

Amygdala Suppression and Failure to Acquire Amygdala-Dependent Fear

Suppression of amygdala learning-dependent plasticity is critical for the acquisition of the paradoxical preference/attachment learning that occurs in pups within the sensitive period (up to PN 10) with odor–pain learning (see Figure 4.1). In contrast, the amygdalae of older pups and adults display learning-induced plasticity that results in fear learning (Sananes & Campbell, 1989; Davis, 1997; Fanselow & LeDoux, 1999; McGaugh, Roozendaal, & Cahill, 1999; Blair, Schafe, Bauer, Rodgrigues, & LeDoux, 2001; Schettino & Otto, 2001; Fanselow & Gale, 2003; Maren, 2003; Pape & Stork, 2003; Pare, Quirk, & LeDoux, 2004; Sevelinges, Gervais, Messaoudi, Granjon, & Mouly, 2004; Sigurdsson, Doyère, Cain, & LeDoux, 2007; Poulos et al., 2009). However, although the young infant rat's amygdala responds to pain and odors, the amygdala does not display learning-related plasticity in rat pups younger than PN 10 (Sullivan et al., 2000b; Wiedenmayer & Barr, 2001; Moriceau, Roth, Okotoghaide, & Sullivan, 2004; Roth & Sullivan, 2005). Instead, odor–shock conditioning that occurs during the sensitive period, which leads to a behavioral preference for the conditioned odor, accesses the same circuitry used during attachment learning tasks—with learning-induced plasticity occurring in the olfactory bulb and anterior piriform cortex (Roth & Sullivan, 2005).

However, even fetal rats can learn to avoid odors supported by malaise conditioning (lithium chloride [LiCl] or strong shock altering the gut; Hennessy, Smotherman, & Levine, 1976; Smotherman, Hennessy, & Levine, 1976; Rudy & Cheatle, 1983; Bermudez-Rattoni, Grijalva, Rusiniak, & Garcia, 1986; Hoffmann, Molina, Kucharski, & Spear, 1987; Hunt, Spear, & Spear, 1991; Shionoya et al., 2006; Raineki, Shionoya, Sander, & Sullivan, 2009). Importantly, unlike adult amygdala-dependent odor–malaise learning (Touzani & Sclafani, 2005), this pup learning does not engage the amygdala until pups approach weaning age (Shionoya et al., 2006; Raineki et al., 2009). Thus, the neurodevelopment of odor–malaise learning shows sharp ontogenetically distinct features from that of pup attachment learning, which dramatically shows the amygdala's lack of function in early life.

The end of the attachment sensitive period and the emergence of amygdala-dependent odor–pain learning emerges around PN 10 (Sullivan et al., 2000b), when pups enter the transitional sensitive period. This corresponds with the emergence of walking and brief periods of time outside the nest (Bolhuis & Honey, 1998; see Figure 4.1). A molecular signal that is critical for pups' transition between the sensitive period and transitional sensitive period is the stress-induced corticosterone (CORT) release that acts on the amygdala. CORT levels are normally low in infant rat pups and do not change in response to most stressors (called the stress hyporesponsive period [SHRP]; Levine, 1962; Guillet & Michaelson, 1978; Henning, 1978; Walker, Sapolsky, Meaney, Vale, & Rivier, 1986; Walker, Scribner, Cascio, & Dallman, 1991; Rosenfeld, Suchecki, & Levine, 1992; Grino, Paulmyer-Lacroix, Faudon, Renard, & Anglade, 1994). Despite this, it is clear that the hypothalamic–pituitary–adrenal (HPA) axis, which is critical for CORT release, is functional during the SHRP, because stressors such as long-term maternal separation or reduced temperatures can acutely increase pups' CORT levels (Walker et al., 1991). In addition, early life stress can induce a precocial end to the sensitive period (Moriceau et al., 2009).

We have shown in our laboratory that during the sensitive period, an acute increase in CORT can transiently engage the amygdala to permit amygdala-dependent fear learning (Moriceau & Sullivan, 2006). In contrast, during the transitional sensitive period (PN 10–PN 15) CORT levels naturally rise in response to stressful stimuli during conditioning and permit fear learning. However, rapid decreases in CORT can reinstate sensitive period-like learning (i.e., attachment; Moriceau et al., 2004, 2009; Moriceau & Sullivan, 2006; Barr et al., 2009). For example, the maternal presence can naturally decrease CORT levels during the transitional sensitive period (Hennessy, Li, & Levine, 1980; Hennessy, Kaiser, & Sachser, 2009; Stanton, Wallstrom, & Levine, 1987; Stanton & Levine, 1990; DeVries, Glasper, & Detillion, 2003) and this leads to a blockade of pups' ability to display amygdala-dependent fear learning (Moriceau & Sullivan, 2006; Shionoya et al., 2006; Upton & Sullivan, 2010; see the transitional sensitive period in Figure 4.1). Specifically, this occurs through social buffering via suppression of NE into the paraventricular nucleus (PVN) of the hypothalamus (Moriceau & Sullivan, 2006; Shionoya, Moriceau, Bradstock, & Sullivan, 2007). Thus, modulating CORT levels dictates whether pups will learn an attachment or an aversion, but as illustrated below, the slow-developing amygdala and CORT also have profound effects on pups' expression of social behavior and social interactions with the attachment figure, the mother (Takahashi, 1994; Barr, 1995; Fitzgerald, 2005; Moriceau & Sullivan, 2006; Moriceau et al., 2006; Shionoya et al., 2007).

Infant Social Behavior and Amygdala Involvement

In humans, the amygdala is implicated in social behavior in adulthood (Thomas et al., 2001; Stone, Baron-Cohen, Calder, Keane, & Young, 2003), as well as during development (Skuse, Morris, & Lawrence, 2006; Tottenham, Hare, & Casey, 2009). Clues to the importance of the amygdala in social behavior have been further supported by research showing that humans with amygdala lesions have social behavior deficits (Adolphs, Tranel, & Damasio, 1998; Adolphs, Sears, & Piven, 2001; Amaral, 2003; see also the Chapters in this volume by Feinstein, Adolphs, & Tranel, Chapter 1; Adolphs, Chapter 10; van Honk, Terburg, Thornton, Stein, & Morgan, Chapter 12; Patin & Hurlemann, Chapter 11) and disorders associated with social behavior deficits, such as autism and Williams syndrome, show amygdala abnormalities (Baron-Cohen et al., 1999; Bachevalier, Malkova, & Mishkin., 2000; Critchley et al., 2000; Howard et al.,

2000; Pierce, Muller, Ambrose, Allen, & Courchesne, 2001; Haas et al., 2009; Paul et al., 2009). Moreover, nonhuman primate studies, in which experimental manipulations can be more controlled, demonstrate that monkeys without amygdalae display inappropriate social behavior, supporting the role of the amygdala in this facet (Kling & Brothers, 1992; Baron-Cohen et al., 2000; Emery et al., 2001; Amaral, 2003; Malkova, Mishkin, Suomi, & Bachevalier, 2010; Bliss-Moreau, Bauman, & Amaral, 2011).

Although the amygdala is also implicated in social behavior in children (Skuse et al., 2006; Tottenham et al., 2009), its role is less clear. Indeed, the first hints that dramatic developmental differences in amygdala function might exist were from the nonhuman primate literature, where amygdala lesions lead to a similar lack of fear response to normally fear-inducing stimuli, but an enhanced response to novel social situations (Amaral, 2002; Amaral, 2003). Further support was derived from the rodent literature in which more precise roles of amygdala nuclei were documented. Social behavior in adult rodents appears to rely on the medial amygdala (Rasia-Filho, Londero, & Achaval, 2000). Specifically, c-Fos activity in the medial amygdala increases following nonsexual encounters and maternal behavior in rodent models (Fleming, Suh, Korsmit, & Rusak, 1994; Kirkpatrick, Kim, & Insel, 1994). Medial amygdala activation is also associated with parental behavior in voles, which is blocked by lesioning this nucleus (Kirkpatrick et al., 1994; Fergusen, Aldag, Insel, & Young, 2001; Fergusen, Young, & Insel, 2002; Gobrogge, Liu, Jia, & Wang, 2007). While the medial amygdala has a prominent role in social behavior, the basolateral, central and cortical amygdala nuclei have also been implicated (Katayama et al., 2009).

We have explored in our laboratory the development of social behavior in rat pups and possible involvement of the amygdala. Using both naturalistic and classical conditioning paradigms (see Figure 4.2), we can disrupt normal development by modeling early-life maltreatment, including the controlled odor–shock conditioning described earlier, and a more ecologically relevant paradigm in which the mother rears her pups with insufficient bedding for nest building, both of which occur from PN 8 to PN 12 (Roth & Sullivan, 2005; Ivy, Brunson, Sandman, & Baram, 2008; Rice, Sandman, Lenjavi, & Baram, 2008). Both models of early-life maltreatment have converging results that demonstrate myriad neurobehavioral modifications across development. Specifically, infant social behavior is tested using both a Y-maze (measuring pups' approach toward a learned maternal odor) and a maternal–pup interaction test (a direct measure of interaction between mother and pup). Interestingly, these tests show that infants with maltreatment display normal social behavior with the mother when tested just a couple of days after maltreatment ends. This was surprising to us, since, as we discuss below, early-life maltreatment results in adult neurobehavioral abnormalities in rats, and this enduring effect of early-life maltreatment is consistent with many other early-life stress paradigms and the clinical literature (Heim, Owens, Plotskey, & Nemeroff, 1997; Heim, Newport, Mletzko, Miller, & Nemeroff, 2008; Caspi et al., 2003; De Kloet, Joels, & Holsboer, 2005; Nemeroff & Vale, 2005). While the human literature also documents difficulties in identifying maltreated children, increased stress during testing of these children (i.e., the Strange Situation test) produces aberrant behavior with the caregiver (Crittenden, 1992; Gunnar, Brodersen, Nachmias, Buss, & Rigatuso, 1996). Thus, we questioned whether stress might uncover neurobehavioral differences with pups following early-life maltreatment. Indeed, an injection of CORT (modeling a heightened stress environment) in pups at PN 13–PN 14 uncovers strong behavioral deficits following early maltreatment (i.e., fewer choices toward a maternal odor and less time nipple attached). Interestingly, pups with social behavior deficits also showed amygdala activation when stressed, suggesting that early-life abusive attachment recruited the amygdala despite pups failing to learn the amygdala-dependent fear (Raineki et al., 2010). This social impairment also predicted later life depressive-like behaviors, suggesting an interesting ontogeny of deficits, in which social behavioral deficits appear prior to those of depression. This is similar to what is found in childhood dysfunctional social behavior that occurs prior to depression (Mason et al., 2004; Letcher, Smart, Sanson, & Toumbourou, 2009; Mazza et al., 2009).

In summary, it is important to note that while social behavior in adults involves the amygdala and can be a behavioral measure used to reveal those adults with early-life trauma, in pups, only periods of heightened stress (CORT) combined with early-life trauma uncover social behavior deficits and heightened amygdala neural activity in this population. This suggests that the amygdala is not involved with social behavior in infancy and its activation can, in fact, impair social behavior at this age. These data converge with nonhuman primate data in which stress, peer rearing, and extensive amygdala lesions indicate considerable social behavior disruption (Bachevalier et al., 2000, 2001; Malkova et al., 2010), whereas amygdala activity may not be essential for infant social behavior during typical rearing (Amaral et al., 2003).

Enduring Consequences of Attachment Quality on Behavior and the Amygdala

The amygdala is one of many brain areas (i.e., including also the hippocampus and prefrontal cortex) involved in emotional regulation (Drevets, 2001; Drevets, Price, & Furey, 2008; Rigucci, Serafini, Pompili, Kotzalidis,

& Tatarelli, 2010; Ritchey, Dolcos, Eddington, Strauman, & Cabeza, 2011). Thus, abnormal function of any of these regions has been implicated in depression and antidepressant action (Berton & Nestler, 2006; Krishnan & Nestler, 2008, 2010). Here we focus on the link between the quality of developmental attachment and the consequences on adult behavioral measures and how the amygdala could play a role in the outcome. The clinical literature draws a strong correlation between the quality of developmental attachment and adult behavior. Specifically, abnormal attachment that occurs during development (possibly as a result of early-life trauma) is highly related to later-life depressive-like symptoms and social behavioral problems. For example, as mentioned earlier, adult depression is often associated with social behavior dysfunction during childhood (Mason et al., 2004; Letcher et al., 2009). These findings are in line with our work in the rat animal model, which demonstrates that following early life trauma, deficits in social behavior emerge prior to depressive-like symptoms (Raineki et al., 2012). In fact, it seems that antisocial behavior in girls is highly predictive of later-life depression, whereas anxiety is also a strong predictor of later-life depression in boys (Mazza et al., 2009). However, in clinical populations, although many findings suggest a relationship between early-life social deficits and later-life depression, how they are related is often unclear. For example, social behavior deficits in humans can enhance stress and anxiety levels on their own, resulting in compromised development. This is a critical factor, because early-life stress is associated with later-life depression (Heim et al., 1997, 2008; Nemeroff & Vale, 2005; Gatt et al., 2009; Savitz & Drevets, 2009) and altered genetic predisposition (Caspi et al., 2003; De Kloet et al., 2005; Nemeroff & Vale, 2005; Brown & Harris, 2008) with the onset of depression associated with a precipitating stressful event (Caspi et al., 2003; Drevets, 2003).

Another dimension to this complex relationship is that both clinical and animal studies have demonstrated that the altered amygdala function is associated with depressive-like symptoms and is a consequence of early-life abuse. For example, patients with depression also show amygdala abnormalities and dysfunctional connectivity with other brain areas (Teicher, Andersen, Polcari, Anderson, & Navalta, 2002; Bremner, 2003; McEwen, 2003; Ressler & Mayberg, 2007; Savitz & Drevets, 2009; Sibille et al., 2009). Furthermore, abuse-related attachment in humans is associated with social behavior problems, later-life depressive-like behavior, and abnormal amygdala activity (Heim & Nemeroff, 1999; Teicher et al., 2002; Teicher et al., 2003).

In fact, studies of animal models agree with the adult clinical literature and demonstrate a link between early-life trauma and the enduring consequences of later-life depressive-like behaviors and amygdala dysfunction. For example, various forms of infant and adolescent stress paradigms result in similar later-life deficits in behavior and amygdala dysfunction (Huang & Lin, 2006; Leussis & Andersen, 2008; Kuramochi & Nakamura, 2009). Indeed, the amygdala, most specifically the baso-lateral nucleus, is primarily involved in the expression of depression-like symptoms in adult rats (Coryell et al., 2009). Our model of early-life abuse is consistent with these results and indicates this as a strong risk factor for the development of depression, among other psychopathologies (see Figure 4.2). Given that using an animal model allows for high experimen-tal control, we are also able to determine a pattern of emergence for the deficits as a direct result of early-life abuse. Specifically, those rats with early-life abuse display social behavioral deficits prior to weaning, then display depressive-like symptoms later, as adolescents. Interestingly, the emergence of amygdala dysfunction is associated in development with the appearance of depressive-like behaviors (Raineki et al., 2012). Further-more, using two common measures of depressive-like behavior, sucrose consumption and forced swim tests, we have found that these deficits per-sist into adulthood (Sevelinges et al., 2011). Finally, a causal link between these behaviors and amygdala function was demonstrated by temporary inactivation of the amygdala via muscimol (a gamma-aminobutyric acid [GABA$_A$] receptor agonist), leading to a normalization of behavior on a forced swim test of depressive-like behavior (Raineki et al., 2012). Thus, using studies in animal models to complement those in humans brings us closer to the development of specific strategies for preventing or reversing resultant psychopathologies in these individuals. These findings broaden the scope of our knowledge of potential underlying mechanisms and lay out a potential ontogenetic pattern of social behavior deficits that may precede later-life mental dysfunction, such as depression.

Implications for Developmental Disorders, Amygdala and Social Behavior

Together, the literature reviewed here suggests that adult social behavior is associated with amygdala activation; this is not the case with infant social behavior with the mother, unless the infant has been reared under stressful conditions and is acutely stressed. As we relate these data to humans, it should be noted that it is unclear exactly when the human amygdala becomes functional, but anatomical markers of maturity can at least provide information on whether the amygdala is potentially suf-ficiently functionally mature. The amygdala experiences major develop-ment progress throughout the first 7 years of life but continues to develop into adolescence (Letcher et al., 2009; Lupien, McEwen, Gunnar, & Heim, 2009; Tottenham et al., 2009). Specifically, much of the architecture of the amygdala is present by birth in humans, and much of structural growth is completed by 4 years of age (Humphrey, 1968; Giedd et al.,

1996; Ulfig, Setzer, & Bohl, 2003). This may be a period of rapid change and likewise heightened vulnerability of the amygdala to environmental influence (Lupien et al., 2009). Thus, similar to what was demonstrated in the previously discussed rodent studies, we might predict that early life is also a sensitive period for the human amygdala. While mechanisms of human attachment may contain more complexities than those found in animal models, it is important to use what we have gained from this work to direct the future studies of developmental disorders and their relation to a functional amygdala.

ACKNOWLEDGMENT

This work was supported by Grant Nos. NIH-DC009910, NIH-MH091451, and T32 MH 67763-10.

REFERENCES

Adolphs, R, Sears, L., & Piven, J. (2001). Abnormal processing of social information from faces in autism. *Journal of Cognitive Neuroscience, 13*, 232–240.

Adolphs, R., Tranel, D., & Damasio, A. (1998). The human amygdala in social judgment. *Nature, 393*, 470–474.

Adriani, W., & Laviola, G. (2004). Windows of vulnerability to psychopathology and therapeutics strategy in the adolescent rodent model. *Behavioural Pharmacology, 15*, 341–352.

Al Ain, S., Belin, S., Schaal, B., & Petris, B. (2012). How does a newly born mouse get to the nipple?: Odor substrates eliciting first nipple grasping and sucking responses. *Developmental Psychobiology, 55*(8), 888–901.

Amaral, D. (2002). The primate amygdala and the neurobiology of social behavior: Implications for understanding social anxiety. *Biological Psychiatry, 51*, 11–17.

Amaral, D. (2003). The amygdala, social behavior, and danger detection. *Annals of the New York Academy of Sciences, 1000*, 337–347.

Amaral, D., Bauman, M., Capitanio, J., Lavenex, P., Mason, W., Mauldin-Jourdain, M., et al. (2003). The amygdala: Is it an essential component of the neural network for social cognition? *Neuropsychologia, 41*, 517–522.

Bachevalier, J., Malkova, L., & Mishkin, M. (2000). The amygdala, social cognition, and autism. In J. Aggleton (Ed.), *The amygdala* (pp. 509–543). New York: Oxford University Press.

Bachevalier, J., Malkova, L., & Mishkin, M. (2001). Effects of selective neonatal medial temporal lobe lesions on socioemotional behaviors in monkeys. *Behavioral Neuroscience, 115*, 545–560.

Baron-Cohen, S., Ring, H., Bullmore, E., Wheelwright, S., Ashwin, C., & Williams S. (2000). The amygdala theory of autism. *Neuroscience and Biobehavioral Reviews, 24*, 355–364.

Baron-Cohen, S., Ring, H., Wheelwright, S., Bullmore, E., Brammer, M.,

Simmons, A., et al. (1999). Social intelligence in the normal and autistic brain: An fMRI study. *European Journal of Neuroscience, 11*, 1891–1989.

Barr, G. (1995). Ontogeny of nociception and antinociception. *NIDA Research Monographs, 158*, 172–201.

Barr, G., Moriceau, S., Shionoya, K., Muzny, K., Gao, P., Wang, S., et al. (2009). Transitions in infant learning are modulated by dopamine in the amygdala. *Nature Neuroscience, 12*, 1367–1369.

Bartels, A., & Zeki, S. (2000). The neural basis of romantic love. *NeuroReport, 11*, 3829–3834.

Bartels, A., & Zeki, S. (2004). The neural correlates of maternal and romantic love. *NeuroImage, 21*, 1155–1166.

Bermudez-Rattoni, F., Grijalva, C., Rusiniak, K. W., & Garcia, J. (1986). Flavor-illness aversions: The role of the amygdala in the acquisition of taste-potentiated odor aversions. *Physiology and Behavior, 38*, 503–508.

Berton, O., & Nestler, E. (2006). New approaches to antidepressant drug discovery: Beyond monoamines. *Nature Reviews Neuroscience, 7*, 137–151.

Blair, H., Schafe, G., Bauer, E., Rodrigues, S., & LeDoux, J. (2001). Synaptic plasticity in the lateral amygdala: A cellular hypothesis of fear conditioning. *Learning and Memory, 8*, 229–242.

Bliss-Moreau, E., Bauman, M., & Amaral, D. (2011). Neonatal amygdala lesions result in globally blunted affect in adult rhesus macaques. *Behavioral Neuroscience, 125*, 848–858.

Bolhuis, J., & Honey, R. (1998). Imprinting, learning and development: From behaviour to brain and back. *Trends in Neuroscience, 21*, 306–311.

Bowlby, J. (1965). *Attachment*. New York: Basic Books.

Brake, S. (1981). Suckling infant rats learn a preference for a novel olfactory stimulus paired with milk delivery. *Science, 211*, 506–508.

Bremner, J. (2003). Long-term effects of childhood abuse on brain and neurobiology. *Child and Adolescent Psychiatric Clinics of North America, 12*, 271–292.

Brown, G., & Harris, T. (2008). Depression and the serotonin trasnporter *5-HTTLPR* polymorphism: A review and a hypothesis concerning gene-environment interaction. *Journal of Affective Disorders, 111*, 1–12.

Brunjes, P., & Alberts, J. (1979). Olfactory stimulation induces filial preferences for huddling in rat pups. *Journal of Comparative and Physiological Psychology, 93*, 548–555.

Camp, L., & Rudy, J. (1988). Changes in the categorization of appetitive and aversive events during postnatal development of the rat. *Developmental Psychobiology, 21*, 25–42.

Campbell, B. (1984). *Reflections on the ontogeny of learning and memory*. Hillsdale, NJ: Erlbaum.

Carew, T. (1996). Molecular enhancement of memory formation. *Neuron, 16*, 5–8.

Carew, T., & Sutton, M. (2001). Molecular stepping stones in memory consolidation. *Nature Neuroscience, 4*, 769–771.

Carvell, G., & Simons, D. (1996). Abnormal tactile experience early in life disrupts active touch. *Journal of Neuroscience, 16*, 2750–2757.

Caspi, A., Sugden, K., Moffitt, T., Taylor, A., Craig, I., Harrington, H., et al. (2003). Influence of life stress on depression: Moderation by a polymorphism in the *5-HTT* gene. *Science, 301*, 386–389.

Caza, P., & Spear, N. (1984). Short-term exposure to an odor increases its subsequent preference in preweanling rats: A descriptive profile of the phenomenon. *Developmental Psychobiology, 17,* 407–422.

Cheslock, S., Varlinskaya, E., Petrov, E., & Spear, N. (2000). Rapid and robust olfactory conditioning with milk before suckling experience: Promotion of nipple attachment in the newborn rat. *Behavioral Neuroscience, 114,* 484–495.

Coopersmith, R., & Leon, M. (1986). Enhanced neural response by adult rats to odors experienced early in life. *Brain Research, 371,* 400–403.

Coryell, M., Wunsch, A., Haenfler, J., Allen, J., Schnizler, M., Ziemann, A., et al. (2009). Acid-sensing ion channel-1a in the amygdala, a novel therapeutic target in depression-related behavior. *Journal of Neuroscience, 29,* 5381–5388.

Crews, F., He, J., & Hodge, C. (2007). Adolescent cortical development: A critical period of vulnerability for addiction. *Pharmacology Biochemistry and Behavior, 86,* 189–199.

Critchley, H., Daly, E., Bullmore, E., Williams, S., Van Amelsvoort, T., Robertson, T., et al. (2000). The functional neuroanatomy of social behaviour: Changes in cerebral blood flow when people with autistic disorder process facial expressions. *Brain, 123,* 2203–2212.

Crittenden, P. (1992). Children's strategies for coping with adverse home environments: An interpretation using attachment theory. *Child Abuse and Neglect, 16,* 329–343.

Davis, M. (1997). Neurobiology of fear responses: The role of the amygdala. *Journal of Neuropsychiatry and Clinical Neurosciences, 9,* 382–402.

DeCasper, A., & Fifer, W. (1980). Of human bonding: newborns prefer their mothers' voices. *Science, 208,* 1174–1176.

De Kloet, E., Joels, M., & Holsboer, F. (2005). Stress and the brain: From adaptation to disease. *Nature Reviews Neuroscience, 6,* 463–475.

DeVries, A., Glasper, E., & Detillion, C. (2003). Social modulation of stress responses. *Physiology and Behavior, 79,* 399–407.

Drevets, W. (2001). Neuroimaging and neuropathological studies of depression: Implications for the cognitive–emotional features of mood disorders. *Current Opinion in Neurobiology, 11,* 240–249.

Drevets, W. (2003). Neuroimaging abnormalities in the amygdala in mood disorders. *Annals of the New York Academy of Sciences, 985,* 420–444.

Drevets, W., Price, J., & Furey, M. (2008). Brain structural and functional abnormalities in mood disorders: Implications for neurocircuitry models of depression. *Brain Structure and Function, 213,* 93–118.

Duveau, A., & Godinot, F. (1988). Influence of the odorization of the rearing environment on the development of odor-guided behavior in rat pups. *Physiology and Behavior, 43,* 265–270.

Emery, N., Capitanio, J., Mason, W., Machado, C., Mendoza, S., & Amaral, D. (2001). The effects of bilateral lesions of the amygdala on dyadic social interactions in rhesus monkeys (*Macaca mulatta*). *Behavioral Neuroscience, 115,* 515–544.

Fanselow, M., & Gale, G. (2003). The amygdala, fear, and memory. *Annals of the New York Academy of Sciences, 985,* 125–134.

Fanselow, M., & LeDoux, J. (1999). Why we think plasticity underlying Pavlovian fear conditioning occurs in the basolateral amygdala. *Neuron, 23,* 229–232.

Fergusen, J., Aldag, J., Insel, T., & Young, L. (2001). Oxytocin in the medial amygdala is essential for social recognition in the mouse. *Journal of Neuroscience, 21*, 8278–8285.

Fergusen, J., Young, L., & Insel, T. (2002). The neuroendocrine basis of social recognition. *Frontiers in Neuroendocrinology, 23*(2), 200–224.

Ferry, B., & McGaugh, J. (2000). Role of amygdala norepinephrine in mediating stress hormone regulation of memory storage. *Acta Pharmacologica Sinica, 21*, 481–493.

Fitzgerald, M. (2005). The development of nociceptive circuits. *Nature Reviews Neuroscience, 6*, 507–520.

Fleming, A., O'Day, D., & Kraemer, G. (1999). Neurobiology of mother–infant interactions: Experience and central nervous system plasticity across development and generations. *Neuroscience and Biobehavioral Reviews, 23*, 673–685.

Fleming, A., Suh, E., Korsmit, M., & Rusak, B. (1994). Activation of Fos-like immunoreactivity in the medial preoptic area and limbic structures by maternal and social interactions in rats. *Behavioral Neuroscience, 108*, 251–260.

Galef, B. J., & Kaner, H. (1980). Establishment and maintenance of preference for natural and artificial olfactory stimuli in juvenile rats. *Journal of Comparative and Physiological Psychology, 94*, 588–595.

Galef, B. J., & Sherry, D. (1973). Mother's milk: A medium for transmission of cues reflecting the flavor of mother's diet. *Journal of Comparative and Physiological Psychology, 83*, 374–378.

Gatt, J., Nemeroff, C., Dobson-Stone, C., Paul, R., Bryant, R., Schofield, P., et al. (2009). Interactions between BDNF Val66Met polymorphism and early life stress predict brain and arousal pathways to syndromal depression and anxiety. *Molecular Psychiatry, 14*, 681–695.

Giedd, J., Vaituzis, A., Hamburger, S., Lange, N., Rajapakse, J., Kaysen, D., et al. (1996). Quantitative MRI of the temporal lobe, amygdala, and hippocampus in normal human development: Ages 4–18 years. *Journal of Comparative Neurology, 366*, 223–230.

Gobrogge, K., Liu, Y., Jia, X., & Wang, Z. (2007). Anterior hypothalamic neural activation and neurochemical associations with aggression in pair-bonded male prairie voles. *Journal of Comparative Neurology, 502*, 1109–1122.

Grino, M., Paulmyer-Lacroix, O., Faudon, M., Renard, M., & Anglade, G. (1994). Blockade of alpha 2-adrenoceptors stimulates basal and stress-induced adrenocorticotropin secretion in the developing rat through a central mechanism independent from corticotropin-releasing factor and arginine vasopressin. *Endocrinology, 135*, 2549–2557.

Guillet, R., & Michaelson, S. (1978). Corticotropin responsiveness in the neonatal rat. *Neuroendocrinology, 27*, 119–125.

Gunnar, M., Brodersen, L., Nachmias, M., Buss, K., & Rigatuso, J. (1996). Stress reactivity and attachment security. *Developmental Psychobiology, 29*, 191–204.

Haas, B., Mills, D., Yam, A., Hoeft, F., Bellugi, U., & Reiss, A. (2009). Genetic influences on sociability: Heightened amygdala reactivity and event-related responses to positive social stimuli in Williams syndrome. *Journal of Neuroscience, 29*, 1132–1139.

Haberly, L. (2001). Parallel-distributed processing in olfactory cortex: New insights from morphological and physiological analysis of neuronal cir-cuitry. *Chemical Senses, 26,* 551–576.

Harlow, H., & Harlow, M. (1965). The affectional system. In A. Schrier, H. Har-low, & F. Stollnitz (Eds.), *Behavior of nonhuman primates* (pp. 287–334). New York: Academic Press.

Haroutunian, V., & Campbell, B. (1979). Emergence of interoceptive and extero-ceptive control of behavior in rats. *Science, 205,* 927–929.

Heim, C., & Nemeroff, C. (1999). The impact of early adverse experiences on brain systems involved in the pathophysiology of anxiety and affective disor-ders. *Biological Psychiatry, 46,* 1509–1522.

Heim, C., Newport, D., Mletzko, T., Miller, A., & Nemeroff, C. (2008). The link between childhood trauma and depression: Insights from HPA axis studies in humans. *Psychoneuroendocrinology, 33,* 693–710.

Heim, C., Owens, M., Plotskey, P., & Nemeroff, C. (1997). The role of early adverse life events in the etiology of depression and posttraumatic stress disorder: Focus on corticotropin-releasing factor. *Annals of the New York Academy of Sciences, 821,* 194–207.

Hennessy, J., Smotherman, W., & Levine, S. (1976). Conditioned taste aversion and the pituitary–adrenal system. *Behavioral Biology, 16,* 413–424.

Hennessy, M., Kaiser, S., & Sachser, N. (2009). Social buffering of the stress response: Diversity, mechanisms, and functions. *Frontiers in Neuroendocrinol-ogy, 40,* 470–482.

Hennessy, M., Li, V., & Levine, S. (1980). Infant responsiveness to maternal cues in mice of two inbred lines. *Developmental Psychobiology, 13,* 77–84.

Henning, S. (1978). Plasma concentrations of total and free corticosterone dur-ing development in the rat. *American Journal of Physiology, 235,* 451–456.

Hensch, T. (2004). Critical period regulation. *Annual Review of Neuroscience, 27,* 549–579.

Hess, E. (1962). Ethology: An approach to the complete analysis of behavior. In R. Brown, E. Galanter, E. Hess, & G. Mendler (Eds.), *New directions in psychology* (pp. 159–199). New York: Holt, Rinehart & Winston.

Higley, E., & Dozier, M. (2009). Nighttime maternal responsiveness and infant attachment at one year. *Attachment and Human Development, 11,* 347–363.

Hofer, M., Fisher, A., & Shair, H. (1981). Effects of infraorbital nerve section on survival, growth, and suckling behaviors of developing rats. *Journal of Com-parative and Physiological Psychology, 95,* 123–133.

Hofer, M., Shair, H., & Singh, P. (1976). Evidence that maternal ventral skin sub-stances promote suckling in infant rats. *Physiology and Behavior, 17,* 131–136.

Hofer, M., & Sullivan, R. (2008). Toward a neurobiology of attachment. In C. Nelson & M. Luciana (Eds.), *Handbook of developmental cognitive neuroscience* (pp. 599–616). Cambridge, MA: MIT Press.

Hoffmann, H., Molina, J., Kucharski, D., & Spear, N. (1987). Further examina-tion of ontogenetic limitations on conditioned taste aversion. *Developmental Psychobiology, 20,* 455–463.

Howard, M., Cowell, P., Boucher, J., Broks, P., Mayes, A., Farrant, A., et al. (2000). Convergent neuroanatomical and behavioural evidence of an amygdala hypothesis of autism. *NeuroReport, 11,* 2931–2935.

Huang, T., & Lin, C. (2006). Role of amygdala MAPK activation on immobility behavior of forced swim test. *Behavioural Brain Research, 173*, 104–111.

Humphrey, T. (1968). The development of the human amygdala during early embryonic life. *Journal of Comparative Neurology, 132*, 135–165.

Hunt, P., Spear, L., & Spear, N. (1991). An ontogenetic comparison of ethanol-mediated taste aversion learning and ethanol-induced hypothermia in pre-weanling rats. *Behavioral Neuroscience, 105*, 971–983.

Insel, T., & Young, L. (2001). The neurobiology of attachment. *Nature Reviews Neuroscience, 2*, 128–136.

Ivy, A., Brunson, K., Sandman, C., & Baram, T. (2008). Dysfunctional nurturing behavior in rat dams with limited access to nesting material: A clinically relevant model for early-life stress. *Neuroscience, 154*, 1132–1142.

Johanson, I., & Hall, W. (1979). Appetitive learning in 1-day-old rat pups. *Science, 205*, 419–421.

Johanson, I., & Teicher, M. (1980). Classical conditioning of an odor preference in 3-day-old rats. *Behavioral Neural Biology, 29*, 132–136.

Johnson, B., Woo, C., Duong, H., Nguyen, V., & Leon, M. (1995). A learned odor evokes an enhanced Fos-like glomerular response in the olfactory bulb of young rats. *Brain Research, 699*, 192–200.

Katayama, T., Jodo, E., Sezuki, Y., Hoshino, K., Takeuchi, S., & Kayama, Y. (2009). Phencyclidine affects firing activity of basolateral amygdala neurons related to social behavior in rats. *Neuroscience, 159*, 335–343.

King, T., & Barr, G. (2003). Functional development of neurokinin peptides substance P and neurokinin A in nociception. *NeuroReport, 14*, 1603–1607.

King, T., Heath, M., Debs, P., Davis, M., Hen, R., & Barr, G. (2000). The development of the nociceptive responses in neurokinin-1 receptor knockout mice. *NeuroReport, 11*, 587–591.

Kirkpatrick, B., Kim, J., & Insel, T. (1994). Limbic system fos expression associated with paternal behavior. *Brain Research, 658*, 112–118.

Kling, A., & Brothers, L. (1992). The amygdala and social behavior. In J. Aggleton (Ed.), *Neurobiological aspects of emotion, memory and mental dysfunction* (pp. 353–377). New York: Wiley.

Krishnan, V., & Nestler, E. (2008). The molecular neurobiology of depression. *Nature, 455*, 894–902.

Krishnan, V., & Nestler, E. (2010). Linking molecules to mood: new insight into the biology of depression. *American Journal of Psychiatry, 167*, 1305–1320.

Kuramochi, M., & Nakamura, S. (2009). Effects of postnatal isolation rearing and antidepressant treatment on the density of serotonergic and noradrenergic axons and depressive behaviors in rats. *Neuroscience, 163*, 448–455.

Landers, M., & Sullivan, R. (1999a). Norepinephrine and associative conditioning in the neonatal rat somatosensory system. *Brain Research: Developmental Brain Research, 114*, 261–264.

Landers, M., & Sullivan, R. (1999b). Vibrissae evoked behavior and conditioning before functional ontogeny of somatosensory vibrissae cortex. *Journal of Neuroscience, 19*, 5131–5137.

Landers, M., & Sullivan, R. (2012). The development and neurobiology of infant attachment and fear. *Developmental Neuroscience, 34*(2–3), 101–114.

Landers, M., & Zeigler, H. (2006). Development of rodent whisking: trigeminal input and central pattern generation. *Somatosensory and Motor Research, 23,* 1–10.

Langdon, P., Harley, C., & McLean, J. (1997). Increased beta adrenoceptor activation overcomes conditioned olfactory learning deficits induced by serotonin depletion. *Brain Research: Developmental Brain Research, 102,* 291–293.

Lecanuet, J., & Schaal, B. (1996). Fetal sensory competencies. *European Journal of Obstetrics and Gynecology and Reproductive Biology, 68,* 1–23.

LeDoux, J. (2000). Emotion circuits in the brain. *Annual Review of Neuroscience, 23,* 155–184.

LeDoux, J. (2003). The emotional brain, fear, and the amygdala. *Cellular and Molecular Neurobiology, 23,* 727–738.

LeDoux, J. (2007). The amygdala. *Current Biology, 17,* R868–R874.

Leon, M. (1975). Dietary control of maternal pheromone in the lactating rat. *Physiology and Behavior, 14,* 311–319.

Leon, M. (1992). The neurobiology of filial learning. *Annual Review of Psychology, 43,* 377–398.

Letcher, P., Smart, D., Sanson, A., & Toumbourou, J. (2009). Psychosocial precursors and correlates a differing internalizing trajectories from 3 to 15 years. *Social Development, 18,* 618–646.

Leussis, M., & Andersen, S. (2008). Is adolescence a sensitive period for depression?: Behavioral and neuroanatomical findings from a social stress model. *Synapse, 62,* 22–30.

Levin, B., Craik, R., & Hand, P. (1988). The role of norepinephrine in adult rat somatosensory cortical metabolism and plasticity. *Brain Research, 443,* 261–271.

Levine, S. (1962). Plasma-free corticosteroid response to electric shock in rats stimulated in infancy. *Science, 135,* 795–796.

Lupien, S., McEwen, B., Gunnar, M., & Heim, C. (2009). Effects of stress throughout the lifespan on the brain, behaviour and cognition. *Nature Reviews Neuroscience, 10,* 434–445.

Maestripieri, D., Tomaszycki, M., & Carroll, K. (1999). Consistency and change in the behavior of rhesus macaque abusive mothers with successive infants. *Developmental Psychobiology, 34,* 29–35.

Malkova, L., Mishkin, M., Suomi, S., & Bachevalier, J. (2010). Long-term effects of neonatal medial temporal ablations on socioemotional behavior in monkeys (*Macaca mulatta*). *Behavioral Neuroscience, 124,* 742–760.

Maren, S. (2003). The amygdala, synaptic plasticity, and fear memory. *Annals of the New York Academy of Sciences, 985,* 106–113.

Marshall, K., Christie, M., Finlayson, P., & Williams, J. (1991). Developmental aspects of the locus coeruleus–noradrenaline system. *Progress in Brain Research, 88,* 173–185.

Mason, W., Kosterman, R., Hawkins, J., Herrenkohl, T., Lengua, L., & McCauley, E. (2004). Predicting depression, social phobia, and violence in early adulthood from childhood behavior problems. *Journal of the American Academy of Child and Adolescent Psychiatry, 43,* 307–315.

Mazza, J., Abbott, R., Fleming, C., Harachi, T., Cortes, R., Park, J., et al. (2009).

Early predictors of adolescent depression. *Journal of Early Adolescence, 29*, 664–692.

McEwen, B. (2003). Early life influences on life-long patterns of behavior and health. *Mental Retardation and Developmental Disabilities Research Reviews, 9*, 149–154.

McGaugh, J. (2006). Make mild moments memorable: Add a little arousal. *Trends in Cognitive Sciences, 10*, 345–347.

McGaugh, J., Roozendaal, B., & Cahill, L. (1999). Modulation of memory storage by stress hormones and the amygdaloid complex. In M. Gazzaniga (Ed.), *Cognitive neuroscience* (pp. 1081–1098). Cambridge, MA: MIT Press.

McLean, J., Darby-King, A., Sullivan, R., & King, S. (1993). Serotonergic influence on olfactory learning in the neonate rat. *Behavioral and Neural Biology, 60*, 152–162.

McLean, J., Harley, C., Darby-King, A., & Yuan, Q. (1999). pCREB in the neonate rat olfactory bulb is selectively and transiently increased by odor preference-conditioned training. *Learning and Memory, 6*, 608–618.

McLean, J., & Shipley, M. (1991). Postnatal development of the noradrenergic projection from locus coeruleus to the olfactory bulb in the rat. *Journal of Comparative Neurology, 304*, 467–477.

Mennella, J. (1995). Mother's milk: A medium for early flavor experiences. *Journal of Human Lactation, 11*, 39–45.

Miller, J., Jagielo, J., & Spear, N. (1989). Age-related differences in short-term retention of separable elements of an odor aversion. *Journal of Experimental Psychology: Animal Behavioral Processes, 15*, 194–201.

Moriceau, S., Roth, T., Okotoghaide, T., & Sullivan, R. (2004). Corticosterone controls the developmental emergence of fear and amygdala function to predator odors in infant rat pups. *International Journal of Developmental Neuroscience, 22*, 415–422.

Moriceau, S., Shionoya, K., Jakups, K., & Sullivan, R. (2009). Early life stress disrupts attachment learning: The role of amygdala corticosterone, locus coeruleus CRF and olfactory bulb NE. *Journal of Neuroscience, 29*, 15745–15755.

Moriceau, S., & Sullivan, R. (2006). Maternal presence serves as a switch between learning fear and attraction in infancy. *Nature Neuroscience, 9*, 1004–1006.

Moriceau, S., Wilson, D., Levine, S., & Sullivan, R. (2006). Dual circuitry for odor–shock conditioning during infancy: Corticosterone switches between fear and attraction via amygdala. *Journal of Neuroscience, 26*, 6737–6748.

Nakamura, S., Kimura, F., & Sakaguchi, T. (1987). Postnatal development of electrical activity in the locus coeruleus. *Journal of Neurophysiology, 58*, 510–524.

Nakamura, S., & Sakaguchi, T. (1990). Development and plasticity of the locus coeruleus: A review of recent physiological and pharmacological experimentation. *Progress in Neurobiology, 34*, 505–526.

Nemeroff, C., & Vale, W. (2005). The neurobiology of depression: Inroads to treatment and new drug discovery. *Journal of Clinical Psychiatry, 66*, 5–13.

Okutani, F., Kaba, H., Takahashi, S., & Seto, K. (1998). The biphasic effects of locus coeruleus noradrenergic activation on dendrodendritic inhibition in the rat olfactory bulb. *Brain Research, 783*, 272–279.

Pape, H., & Stork, O. (2003). Genes and mechanisms in the amygdala involved in the formation of fear memory. *Annals of the New York Academy of Sciences, 985*, 92–105.

Pare, D., Quirk, G., & LeDoux, J. (2004). New vistas on amygdala networks in conditioned fear. *Journal of Neurophysiology, 92*, 1–9.

Paul, B., Snyder, A., Haist, F., Raichle, M., Bellugi, M., & Stiles, J. (2009). Amygdala response to faces parallels social behavior in Williams syndrome. *Social Cognitive and Affective Neuroscience, 4*, 278–285.

Pederson, P., Williams, C., & Blass, E. (1982). Activation and odor conditioning of suckling behavior in 3-day-old albino rats. *Experimental Psychology: Animal Behavioral Processes, 8*, 329–341.

Pierce, K., Muller, R., Ambrose, J., Allen, G., & Courchesne, E. (2001). Face processing occurs outside the fusiform "face area" in autism: Evidence from functional MRI. *Brain, 124*, 2059–2073.

Polan, J., & Hofer, M. (1998). Olfactory preference for mother over home nest shaving by newborn rats. *Developmental Psychobiology, 33*, 5–20.

Poulos, A., Li, V., Sterlace, S., Tokushige, F., Ponnusamy, R., & Fanselow, M. (2009). Persistence of fear memory across time requires the basolateral amygdala complex. *Proceedings of the National Academy of Sciences USA, 106*, 11737–11741.

Raineki, C., Moriceau, S., & Sullivan, R. (2010). Developing a neurobehavioral animal model of infant attachment to an abusive caregiver. *Biological Psychiatry, 67*, 1137–1145.

Raineki, C., Rincon Cortes, M., Belnoue, L., & Sullivan, R. (2012). Effects of early-life abuse differ across development: Infant social behavior deficits are followed by adolescent depressive-like behaviors mediated by the amygdala. *Journal of Neuroscience, 32*, 7758–7765.

Raineki, C., Shionoya, K., Sander, K., & Sullivan, R. (2009). Ontogeny of odor–LiCl vs odor–shock learning: Similar behaviors but divergent ages of amygdala functional emergence. *Learning and Memory, 16*(2), 114–121.

Rajecki, D., Lamb, M., & Obmascher, P. (1978). Towards a general theory of infantile attachment: A comparative review of aspects of the social bond. *Brain Sciences, 3*, 417–464.

Rangel, S., & Leon, M. (1995). Early odor preference training increases olfactory bulb norepinephrine. *Brain Research: Developmental Brain Research, 85*, 187–191.

Rasia-Filho, A., Londero, R., & Achaval, M. (2000). Functional activities of the amygdala: An overview. *Journal of Psychiatry and Neuroscience, 25*, 14–23.

Ressler, K., & Mayberg, H. (2007). Targeting abnormal neural circuits in mood and anxiety disorders: From the laboratory to the clinic. *Nature Neuroscience, 10*, 1116–1124.

Rice, C., Sandman, C., Lenjavi, M., & Baram, T. (2008). A novel mouse model for acute and long-lasting consequences of early life stress. *Endocrinology, 149*, 4892–4900.

Rigucci, S., Serafini, G., Pompili, M., Kotzalidis, G., & Tatarelli R. (2010). Anatomical and functional correlates in major depressive disorders: The contribution of neuroimaging studies. *World Journal of Biological Psychiatry, 11*, 165–180.

Ritchey, M., Dolcos, F., Eddington, K., Strauman, T., & Cabeza, R. (2011). Neural correlates of emotional processing in depression: Changes with cognitive behavioral therapy and predictors of treatment response. *Journal of Psychiatric Research, 45,* 577–587.

Rosen, K., & Burke, P. (1999). Multiple attachment relationships within families: Mothers and fathers with two young children. *Developmental Psychology, 35,* 436–444.

Rosenfeld, P., Suchecki, D., & Levine, S. (1992). Multifactorial regulation of the hypothalamic–pituitary–adrenal axis during development. *Neuroscience and Biobehavioral Reviews, 16,* 553–568.

Roth, T., & Sullivan, R. (2005). Memory of early maltreatment: Neonatal behavioral and neural correlates of maternal maltreatment within the context of classical conditioning. *Biological Psychiatry, 57,* 823–831.

Roth, T., Wilson, D., & Sullivan, R. (2004). Neurobehavioral development of infant learning and memory: Designed for attachment. In J. Slater, C. Snowdon, & T. Ropers (Eds.), *Advances in the study of behavior* (pp. 103–123). San Diego: Elsevier/Academic Press.

Rudy, J., & Cheatle, M. (1977). Odor-aversion learning in neonatal rats. *Science, 198,* 845–846.

Rudy, J., & Cheatle, M. (1983). Odor-aversion learning by rats following LiCl exposure: Ontogenetic influences. *Developmental Psychobiology, 16,* 13–22.

Salzen, E. (1970). Imprinting and environmental learning. In D. Aronson & J. Rosenblatt (Eds.), *Development and evolution of behavior* (pp. 158–178). San Francisco: Freeman.

Sananes, C., & Campbell, B. (1989). Role of the central nucleus of the amygdala in olfactory heart rate conditioning. *Behavioral Neuroscience, 103,* 519–525.

Sanchez, M., Ladd, C., & Plotskey, P. (2001). Early adverse experience as a developmental risk factor for later psychopathology: Evidence from rodent and primate models. *Development and Psychopathology, 13,* 419–449.

Savitz, J., & Drevets, W. (2009). Bipolar and major depressive disorder: Neuroimaging the developmental–degenerative divide. *Neuroscience and Biobehavioral Reviews, 33,* 699–771.

Schaal, B., Marlier, L., & Soussignan, R. (1995). Responsiveness to the odour of amniotic fluid in the human neonate. *Biology of the Neonate, 67,* 397–406.

Schettino L, Otto T. 2001. Patterns of fos expression in the amygdala and ventral perirhinal cortex induced by training in an olfactory fear conditioning paradigm. *Behavioral Neuroscience, 115,* 1257–1272.

Schleidt, M., & Genzel, C. (1990). The significance of mother's perfume for infants in the first weeks of their life. *Ethology and Sociobiology, 11,* 145–154.

Schwob, J., & Price, J. (1984). The development of axonal connections in the central olfactory system of rats. *Journal of Comparative Neurology, 223,* 177–202.

Sevelinges, Y., Gervais, R., Messaoudi, B., Granjon, L., & Mouly, A. (2004). Olfactory fear conditioning induces field potential potentiation in rat olfactory cortex and amygdala. *Learning and Memory, 11,* 761–769.

Sevelinges, Y., Levy, F., Mouly, A., & Ferreira, G. (2009). Rearing with artificially scented mothers attenuates conditioned odor aversion in adulthood but not its amygdala dependency. *Behavioural Brain Research, 198,* 313–320.

Sevelinges, Y., Mouly, A., Raineki, C., Moriceau, S., Forest, C., & Sullivan, R. (2011). Adult depression-like behavior, amygdala dysfunction and olfactory cortex functions are restored by odor previously paired with shock during infant's sensitive period attachment learning. *Developmental Cognitive Neuroscience, 1*, 77–87.

Shionoya, K., Moriceau, S., Bradstock, P., & Sullivan, R. (2007). Maternal attenuation of hypothalamic paraventricular nucleus norepinephrine switches avoidance learning to preference learning in preweanling rat pups. *Hormones and Behavior, 52*, 391–400.

Shionoya, K., Moriceau, S., Lunday, L., Miner, C., Roth, T., & Sullivan, R. (2006). Development switch in neural circuitry underlying odor–malaise learning. *Learning and Memory, 13*, 801–808.

Shipley, M., Halloran, F., & de la Torre, J. (1985). Surprisingly rich projection from locus coeruleus to the olfactory bulb in the rat. *Brain Research, 329*, 294–299.

Sibille, E., Wang, Y., Joeyen-Waldorf, J., Gaiteri, C., Surget, A., Oh, S., et al. (2009). A molecular signature of depression in the amygdala. *American Journal of Psychiatry, 166*, 1011–1024.

Sigurdsson, T., Doyère, V., Cain, C. K., & LeDoux, J. (2007). Long-term potentiation in the amygdala: A cellular mechanism of fear learning and memory. *Neuropharmacology, 52*, 215–227.

Simpson, K., Wang, L., Kirifides, M., Lin, R., & Waterhouse, D. (1997). Lateralization and functional organization of the locus coeruleus projection to the trigeminal somatosensory pathway in rat. *Journal of Comparative Neurology, 385*, 135–147.

Singh, P., & Tobach, E. (1975). Olfactory bulbectomy and nursing behavior in rat pups (Wistar DAB). *Developmental Psychobiology, 8*, 151–164.

Skuse, D., Morris, J., & Lawrence, K. (2006). The amygdala and development of the social brain. *Annals of the New York Academy of Sciences, 1008*, 91–101.

Smotherman, W., Hennessy, J., & Levine, S. (1976). Plasma corticosterone levels during recovery from LiCl produced taste aversions. *Behavioral Biology, 16*, 401–412.

Stanton, M., & Levine, S. (1990). Inhibition of infant glucocorticoid stress response: Specific role of maternal cues. *Developmental Psychobiology, 23*, 411–426.

Stanton, M., Wallstrom, J., & Levine, S. (1987). Maternal contact inhibits pituitary–adrenal stress responses in preweanling rats. *Developmental Psychobiology, 20*, 131–145.

Stone, V., Baron-Cohen, S., Calder, A., Keane, J., & Young, A. (2003). Acquired theory of mind impairments in individuals with bilateral amygdala lesions. *Neuropsychologia, 41*, 209–220.

Stovall, K., & Dozier, M. (2000). The development of attachment in new relationships: Single subject analyses for 10 foster infants. *Development and Psychopathology, 12*, 133–156.

Sullivan, R., Brake, S., Hofer, M., & Williams, C. (1986). Huddling and independent feeding of neonatal rats can be facilitated by a conditioned change in behavioral state. *Developmental Psychobiology, 19*, 625–635.

Sullivan, R., & Holman, P. (2010). Transitions in sensitive period attachment learning in infancy: The role of corticosterone. *Neuroscience and Biobehavioral Reviews, 34*, 835–844.

Sullivan, R., Landers, M., Flemming, J., Vaught, C., Young, T., & Polan, J. (2003). Characterizing the functional significance of the neonatal rat vibrissae prior to the onset of whisking. *Somatosensory and Motor Research, 20*, 157–162.

Sullivan, R., Landers, M., Yeaman, B., & Wilson, D. (2000a). Good memories of bad events in infancy. *Nature, 407*, 38–39.

Sullivan, R., & Leon, M. (1986). Early olfactory learning induces an enhanced olfactory bulb response in young rats. *Brain Research, 392*, 278–282.

Sullivan, R., Stackenwalt, G., Nasr, F., Lemon, C., & Wilson, D. (2000b). Association of an odor with activation of olfactory bulb noradrenergic B receptors or locus coeruleus stimulation is sufficient to produce learned approach response to that odor in neonatal rats. *Behavioral Neuroscience, 114*, 957–962.

Sullivan, R., & Toubas, P. (1998). Clinical usefulness of maternal odor in newborns: Soothing and feeding preparatory responses. *Biology of the Neonate, 74*, 402–408.

Sullivan, R., & Wilson, D. (1991). Neural correlates of conditioned odor avoidance in infant rats. *Behavioral Neuroscience, 105*, 307–312.

Sullivan, R., & Wilson, D. (1994). The locus coeruleus, norepinephrine, and memory in newborns. *Brain Research Bulletin, 35*, 467–472.

Sullivan, R., Wilson, D., & Leon, M. (1989). Norepinephrine and learning-induced plasticity in infant rat olfactory system. *Journal of Neuroscience, 9*, 3998–4006.

Sullivan, R., Wilson, D., Wong, R., Correa, A., & Leon, M. (1990). Modified behavioral and olfactory bulb responses to maternal odors in preweanling rats. *Brain Research: Developmental Brain Research, 53*(2), 243–247.

Sullivan, R., Zyzak, D., Skierkowski, P., & Wilson, D. (1992). The role of olfactory bulb norepinephrine in early olfactory learning. *Brain Research: Developmental Brain Research, 70*, 279–282.

Suomi, S. (1997). Early determinants of behaviour: evidence from primate studies. *British Medical Bulletin, 53*, 170–184.

Takahashi, L. (1994). Organizing action of corticosterone on the development of behavioral inhibition in the preweanling rat. *Brain Research: Developmental Brain Research, 81*, 121–127.

Tao, X., Finkbeiner, S., Arnold, D., Shaywitz, A., & Greenberg, M. (1998). Ca^{2+} influx regulates BDNF transcription by a CREB family transcription factor-dependent mechanism. *Neuron, 20*, 709–726.

Teicher, M., Andersen, S., Polcari, A., Anderson, C., & Navalta, C. (2002). Developmental neurobiology of childhood and trauma. *Psychiatric Clinics of North America, 25*, 397–426.

Teicher, M., Andersen, S., Polcari, A., Anderson, C., Navalta, C., & Kim, D. (2003). The neurobiological consequences of early stress and childhood maltreatment. *Neuroscience and Biobehavioral Reviews, 27*, 33–44.

Teicher, M., & Blass, E. (1977). First suckling response of the newborn albino rat: The roles of olfaction and amniotic fluid. *Science, 198*, 635–636.

Teicher, M., Flaum, L., Williams, M., Eckhert, S., & Lumia, A. (1978). Survival, growth and suckling behavior of neonatally bulbectomized rats. *Physiology and Behavior, 21*, 553–561.

Terry, L., & Johanson, I. (1996). Effects of altered olfactory experiences on the development of infant rats' responses to odors. *Developmental Psychobiology, 29*, 353–377.

Thomas, K., Drevets, W., Dahl, R., Ryan, N., Birmaher, B., Eccard, C., et al. (2001). Amygdala response to fearful faces in anxious and depressed children. *Archives of General Psychiatry, 58*, 1057–1063.

Tottenham, N., Hare, T., & Casey, B. (2009). A developmental perspective on human amygdala function. In E. Phelps & P. Whalen (Eds.), *The human amygdala* (pp. 107–117). New York: Guilford Press.

Touzani, K., & Sclafani, A. (2005). Critical role of amygdala in flavor but not taste preference learning in rats. *European Journal of Neuroscience, 22*, 1767–1774.

Ulfig, N., Setzer, M., & Bohl, J. (2003). The ontogeny of the human amygdala. *Annals of the New York Academy of Sciences, 985*, 22–33.

Upton, K., & Sullivan, R. (2010). Defining age limits of the sensitive period for attachment learning in rat pups. *Developmental Psychobiology, 52*, 453–464.

Varendi, H., Porter, R., & Winberg, J. (1996). Attractiveness of amniotic fluid odor: Evidence of prenatal olfactory learning? *Acta Paediatrica, 85*, 1223–1227.

Vervoort, T., Goubert, L., Eccleston, C., Verhoeven, K., De Clercq, A., Buysse, A., et al. (2008). The effects of parental presence upon the facial expression of pain: The moderating role of child pain catastrophizing. *Pain, 138*, 277–285.

Walker, C., Sapolsky, R., Meaney, M., Vale, W., & Rivier, C. (1986). Increased pituitary sensitivity to glucocorticoid feedback during the stress nonresponsive period in the neonatal rat. *Endocrinology, 119*, 1816–1821.

Walker, C., Scribner, K., Cascio, C., & Dallman, M. (1991). The pituitary-adrenocortical system of neonatal rats is responsive to stress throughout development in a time-dependent and stressor-specific fashion. *Endocrinology, 128*, 1385–1395.

Weldon, D., Travis, M., & Kennedy, D. (1991). Post training D1 receptor blockade impairs odor conditioning in neonatal rats. *Behavioral Neuroscience, 105*, 450–458.

Welker, W. (1964). Analysis of sniffing of the albino rat. *Behaviour, 12*, 223–244.

Wiedenmayer, C., & Barr, G. (2001). Developmental changes in c-Fos expression to an age-specific social stressor in infant rats. *Behavioural Brain Research, 126*, 147–157.

Wilson, D., & Sullivan, R. (1991). Olfactory associative conditioning in infant rats with brain stimulation as reward: II. Norepinephrine mediates a specific component of the bulb response to reward. *Behavioral Neuroscience, 105*, 843–849.

Wilson, D., & Sullivan, R. (1994). Neurobiology of associative learning in the neonate: Early olfactory learning. *Behavioral and Neural Biology, 61*, 1–18.

Wilson, D., Sullivan, R., & Leon, M. (1987). Single-unit analysis of postnatal olfactory learning: Modified olfactory bulb output response patterns to learned attractive odors. *Journal of Neuroscience, 7*, 3154–3162.

Winzer-Serhan, U., Raymon, H., Broide, R., Chen, Y., & Leslie, F. (1997). Expression of alpha-2 adrenoceptors during rat brain development: 2. Alpha 2C messenger RNA expression and [^{3}H]rauwolscine binding. *Neuroscience, 76*, 261–272.

Woo, C., Coopersmith, R., & Leon, M. (1987). Localized changes in olfactory bulb morphology associated with early olfactory learning. *Journal of Comparative Neurology, 263,* 113–125.

Yuan, Q., Harley, C., Darby-King, A., Neve, R., & McLean, J. (2003). Early odor preference learning in the rat: Bidirectional effects of cAMP response element-binding protein (CREB) and mutant CREB support a causal role for phosphorylated CREB. *Journal of Neuroscience, 23,* 4760–4765.

Yuan, Q., Harley, C., McLean, J., & Knopfel T. (2002). Optical imaging of odor preference memory in the rat olfactory bulb. *Journal of Neurophysiology, 87,* 3156–3159.

Zhang, J., Okutani, F., Inoue, S., & Kaba, H. (2003). Activation of the cyclic AMP response element-binding protein signaling pathway in the olfactory bulb is required for the acquisition of olfactory aversive learning in young rats. *Neuroscience, 117,* 707–713.

CHAPTER 5

Foraging in the Face of Fear

Novel Strategies for Evaluating Amygdala Functions in Rats

JEANSOK J. KIM

JUNE-SEEK CHOI

HONGJOO J. LEE

Fear is a defensive mechanism that plays an important role in our lives: It activates organized bodily–behavioral responses that help minimize our exposure to risks. This chapter presents a novel ethobehavioral paradigm to explore foraging behavior in laboratory rats in quantifiable "approach food–avoid predator" situations that simulate the environments in which the adaptive functions of fear evolved. Specifically, animals seeking food in a seminaturalistic apparatus, consisting of a nest and an open area, encountered a "predatory" robot executing a programmed set of threatening actions. All rats instinctively and robustly reacted to the looming robot by fleeing into the safety of the nest and freezing (fear responses). Afterward, the animals emerged from the nest and cautiously approached the food until the surging robot reevoked fear responses. With repeated encounters, however, the success of seizing the food correlated positively with the food-to-robot distance, suggesting that rats use a spatial (or distance) gradient of fear from the locus of the threat. Further experiments revealed that the amygdala bidirectionally regulates rats' foraging behavior in risky environments. Researching fear from functional, mechanistic, and phylogenetic perspectives will likely provide a deeper understanding of this fundamental emotion.

In order for the defense reaction to take place, the organism must
always receive an injury. This is bad biological economy. Clearly
a corrective accessory mechanism is needed. This exists in the
substitution-of-stimulus tendency characteristic of redintegration.
                                              —HULL (1929, p. 500)

No real-life predator is going to present cues before it attacks . . . [or give]
enough trials for the necessary learning to occur. . . . What keeps animals
alive in the wild is that they have very effective *innate* defensive reactions
which occur when they encounter any kind of new or sudden stimulus.
                                              —BOLLES (1970, pp. 32–33)

Contemporary Views of Fear

Fear is a neural–behavioral system that evolved because of its evolutionary success in defending animals, including humans, from threats such
as predators, conspecific aggression, and unfamiliar situations. Fear of
certain stimuli and situations are innate (i.e., unlearned). For example,
naive rats and monkeys display fear behavior to a cat (D. C. Blanchard &
Blanchard, 1972)[1] and a rubber snake (Amaral et al., 2003; Klüver & Bucy,
1939), respectively, and infants cry when scared by loud noises (Watson
& Rayner, 1920) and avoid visual cliffs with maturing depth perception
(Walk, 1966). The fear system also supports rapid, lasting learning so animals can adapt to new dangers in their environments.

The contemporary models of fear have largely been shaped by
learned or acquired fear based on many decades of Pavlovian (classical)
and instrumental (avoidance) fear conditioning research (Fanselow &
LeDoux, 1999; Hull, 1929; McGaugh, 2000; Mowrer, 1951; Rescorla &
Solomon, 1967; Watson & Rayner, 1920). It is generally agreed that during Pavlovian fear conditioning, information about the initially innocu-
ous conditioned stimulus (CS; e.g., tones, lights, contexts) and the reflexively aversive unconditioned stimulus (US; e.g., electric shocks) converge
in the amygdala, resulting in associative (or Hebbian) synaptic changes—
such as long-term potentiation (LTP)—that strengthen the CS afferents to
amygdalar neurons (Fanselow & LeDoux, 1999; Kim et al., 2007; Maren,
2011; Paré, Quirk, & LeDoux, 2004). As Clark Hull (1929) asserted over
80 years ago (see chapter opening quotation), fear conditioning to stimuli

---

[1]The late Robert J. Blanchard, who passed away November 24, 2013, was a pioneer
in the field of fear research. He and his spouse, D. Caroline Blanchard, popularized
the freezing response as a reliable measure of innate and learned fear, which is the
leading behavioral assay of fear in rats and mice, and implicated the functions of
the amygdala and hippocampus in fear conditioning in the early 1970s. Their work
has profoundly influenced and inspired generations of fear researchers, including
ourselves.

associated with the source of injury is believed to occur in nature to fore-warn animals about future harm that can be fatal. Different types of CS information reach distinct amygdalar nuclei, where the crucial CS–US associations are thought to take place, that is, the lateral nucleus for tone CSs via the auditory thalamus (Quirk, Repa, & LeDoux, 1995; Romanski & LeDoux, 1992), the basolateral complex for light CSs via the visual thal-amus (Shi & Davis, 2001), and the basal nucleus for contextual CSs via the hippocampus (Maren & Fanselow, 1995). These nuclei are interconnected with the central nucleus (Barton, Aggleton, & Grenyer, 2003), which is the main amygdaloid output structure that projects to downstream auto-nomic and somatomotor centers triggering specific components of the fear response, such as cardiovascular changes, freezing, and potenti-ated startle (Campeau & Davis, 1995; Fanselow, 1984; Helmstetter, 1992; Kapp, Frysinger, Gallagher, & Haselton, 1979). In recent years, infralim-bic (IL) and prelimbic (PL) regions of the medial prefrontal cortex have been postulated to exert "top-down" control of the amygdala, namely, the IL-intercalated cells of the amygdala pathway's importance in the extinc-tion of conditioned fear (Laurent & Westbrook, 2009; Mueller, Porter, & Quirk, 2008; Pape & Paré, 2010), while the PL-lateral amygdalar pathway is necessary in the expression of conditioned fear responses (Corcoran & Quirk, 2007; S. C. Kim, Jo, Kim, Kim, & Choi, 2010). The hippocampus is also implicated when spatial–contextual information influences fear conditioning (J. J. Kim & Fanselow, 1992; Phillips & LeDoux, 1992), such as renewal (Orsini, Kim, Knapska, & Maren, 2011) and occasion setting (Yoon, Graham, & Kim, 2011). Thus, afferents to and efferents from dif-ferent amygdalar nuclei seem to be important in responding to specific CS events, and in regulating and coordinating fear responses. Other stud-ies employing the instrumental avoidance learning paradigms (Amora-panth, LeDoux, & Nader, 2000; Choi, Cain, & LeDoux, 2010; Killcross, Robbins, & Everitt, 1997) further support the view that the amygdala, as a collection of distinctive nuclei, does not contain a single, unified locus of learned fear behavior. However, alternative views posit that the amygdala is not the repository of fear memory but is instead critical in modulat-ing fear (and other) memory traces that develop in other parts of the brain (McGaugh, 2004; McGaugh, Cahill, & Roozendaal, 1996; Parent, McGaugh, & Tomaz, 1992).

While fear-conditioning research has generated a wealth of data, the research is, to a large degree, based on assessing specific responses (e.g., freezing, heart rate, respiration rate, startle, hypoalgesia, 22-kHz ultra-sonic vocalization [USV], active–passive avoidance) in small experimental chambers that restrict the animal's repertoire of behavior; therefore, the research may provide an incomplete picture of fear. If so, it is essential to consider the utility of the circuits, neural activity, synaptic plasticity, and cellular–molecular mechanisms discovered from fear conditioning studies to natural conditions in which the adaptive functions of innate fear evolved (Darwin, 1872).[2] There are behavioral paradigms that make use of naturalistic situations, such as introducing a cat or predatory odors to rats living in visible burrow systems (Blanchard, Blanchard, Agullana, & Weiss, 1991a) and placing rodents in exposed settings, such as open fields or elevated plus mazes (Basso, Beattie, & Bresnahan, 1995; Pellow, Chopin, File, & Briley, 1985); these behavioral assays have become valuable in psychopharmacology and psychopathology research. More recently, rats infected with the *Toxoplasma gondii* parasite have been reported to exhibit attraction, rather than aversion, to cat urine (Berdoy, Webster, & Macdonald, 2000; Vyas, Kim, Giacomini, Boothroyd, & Sapolsky, 2007). Overall, the evolutionarily conserved role of fear in innately guiding behavior in dangerous (risky) situations has largely been overlooked in contemporary fear research.

Novel Risky Foraging Paradigm

Based on the premise that fear evolved to influence risky decisions of foragers in "approach–avoid" conflicts (Bolles, 1970; Coleman, Brown, Levine, & Mellgren, 2005; Stephens, Brown, & Ydenberg, 2007), we have developed a relatively simple, seminaturalistic preparation to investigate a rat's foraging behavior when confronted with an artificial predator—dubbed ROBOGATOR, assembled from a commercially available LEGO Mindstorms robotics kit—programmed to surge toward the animal that is seeking food (Figure 5.1; Choi & Kim, 2010). In this task, hunger-motivated rats underwent successive habituation, baseline, and test phases in a custom-made foraging apparatus; the animal's movement was recorded using the ANY-maze video tracking system (Stoelting Co.). From the time-stamped Cartesian coordinate data, a number of dependent variables (e.g., movement speed/distance/pattern, time spent in designated areas, freezing) can be extracted. The *habituation phase* involved placing each rat in the nesting area equipped with a water bottle, from which food pellets were available for consumption. During the *baseline phase* (no food pellets in the nest), the gateway to the foraging area was remotely opened, and each rat was allowed to explore for food pellets placed at varying distances (three trials/day) from the acclimated nest (Figure 5.2A). At first, each animal cautiously exited the nest

---

[2]Presumably, even in adult predatory animals that are not preyed upon (e.g., lions), the amygdala–fear system functions similarly, since they may have once been prey in their evolutionary history, as young cubs they were subjected to predation, and they face conspecific aggression over resources and mates.

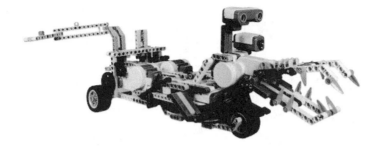

FIGURE 5.1. Artificial predatory robot. The Robogator on wheels (about 66 cm long, 18 cm wide, 15 cm high) was programmed to surge 23 cm at a velocity of 75 cm/second, snap its jaws once, and return to its starting position. The program can be initiated with either a wireless transmitter or a Bluetooth signal, when the animal enters a predefined zone, via video tracking, to the robot.

and explored the foraging area. Upon procuring the pellet, which was sized so as to deter the animal from eating in an open space, the animal instinctively returned to the nest to consume it. By baseline day 2, each rat readily entered the foraging area seeking the pellet, and upon returning to the nest and consuming it, the animal usually prompted the next trial by scratching the gate (Figure 5.2B). In the *test phase,* the Robogator was placed at the opposite end of the open field (Figure 5.3). As the rat emerged from the nest and approached the pellet zone, the Robogator executed its programmed action: It surged a fixed distance (~23 cm) at a set velocity (~75 cm/second), snapped its jaws, then returned to its starting position. In response, the rat instantly fled into the safety of the nest and froze in the corner, demonstrating innate fear responses. This was followed by the rat's displays of a stretched posture while anchored inside the nest opening as it scanned the outside area (risk assessment), before cautiously venturing out, pausing, then moving toward the food, until the looming Robogator retriggered the rat's fear responses.

The Amygdala and Risky Foraging

Lesions of the Amygdala

To test the function of the amygdala in risky foraging behavior, rats were implanted with lesion electrodes in their amygdalae (Choi & Kim, 2010). On robot test day 1, all rats displayed fear behavior to the looming Robogator, as described previously. Whether the rat attained the food pellet depended on the nest-to-food distance; none of the rats procured the pellet placed ~76 cm from the nest within the 3-minute allotted time, but they

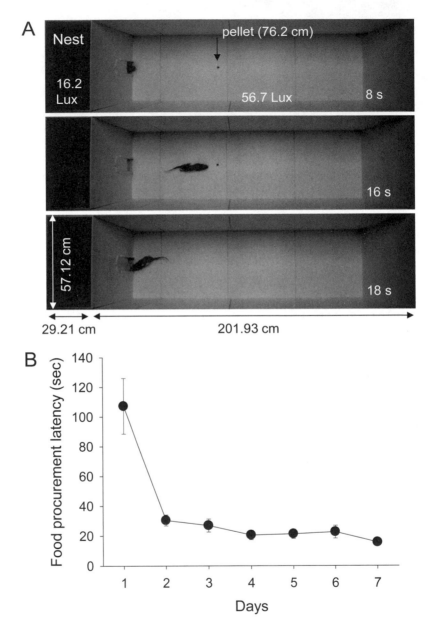

FIGURE 5.2. A seminaturalistic foraging task. (A) Baseline days. Time-lapse photos of a rat emerging from a nest into a foraging area to search for a food pellet placed at variable distances from the nest. Once the animal instinctively returned with the food to the nest, the gateway closed until the next trial. (B) Group mean (+ *SEM* [standard error of the mean]) latencies to procure pellets across the baseline days.

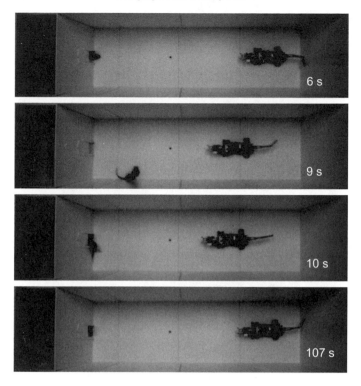

FIGURE 5.3. Robot test day. Snapshots show the rat foraging for a pellet when confronted with the Robogator for the first time. Each time the animal approached the vicinity of the pellet, the Robogator executed a programmed set of actions. The rat instinctively fled to the nesting area and froze.

succeeded at distances ≤ ~25 cm (Figure 5.4A). Hence, with experience, rats seemed to form spatial gradients of fear or defensive distances from the source of threat. Shortly afterward, the animals received electrolytic lesions to their amygdalae bilaterally under light halothane anesthesia. On robot test day 2, all the rats were able to obtain pellets placed ≥ ~101 cm. Instead of fleeing, they paused briefly before the surging Robogator, snatched the pellet, and returned to the nest. Obviously, the lack of fear would be fatal to foraging animals in the natural environment. Perhaps the amygdala-lesioned animals' willingness to forage at unsafe distances is analogous to behaviors exhibited by patients with Urbach–Wiethe disease (focal amygdalar lesions; in this volume, cf. Feinstein, Adolphs, & Tranel, Chapter 2; Adolphs, Chapter 10; Patin & Hurlemann, Chapter 11; van Honk, Terburg, Thornton, Stein, & Morgan, Chapter 12), such as their willingness to accept risky financial gambles (De Martino, Camerer, & Adolphs, 2010).

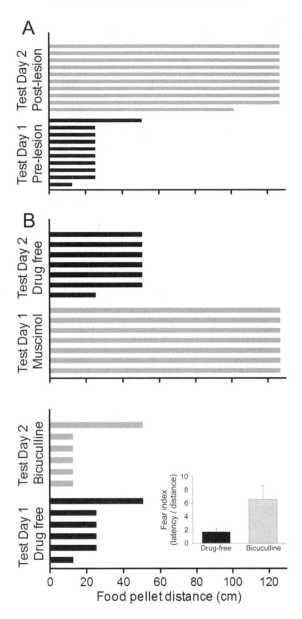

FIGURE 5.4. Limits of foraging distance. (A) The successful foraging distance for each rat before (black horizontal bars; test day 1) and after (gray bars; test day 2) amygdalar lesions. (B) Successful foraging distances under intra-amygdalar muscimol (gray; test day 1) and drug-free (black; test day 2) conditions. (C) Successful foraging distances under drug-free (black; test day 1) and with intra-amygdalar bicuculline (gray; test day 2) conditions. Inset shows fear index between drug-free and bicuculline test. Adapted with permission from Choi and Kim (2010).

Reversible Inactivation of the Amygdala

To clarify whether the lesion effects involved intrinsic neurons or fibers coursing through the amygdala, and whether the initial exposure to the Robogator on day 1 might have reduced fear on test day 2 (e.g., habituation), rats cannulated in the amygdala were infused with the gamma-aminobutryic acid $(GABA)_A$ receptor agonist muscimol before their first encounter with the Robogator. Amygdala-inactivated rats behaved similarly to amygdala-lesioned rats; that is, they briefly paused before the surging Robogator, seized the food pellet placed afar, and returned to the nest (Figure 5.4B). When retested with the Robogator next day (drug free), the rats were unable to procure the pellet placed ~76 cm (akin to lesioned rats), but they were successful with pellets placed ≤ ~50 cm. The fact that these rats were more successful in attaining pellets placed ~50 cm on day 2 (compared to prelesioned rats on day 1) suggests that some learning in the absence of a functional amygdala (e.g., familiarity with the Robogator's fixed pursuit distance/speed) occurred on day 1. Nonetheless, the inability to obtain food pellets beyond some distance (in both amygdala-lesioned rats and inactivated rats) from the nest suggests that rats have an instinctive defensive space (Choi & Kim, 2010). A well-demarcated safety margin of personal space has also been demonstrated in humans (Sambo & Iannetti, 2013).

Disinhibition of the Amygdala

The $GABA_A$ receptor antagonist bicuculline was used to test whether disinhibition of amygdalar neurons from endogenous GABA-mediated inhibition would exacerbate fear of the Robogator. Previous studies have found that bicuculline infusions into the amygdala produce anxiogenic responses (Fanselow & Kim, 1992; Sanders & Shekhar, 1995; Soltis, Cook, Gregg, & Sanders, 1997). Following the bicuculline infusion, rats showed increased latencies and shortened distances to secure pellets compared to the drug-free condition on the previous day, indicating that intra-amygdalar bicuculline exacerbates animals' fear of foraging (Figure 5.4C). Thus, an overactive amygdala producing aggravated fear would likewise be maladaptive to foraging animals in the natural environment.

c-Fos Expression

Neuronal activity following Robogator exposure was assessed via the expression of the c-Fos proto-oncogene in the amygdala, hippocampus, and medial prefrontal cortex (mPFC), three structures implicated in fear learning and extinction. After the 3-minute foraging time with the Robogator, during which none of the rats secured the pellet placed ~76 cm from the nest, the brains were extracted ~90 minutes later. Relative to the control rats that foraged free from the Robogator, these rats showed selectively increased labeled cells in the basolateral complex of the amygdala, infralimbic region of the mPFC, and CA1 region of the hippocampus (Figure 5.5). These c-Fos patterns show that the amygdala, mPFC, and hippocampus are not homogeneously reactive to the innate fear produced by the Robogator. Future research on how these brain regions interact and coordinate risky foraging behavior may have relevance toward understanding risky decision making in humans.

Amygdalar Stimulation

Because exposure to the Robogator increased the c-Fos expression (an index of neuronal activity) in the rats' amygdalae, we recently investigated whether stimulation of the amygdala per se might impact foraging behavior in rats (Kim et al., 2013). Here, when the rat came near the food pellet placed ~76 cm from the nest, mild electrical currents were briefly delivered to the amygdala bilaterally via chronically implanted stimulating electrodes (Figure 5.6). Amygdalar stimulation was sufficient to cause the rats to flee to the safety of the nest. Although these rats made more attempts to obtain the pellet than those tested with the Robogator, each time their amygdalae were stimulated, the animals constantly fled into the nest. Even when the pellet was placed at a short nest–food distance of ~25 cm, so that many rats successfully procured the pellet in spite of the looming Robogator, amygdalar stimulation was just as effective in producing the fleeing behavior. This suggests that electrical (artificial) stimulation activates the amygdala equally (evoking the same intensity of fear) regardless of the nest–food distance, whereas the amygdala is naturally less activated when the external threat is remote, permitting the animal to obtain the pellet placed near the nest. Other unexpected findings were that rats with periaqueductal gray (PAG) lesions still fled in response to amygdala stimulation, and that the same amygdalar stimulation parameter evoked very different fear behaviors in rats when placed in standard test cage (freezing and USV) rather than foraging (fleeing) settings. This indicates that the context in which brain stimulation occurs can vary the expression of fear, and possibly other responses.

Foraging under a Conditional Threat

We examined whether rats can discern 'conditional' threats and modify their behavior accordingly (Figure 5.7). During the baseline, all rats implanted with lesion electrodes in their amygdalae showed a strong bias toward chocolate-flavored pellets over concurrently available, equidistantly placed regular pellets. During the test day, each time a rat

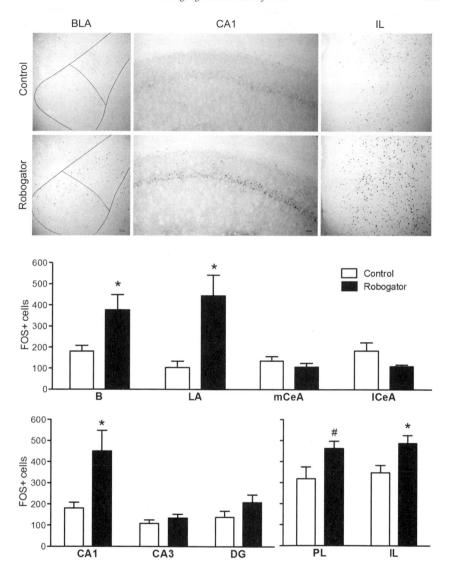

FIGURE 5.5. Robot exposure and c-Fos expression. Experiencing the Robogator for 3 minutes produced differential c-Fos reactivity in amygdala, mPFC, and hippocampus compared to control experience (i.e., exposure to the foraging area without the Robogator). B, basal nucleus of the amygdala; LA, lateral nucleus of the amygdala; mCeA, medial central nucleus of the amygdala; lCeA, lateral central nucleus of the amygdala; PL, prelimbic region of mPFC; IL, infralimbic region of mPFC.

approached the chocolate pellet, the Robogator surged forward, causing the animal to flee to the nest. When the animal inched toward the regular pellet, the Robogator was stationary. After attaining the regular pellet, the rats' subsequent foraging was biased toward the regular pellet (indicating exploitation). Occasionally, they veered toward the chocolate pellet (indicative of exploration), but their attempts were thwarted by the Robogator. Following amygdalar lesions, however, animals immediately reverted to chocolate pellets despite the Robogator's surge. These results indicate that fear shifts a rat's foraging behavior from preferred (but risky) food to less preferred (albeit safe) food, an adaptive behavior abolished by lesions to the amygdala.

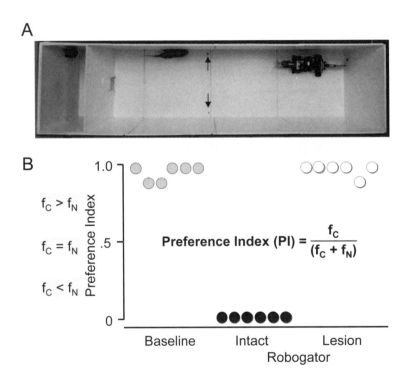

FIGURE 5.6. Foraging under conditional threat. (A) In baseline trials, the animal was allowed to choose freely between chocolate pellets and normal pellets placed on opposite sides of the foraging area, equidistant from the nest. In test trials, every time the rat approached the chocolate pellet (top arrow), the Robogator surged. When the rat approached the normal pellet (bottom arrow), the Robogator remained stationary. (B) Successful procurement of pellets during the baseline (gray circle) and in the presence of the Robogator (black circle = before amygdalar lesions; open circle = after amygdalar lesions). The f_C and f_N denote frequencies of procuring chocolate and normal pellets, respectively.

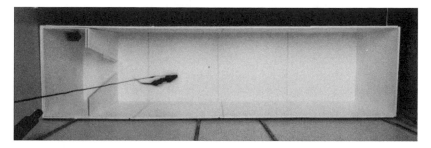

FIGURE 5.7. Amygdalar stimulation in the foraging apparatus. In baseline trials, animals were acclimatized to the tether cable connection and allowed to procure a normal pellet placed at various distances. In test trials, each time the rat neared the pellet, its amygdalae were stimulated bilaterally. Adapted with permission from Kim et al. (2013).

Biological Signals of Threat and Risk Assessment

The "cost–benefit" of attaining resources while avoiding predation is a primal decision problem faced by all foraging animals (Stephens et al., 2007; Stephens & Krebs, 1986). As Robert Bolles (1970) stated (see chapter opening quotation), the innate fear (defensive) system evolved to serve a fundamental protective function in animals in nature. However, it is implausible that animals are born with their genes supplying neural percepts of all potential predators, such as LEGO-assembled robots, with which rats have no evolutionary history. Presumably, rats are instinctively reacting to certain aspects of the Robogator that have qualities of evolutionarily reliable indicators (i.e., sign stimuli) of danger and are using those indicators to guide future foraging decisions. We found that the looming motion of the entity is the crucial factor that evoked fear in rats. With repeated encounters with the Robogator placed at a fixed location but moving forward or backward (same short distance at constant velocity, producing the same sound), the rats' fear of the Robogator gradually was reduced to backward but not forward motion (Figure 5.8). Hence, rats are capable of detecting the directional movement of potential threats—when the approaching entity is a sign stimulus of danger—and adjusting their behavior accordingly. This is not unlike how naive domestic chicks elicit an escape response to a silhouette moving in a direction that produces a "hawk" shadow, but not when the silhouette produces a "goose" shadow in the opposite direction (Schleidt, Shalter, & Moura-Neto, 2011; Spalding, 1954). Humans also step back and try to ward off insects flying directly toward them. Additional tests indicated that a foraging rat's fear behavior correlates with the robot's velocity, the robot's pursuit distance, and the robot's stature (controlling for velocity and pursuit distance). The latter

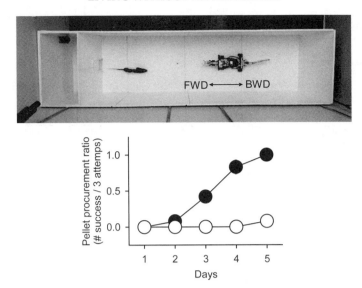

FIGURE 5.8. Foraging under directional threat. Top: In test trials, each time the rat approached the pellet, the Robogator either surged forward (FWD) or backward (BWD) at the same velocity and distance from the start position, snapped its jaws once, and returned to its original position. Bottom: Animals were subjected to three FWD (black circle) and three BWD (open circle) trials, and the order was counterbalanced each day for 5 consecutive days.

observation suggests that a larger looming entity evokes stronger fear because a rat's visual system is binocularly sensitive to visual stimuli above the animal's head (Wallace et al., 2013). Also, though we have not tested this yet, we predict that a robot moving at random velocity and pursuit distance is likely to produce stronger fear than the same robot moving at a fixed velocity and pursuit, because unpredictability represents risk.

Bolles's (1970) species-specific defense reactions and Bolles and Fanselow's (1980) predatory imminence continuum hypotheses propose that fear is an evolutionarily conserved set of mechanistic–heuristic logic that allows animals to adapt to dynamic environments (Blanchard, Blanchard, Rodgers, & Weiss, 1991b; Darwin, 1872; Fanselow & Lester, 1988). Obviously, an innate fear of threats eliminates the danger of trial-and-error learning. Therefore, we should not expect foraging rats to make accurate risk assessments of danger initially, but with experience with the same predator, the animals use estimates of ongoing situations to guide their behavior. Consistent with this view, with repeat encounters with the Robogator surging at a fixed velocity and distance, rats were able to procure pellets placed near the nest. If the pellets were placed afar, rats failed to secure them, because the predation risk became stronger and the rats had insufficient encounters to assess the risk. These observations suggest that fear influences the fundamental decision problem of foraging via assessing the risk associated with the food distance relative to the location of potential threat to form a spatial or distance gradient of fear, which we have incorporated into a quantitative model:

$$F = \frac{D_{predator}}{V_{predator}} - \frac{D_{rat}}{V_{rat} * M}$$

This simple model posits that a rat's likelihood of foraging (F) can be estimated from the time required for the animal to reach the food and carry it back to the safe nest (denoted by the animal's distance to food and velocity) subtracted from the time required for the predator to intersect with the prey (denoted by the predator's pursuit distance and velocity). Thus, larger F values correspond to lower risks (or higher margins of safety) of foraging. The variable M represents modulatory factors, such as hunger. For instance, hunger will increase the animal's risk taking to forage, whereas satiety will make the animal more risk averse (Figure 5.9). Note that the model has a built-in nonlinear relationship if exponential values are used. A useful analogy of the model would be jaywalking behavior in humans. If the approaching car is far away (large distance) and/or moving slowly (low velocity), most people will jaywalk. However, if the approaching car is very near (short distance) and/or moving fast (high velocity), most people will not risk jaywalking. The proposed model

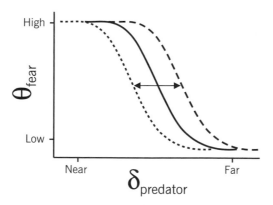

FIGURE 5.9. A hypothetical model of foraging likelihood. The threshold of fear (θ_{fear}) varies as a function of the predator's distance ($\delta_{predator}$) from the animal: near = high fear and far = low fear. This fear–distance relationship can be modulated by the animal's state, such as hunger. The dotted and dashed lines represent decrease and increase likelihood foraging, respectively.

can account for the findings that most rats were unable to acquire pellets placed afar (~76 cm) from the nest but were successful when pellets were placed nearby (~25 cm), and on how the robot's velocity and pursuit distance can affect a rat's foraging behavior. As mentioned earlier, humans also exhibit a "safety margin" or defensive peripersonal space (Graziano & Cooke, 2006), and a recent study indicated that the defensive space of the face between 20 and 40 cm correlated positively with anxiety (Sambo & Iannetti, 2013).

Conclusion

Our novel animal model of risky foraging using artificial predators offers a means to study the functional aspects of fear—namely, the evolutionarily conserved roles of fear in guiding behavior and shaping decisions—that have largely been overlooked in contemporary neurobiological fear research. In essence, the Robogator effectively mimics a naturalistic threat, because its size is relatively larger than that of the rat, and its shape (with eyes, a moving jaw, and a tail) and surging action simulate a predatory strike. Moreover, using a programmable robotic predator has several advantages over using a real predatory animal, such as a cat, because the robot's actions are completely controllable, scalable (e.g., the size of the robot and its movement distance and velocity are proportional to the rat's fear), consistent across trials and rats, and they pose no physical harm despite being capable of eliciting robust fear responses. Other features of predators, such as odor (Dielenberg & McGregor, 2001), can be easily incorporated into the behavioral paradigm. This "approach-avoid" conflict paradigm will expand the current understanding of fear, because it imparts the ecological relevance to examine critically current neural models of fear, which are largely based on fear conditioning. This research also extends into the general field of decision making and has broad translational relevance to anxiety disorders, which are linked to alterations in sets of behaviors coupled to "risk assessment" (American Psychiatric Association, 2013; Craske et al., 2011; Öhman & Mineka, 2001; Seligman, 1971), which is not directly investigated in fear conditioning studies.

ACKNOWLEDGMENTS

This work was supported by National Institutes of Health Grant Nos. MH64457 and MH099073 (to Jeansok J. Kim) and the National Research Foundation of Korea grant from the Korean Government (No. MEST 2012R1A2A4A01008836) to June-Seek Choi.

REFERENCES

Amaral, D. G., Capitanio, J. P., Jourdain, M., Mason, W. A., Mendoza, S. P., & Prather, M. (2003). The amygdala: Is it an essential component of the neural network for social cognition? *Neuropsychologia, 41*(2), 235–240.

American Psychiatric Association. (2013). *Diagnostic and statistical manual of mental disorders* (5th ed.). Arlington, VA: Author.

Amorapanth, P., LeDoux, J. E., & Nader, K. (2000). Different lateral amygdala outputs mediate reactions and actions elicited by a fear-arousing stimulus. *Nature Neuroscience, 3*(1), 74–79.

Barton, R. A., Aggleton, J. P., & Grenyer, R. (2003). Evolutionary coherence of the mammalian amygdala. *Proceedings of the Royal Society of London B: Biological Sciences, 270*(1514), 539–543.

Basso, D. M., Beattie, M. S., & Bresnahan, J. C. (1995). A sensitive and reliable locomotor rating scale for open field testing in rats. *Journal of Neurotrauma, 12*(1), 1–21.

Berdoy, M., Webster, J. P., & Macdonald, D. W. (2000). Fatal attraction in rats infected with *Toxoplasma gondii*. *Proceedings of the Royal Society of London B: Biological Sciences, 267*(1452), 1591–1594.

Blanchard, D. C., & Blanchard, R. J. (1972). Innate and conditioned reactions to threat in rats with amygdaloid lesions. *Journal of Comparative and Physiological Psychology, 81*(2), 281–290.

Blanchard, R. J., Blanchard, D. C., Agullana, R., & Weiss, S. M. (1991a). Twenty-two kHz alarm cries to presentation of a predator, by laboratory rats living in visible burrow systems. *Physiology and Behavior, 50*(5), 967–972.

Blanchard, R. J., Blanchard, D. C., Rodgers, J., & Weiss, S. M. (1991b). The characterization and modelling of antipredator defensive behavior. *Neuroscience and Biobehavioral Reviews, 14*(4), 463–472.

Bolles, R. C. (1970). Species-specific defense reactions and avoidance learning. *Psychological Review, 77*(1), 32–48.

Bolles, R. C., & Fanselow, M. S. (1980). A perceptual–defensive–recuperative model of fear and pain. *Behavioral and Brain Sciences, 3*(2), 291–301.

Campeau, S., & Davis, M. (1995). Involvement of the central nucleus and basolateral complex of the amygdala in fear conditioning measured with fear-potentiated startle in rats trained concurrently with auditory and visual conditioned stimuli. *Journal of Neuroscience, 15*(3), 2301–2311.

Choi, J. S., Cain, C. K., & LeDoux, J. E. (2010). The role of amygdala nuclei in the expression of auditory signaled two-way active avoidance in rats. *Learning and Memory, 17*(3), 139–147.

Choi, J. S., & Kim, J. J. (2010). Amygdala regulates risk of predation in rats foraging in a dynamic fear environment. *Proceedings of the National Academy of Sciences USA, 107*(50), 21773–21777.

Coleman, S. L., Brown, V. R., Levine, D. S., & Mellgren, R. L. (2005). A neural network model of foraging decisions made under predation risk. *Cognitive, Affective, and Behavioral Neuroscience, 5*(4), 434–451.

Corcoran, K. A., & Quirk, G. J. (2007). Activity in prelimbic cortex is necessary for the expression of learned, but not innate, fears. *Journal of Neuroscience, 27*(4), 840–844.

Craske, M. G., Rauch, S. L., Ursano, R., Prenoveau, J., Pine, D. S., & Zinbarg, R. E. (2011). What is an anxiety disorder? *FOCUS, 9*(3), 369–388.

Darwin, C. (1872). *The expression of the emotions in man and animals.* London: J. Murray.

De Martino, B., Camerer, C. F., & Adolphs, R. (2010). Amygdala damage eliminates monetary loss aversion. *Proceedings of the National Academy of Sciences USA, 107*(8), 3788–3792.

Dielenberg, R. A., & McGregor, I. S. (2001). Defensive behavior in rats towards predatory odors: a review. *Neuroscience and Biobehavioral Reviews, 25*(7), 597–609.

Fanselow, M. S. (1984). What is conditioned fear? *Trends in Neurosciences, 7*(12), 460–462.

Fanselow, M. S., & Kim, J. J. (1992). The benzodiazepine inverse agonist DMCM as an Unconditional Stimulus for Fear-Induced Analgesia—Implications for the role of GABA-A receptors in fear-related behavior. *Behavioral Neuroscience, 106*(2), 336–344.

Fanselow, M. S., & LeDoux, J. E. (1999). Why we think plasticity underlying Pavlovian fear conditioning occurs in the basolateral amygdala. *Neuron, 23*(2), 229–232.

Fanselow, M. S., & Lester, L. S. (1988). A functional behavioristic approach to aversively motivated behavior: Predatory imminence as a determinant of the topography of defensive behavior. In R. C. Bolles & M. D. Beecher (Eds.), *Evolution and learning* (pp. 185–212). Hillsdale, NJ: Erlbaum.

Graziano, M. S., & Cooke, D. F. (2006). Parieto-frontal interactions, personal space, and defensive behavior. *Neuropsychologia, 44*(6), 845–859.

Helmstetter, F. J. (1992). The amygdala is essential for the expression of conditional hypoalgesia. *Behavioral Neuroscience, 106*(3), 518–528.

Hull, C. L. (1929). A functional interpretation of the conditioned reflex. *Psychological Review, 36*, 498–511.

Kapp, B. S., Frysinger, R. C., Gallagher, M., & Haselton, J. R. (1979). Amygdala central nucleus lesions: effect on heart rate conditioning in the rabbit. *Physiology and Behavior, 23*(6), 1109–1117.

Killcross, S., Robbins, T. W., & Everitt, B. J. (1997). Different types of fear-conditioned behaviour mediated by separate nuclei within amygdala. *Nature, 388*(6640), 377–380.

Kim, E. J., Horovitz, O., Pellman, B. A., Tan, L. M., Li, Q. L., Richter-Levin, G., et al. (2013). Dorsal periaqueductal gray–amygdala pathway conveys both innate and learned fear responses in rats. *Proceedings of the National Academy of Sciences USA, 110*(36), 14795–14800.

Kim, J. J., & Fanselow, M. S. (1992). Modality-specific retrograde-amnesia of fear. *Science, 256*(5057), 675–677.

Kim, J. J., Lee, H. J., Welday, A. C., Song, E., Cho, J., Sharp, P. E., et al. (2007). Stress-induced alterations in hippocampal plasticity, place cells, and spatial memory. *Proceedings of the National Academy of Sciences USA, 104*(46), 18297–18302.

Kim, S. C., Jo, Y. S., Kim, I. H., Kim, H., & Choi, J.-S. (2010). Lack of medial prefrontal cortex activation underlies the immediate extinction deficit. *Journal of Neuroscience, 30*(3), 832–837.

Klüver, H., & Bucy, P. C. (1939). Preliminary analysis of functions of the temporal lobes in monkeys. *Archives of Neurology and Psychiatry, 42*(6), 979–1000.

Laurent, V., & Westbrook, R. F. (2009). Inactivation of the infralimbic but not the prelimbic cortex impairs consolidation and retrieval of fear extinction. *Learning and Memory, 16*(9), 520–529.

Maren, S. (2011). Seeking a spotless mind: Extinction, deconsolidation, and erasure of fear memory. *Neuron, 70*(5), 830–845.

Maren, S., & Fanselow, M. S. (1995). Synaptic plasticity in the basolateral amygdala induced by hippocampal formation stimulation *in vivo. Journal of Neuroscience, 15*(11), 7548–7564.

McGaugh, J. L. (2000). Memory—A century of consolidation. *Science, 287*(5451), 248–251.

McGaugh, J. L. (2004). The amygdala modulates the consolidation of memories of emotionally arousing experiences. *Annual Review of Neuroscience, 27,* 1–28.

McGaugh, J. L., Cahill, L., & Roozendaal, B. (1996). Involvement of the amygdala in memory storage: Interaction with other brain systems. *Proceedings of the National Academy of Sciences USA, 93*(24), 13508–13514.

Mowrer, O. H. (1951). Two-factor learning theory: summary and comment. *Psychological Review, 58*(5), 350–354.

Mueller, D., Porter, J. T., & Quirk, G. J. (2008). Noradrenergic signaling in infralimbic cortex increases cell excitability and strengthens memory for fear extinction. *Journal of Neuroscience, 28*(2), 369–375.

Öhman, A., & Mineka, S. (2001). Fears, phobias, and preparedness: Toward an evolved module of fear and fear learning. *Psychological Review, 108*(3), 483–522.

Orsini, C. A., Kim, J. H., Knapska, E., & Maren, S. (2011). Hippocampal and prefrontal projections to the basal amygdala mediate contextual regulation of fear after extinction. *Journal of Neuroscience, 31*(47), 17269–17277.

Pape, H.-C., & Paré, D. (2010). Plastic synaptic networks of the amygdala for the acquisition, expression, and extinction of conditioned fear. *Physiological Reviews, 90*(2), 419–463.

Paré, D., Quirk, G. J., & LeDoux, J. E. (2004). New vistas on amygdala networks in conditioned fear. *Journal of Neurophysiology, 92*(1), 1–9.

Parent, M. B., McGaugh, J. L., & Tomaz, C. (1992). Increased training in an aversively motivated task attenuates the memory-impairing effects of posttraining N-methyl-D-aspartate-induced amygdala lesions. *Behavioral Neuroscience, 106*(5), 789–797.

Pellow, S., Chopin, P., File, S. E., & Briley, M. (1985). Validation of open:closed arm entries in an elevated plus-maze as a measure of anxiety in the rat. *Journal of Neuroscience Methods, 14*(3), 149–167.

Phillips, R. G., & LeDoux, J. E. (1992). Differential contribution of amygdala and hippocampus to cued and contextual fear conditioning. *Behavioral Neuroscience, 106*(2), 274–285.

Quirk, G. J., Repa, J. C., & LeDoux, J. E. (1995). Fear conditioning enhances short-latency auditory responses of lateral amygdala neurons: Parallel recordings in the freely behaving rat. *Neuron, 15*(5), 1029–1039.

Rescorla, R. A., & Solomon, R. L. (1967). Two-process learning theory:

Relationships between Pavlovian conditioning and instrumental learning. *Psychological Review, 74*(3), 151–182.

Romanski, L. M., & LeDoux, J. E. (1992). Equipotentiality of thalamo–amygdala and thalamo–cortico–amygdala circuits in auditory fear conditioning. *Journal of Neuroscience, 12*(11), 4501–4509.

Sambo, C. F., & Iannetti, G. D. (2013). Better safe than sorry?: The safety margin surrounding the body is increased by anxiety. *Journal of Neuroscience, 33*(35), 14225–14230.

Sanders, S. K., & Shekhar, A. (1995). Regulation of anxiety by GABA(a) receptors in the rat amygdala. *Pharmacology Biochemistry and Behavior, 52*(4), 701–706.

Schleidt, W., Shalter, M. D., & Moura-Neto, H. (2011). The hawk/goose story: The classical ethological experiments of Lorenz and Tinbergen, revisited. *Journal of Comparative Psychology, 125*(2), 121–133.

Seligman, M. E. (1971). Phobias and preparedness. *Behavior Therapy, 2*(3), 307–320.

Shi, C., & Davis, M. (2001). Visual pathways involved in fear conditioning measured with fear-potentiated startle: Behavioral and anatomic studies. *Journal of Neuroscience, 21*(24), 9844–9855.

Soltis, R. P., Cook, J. C., Gregg, A. E., & Sanders, B. J. (1997). Interaction of GABA and excitatory amino acids in the basolateral amygdala: Role in cardiovascular regulation. *Journal of Neuroscience, 17*(23), 9367–9374.

Spalding, D. A. (1954). Instinct: With original observations on young animals. *British Journal of Animal Behaviour, 2*(1), 2–11.

Stephens, D. W., Brown, J. S., & Ydenberg, R. C. (2007). *Foraging: Behavior and ecology.* Chicago: University of Chicago Press.

Stephens, D. W., & Krebs, J. R. (1986). *Foraging theory.* Princeton, NJ: Princeton University Press.

Vyas, A., Kim, S.-K., Giacomini, N., Boothroyd, J. C., & Sapolsky, R. M. (2007). Behavioral changes induced by Toxoplasma infection of rodents are highly specific to aversion of cat odors. *Proceedings of the National Academy of Sciences, 104*(15), 6442–6447.

Walk, R. D. (1966). The development of depth perception in animals and human infants. *Monographs of the Society for Research in Child Development, 31*(5), 82–108.

Wallace, D. J., Greenberg, D. S., Sawinski, J., Rulla, S., Notaro, G., & Kerr, J. N. (2013). Rats maintain an overhead binocular field at the expense of constant fusion. *Nature, 498*(7452), 65–69.

Watson, J. B., & Rayner, R. (1920). Conditioned emotional reactions. *Journal of Experimental Psychology, 3*(1), 1–14.

Yoon, T., Graham, L. K., & Kim, J. J. (2011). Hippocampal lesion effects on occasion setting by contextual and discrete stimuli. *Neurobiology of Learning and Memory, 95*(2), 176–184.

CHAPTER 6

Lifetime Consequences of Early Amygdala Damage in Rhesus Monkeys

ELIZA BLISS-MOREAU
GILDA MOADAB
DAVID G. AMARAL

Studies in nonhuman animals and human patients in which the amygdala is damaged suggest a potentially critical role in social and affective processing for the small neural structure buried deep within the temporal lobe. Despite dozens of studies, questions remain about its importance for the development of normal socioemotional processing. To answer these questions, we studied the social and affective lives of a cohort of rhesus macaques (*Macaca mulatta*) that received neurotoxic lesions of the amygdala at 2 weeks of age and were subsequently raised with their mothers in small social groups. For more than a decade we tracked their spontaneous social behaviors in multiple social contexts and their affective behaviors in response to provocative stimuli (e.g., toy snakes, novel objects, videos of conspecifics). Animals with amygdala damage developed species-typical social and affective behavioral repertoires. Although they were hypersocial (in terms of generating more frequent social signals) early in life, their social behavior normalized over time, such that it was indistinguishable from nonoperated animals as adults. In contrast, the magnitude of their affective responses to provocative stimuli was consistently blunted across the course of their lives. We detail in this chapter these animals' life histories, the patterns of their behavior over the course of development, and the implications for understanding the role of the amygdala in the development of normal social and affective behavior.

As the "decade of the brain" came to a close in 1999, our research group embarked on what would become more than a decade-long project studying the social and affective lives of rhesus monkeys with early amygdala damage. Theory placed the amygdala[1] at the center of the "social brain" (Brothers, 1990), casting it as a critical linchpin in the generation and regulation of normal social behavior. Early studies by Kling and colleagues, for example, demonstrated that damage to the amygdala and medial temporal lobe resulted in radically deregulated social processing (Dicks, Myers, & Kling, 1969; Kling & Cornell, 1971). Another body of research, stemming from the seminal studies of Klüver and Bucy, demonstrated that removal of the amygdala led to a blunted emotional response to normally threatening stimuli (Klüver & Bucy, 1939). These findings were quickly confirmed by several laboratories, and Weiskrantz (1956) and colleagues demonstrated that the alteration in emotional response was due largely to damage of the amygdala, rather than tissues surrounding it. Whether the amygdala was critical for the normal development of social and affective behavior remained an open question when we began our longitudinal study.

Our main purpose in this chapter is to report on the life histories of eight rhesus macaques that received specific, complete, neurotoxic lesions to the amygdala at 2 weeks of age and eight sham-operated control peers with whom they were raised. We begin by setting the scientific stage for the experiment. In particular, we discuss studies carried out in adult rhesus monkeys that raised a number of questions concerning the role of the amygdala in social behavior. We describe the theories and studies that fueled our developmental hypotheses, the potential pitfalls we faced, and the methodological innovations we undertook to meet them. We describe innovative practices related to the rearing and social housing conditions of our monkey subjects and the general approach to their study. We then review two types of data that we collected throughout their lives, relating to their social behavior and processing of affective value (or valence), including responding to threat-provoking objects. We conclude by presenting what we believe to be the "take-home" message from this series of experiments and discussing the opportunities for long-term study of nonhuman primates.

---

[1]We and others have promoted the view that the "amygdala" is a complex structure made up of at least 13 nuclei and cortical regions; therefore, it should be rightfully called the amygdaloid complex (Amaral, Price, Pitkänen, & Carmichael, 1992). Since most of the research related to amygdala function in monkeys and humans has not evaluated the effects of damage to specific nuclei, and because the word "amygdala" is certainly more euphonious than "amygdaloid complex," we use the term "amygdala" as synonymous with "amygdaloid complex" in this chapter.

The Social Brain at the Dawn of the 21st Century

The end of the 20th century witnessed a renewed interest in understanding the neurobiology of social processing. Of particular impact were a few major reviews that set the stage for focusing on the relationship between social experience and neurobiology. From an evolutionary perspective, Dunbar (1998) argued that the large brains that are characteristic of primates evolved to meet the cognitive demands of living in large social groups. Brothers (1990) argued that a core set of neuroanatomical structures were critical for the social processing essential for primate group life. That list of structures included the amygdala. At the time, our group had already been engaged in studies of the normal neuroanatomy of the nonhuman primate amygdala (Stefanacci & Amaral, 2000; Stefanacci, Suzuki, & Amaral, 1996; Pitkänen & Amaral, 1998; Amaral et al., 1992; Amaral & Price, 1984; Price & Amaral, 1981). A natural progression of that work led to an investigation of the function of the amygdala in general and of its nuclei in particular. As we see below, the expertise gained from making minute injections of tracer substances into different nuclei of the amygdala facilitated our efforts at making selective lesions.

A Short History of Studies of Bilateral Amygdala Lesions in Adult Rhesus Monkeys

Like many who had come before (Klüver & Bucy, 1939; Rosvold, Mirsky, & Pribram, 1954; Mirsky, 1960; Dicks et al., 1969; Kling, 1974; for a review, see Amaral, Chapter 3, this volume), we started investigating the role of the amygdala in social and affective processing in adult rhesus macaques. Previous research had, for the most part, created either large lesions (of the entire medial temporal lobe) or used aspiration lesions of the amygdala that inescapably damaged fibers of passage through the amygdala (Rosvold et al., 1954; Mirsky, 1960; Myers & Swett, 1970; Kling, 1974). Those studies documented changes in social behavior, dominance status, and or, responsivity to other monkeys and humans following amygdala or medial temporal lobe damage (also see the Feinstein, Adolphs, & Tranel, Chapter 1, this volume). Some studies had disastrous consequences. Monkeys with amygdala damage did not fare well when released back to Cayo Santiago, an island off of the south coast of Puerto Rico that is home to a research station and groups of free-ranging macaques. Two adults that received damage to the amygdala and uncus never rejoined their social groups, were subjected to substantial wounding from conspecifics, and perished rapidly (Dicks et al., 1969). In a subsequent study, four additional males received damage to the amygdala only (sparing the uncus). Of these four, two young animals (2 and 3 years of age) did appear to rejoin their social groups and behave relatively normally, whereas two older animals (4 and 9 years of age) with amygdala damage perished within a month of release (Dicks et al., 1969). In a third study, animals with medial temporal lobe damage were released back into their groups on Cayo Santiago, and all perished between 1 and 32 weeks after release (Myers & Swett, 1970). These findings worried us that animals with amygdala damage might not survive in social housing.

Our neuroanatomical studies also pointed to potential problems with the lesion strategies employed in the earlier studies. For example, we found that projections from other regions of the temporal lobe often traveled within or adjacent to the amygdala en route to the frontal lobe. Existing studies on behavior following damage to the amygdala used lesion techniques that damaged or altogether eliminated those "fibers of passage." So it was not entirely clear whether the behavioral consequences of "amygdala" damage were due to damage of the amygdala per se or damage of fibers of passage, or both! In fact, existing evidence pointed to a reduced impact on affective behavior of lesions that spared fibers of passage through the amygdala, as compared to those that did not (Meunier, Bachevalier, Murray, Malkova, & Mishkin, 1999).

The California National Primate Research Center: An Ideal Facility for Studying Nonhuman Primate Socioaffective Behavior

The California National Primate Research Center (CNPRC) (*www.cnprc. ucdavis.edu*) is one of the eight National Institutes of Health (NIH)-funded national primate centers (*http://nprcresearch.org*). The primate center system was established in the early 1960s by the NIH with direct congressional funding (Dukelow & Whitehair, 1995). The CNPRC was established in 1962 as the National Center for Primate Biology, on 300 acres of land at the periphery of the University of California (UC), Davis campus. Early on, the CNPRC's focus was on breeding and rearing healthy animals for biomedical research. As a result of the Center's early focus on managing large numbers of healthy animals, it has had a long-standing commitment to advancing the care and welfare of captive animals. Like our subjects, the majority of the approximately 5,000 nonhuman primates at the CNPRC are rhesus monkeys (*Macaca mulatta*).

In 1972, after investment from the School of Medicine and School of Veterinary Medicine, the CNPRC envisioned its focus in terms of key research areas that continue to be strengths today—infectious disease, respiratory disease, reproductive and regenerative medicine, and neuroscience, psychological, and behavioral research. These research units are supported by a number of core service units that are able to provide standardized assessments of genetics, endocrine function, pathogen detection, and so on. A large proportion of the infants born at the center are behaviorally phenotyped at 3 months of age via the biobehavioral assessment program run by Dr. John Capitanio (e.g., Capitanio, Mendoza, Mason, & Maninger, 2005; Vandeleest & Capitanio, 2012; see Golub, Hogrefe, Widamen, & Capitanio, 2009 for methodological details about the program) allowing for the selection of animals based on standardized behavioral parameters. A world-class team of primate veterinarians and animal health technicians ensures the health and welfare of research and colony animals. The Center maintains a standardized database of animal information that includes information from core services (e.g., genetic information including maternal and paternal lineages, behavioral information regarding pairing history), the medical team, and the biobehavioral assessment program. This feature allows for the selection of experimental animals that meet particular criteria.

Monkeys at the CNPRC are housed primarily in three sorts of environments. More than half of the colony lives outdoors in large chain-link field enclosures that are 0.5 hectares in size and at least 10 feet high. The enclosures include a variety of ground substrates such as pebbles, gravel, grass and dirt, and objects on which to climb (e.g., human-made perches, trees, children's play gyms, swings, covered raised shelters). Each cage can house between 50 and 200 monkeys, typically in natal family structures. A small proportion of animals are housed in small outdoor pens with between eight and 30 animals. These pens are primarily used for social housing of young weaned monkeys and controlled breeding. As with the larger field corrals, they include a mix of ground substrates and objects on which to climb. Additional monkeys live indoors in a mix of standard primate caging and social group housing. The flexibility of housing options available to monkeys at the CNPRC allowed us to rear our subjects socially and house them in a variety of social settings across their lives, as described below.

Our Studies of Bilateral Amygdalectomy in Adult Rhesus Monkeys

In 1996, we initiated a study of adult animals with amygdala damage and made a number of methodological choices to build on previous work (Emery et al., 2001; Mason, Capitanio, Machado, Mendoza, & Amaral, 2006; Machado et al., 2008a). Our first advancement was with regard to the surgical techniques used to create amygdala damage. We used a neurotoxin, ibotenic acid, to remove amygdala neurons selectively without damaging fibers of passage. Ibotenic acid is found naturally in the mushroom *Amanita muscaria* and is a glutamate agonist in the brain. Ibotenic acid may cause neuronal death through excitotoxic and other metabolic processes, since it is toxic not only to the central nervous system but also to many other body organs. The demonstrated benefit of this neurotoxin is that it removes neurons within the amygdala without damaging fibers running through the amygdala (Jarrard, 1989; Meunier et al., 1999).

Our second class of advancements focused on the animals selected for the study and the behavioral evaluations. Our primary goal was to carry out studies that were as naturalistic as possible. To that end, we selected adult animals from the large field corrals to ensure that they had been reared as normally/naturalistically as possible. In collaboration with primatologists and behavioral biologists at the CNPRC, including Drs. Bill Mason, Sally Mendoza, and John Capitanio, we designed experiments that allowed the monkeys to show us what they could and could not do. Animals were presented with an experience (e.g., either a conspecific, or an object), and we recorded their spontaneous behaviors using a catalog of behaviors that included nearly all species-typical social and affective behaviors. Behavioral catalogs of this sort are called "ethograms." We introduced animals to other social partners in a controlled and protected fashion. Animals with amygdala lesions were first exposed to "interaction partners" behind a metal grill for a number of meetings before they were allowed unrestricted access to those animals. This sort of stepwise introduction has been previously used at zoos successfully to build new social relationships (a procedure called a "howdy" in zoos; Powell, 2010). We followed this procedure due to the earlier evidence that other animals would aggress against amygdala-lesioned animals.

With these methodological considerations in mind, we created neurotoxic damage to the bilateral amygdala of a cohort of male adult rhesus monkeys. Based on the extant literature, we expected that adult amygdala damage would severely disrupt social behavior. In particular, we hypothesized that animals would be either antisocial or inappropriately social and perhaps the targets of aggression by their peers.

As it turned out, we had nothing to be worried about with regard to aggression against the lesioned animals. In fact, amygdala-lesioned animals were not only capable of executing social behaviors but they were also hypersocial! This hypersociality manifested both when these animals interacted with a single social partner (Emery et al., 2001) and in small groups (Machado et al., 2008a). Compared to control animals, amygdala-lesioned animals spent more time in proximity to other animals and generated a greater number of sexual behaviors and positive social signals (e.g., more cooing, presenting for sex, presenting for grooming, approaching; Emery et al., 2001; Machado et al., 2008a). Amygdala-lesioned animals generated social behaviors all of the time, even when to do so was inappropriate by normal monkey standards. Perhaps ironically, this made them preferred social partners. This pattern of effects made us wonder whether our neurosurgeries had actually been successful. Following social behavior testing, we evaluated the adult animals with novel objects and threat-related objects. We observed that compared to control animals, amygdala-lesioned animals' responsivity to the objects was severely blunted (Mason et al., 2006). Together, these findings supported the idea that damage to the adult amygdala blunted affective but not social processing. This patterns of findings suggested to us that the operated animals were insensitive to threat, leading to lack of responses to potentially threatening stimuli and abnormal willingness to approach and interact with novel conspecifics.

Would Social Behavior Be Impacted if Lesions Were Performed in Neonates?: A Historical Context

The adult studies (Emery et al., 2001; Mason et al., 2006; Machado et al., 2008a), provided compelling evidence that the amygdala is not essential for a normal repertoire of social behaviors. However, it was still conceivable that the amygdala plays an organizational role during early development and establishes all of the requisite, social knowledge (perhaps stored in other brain regions) for normal conspecific social interactions. Thus, a logical next question was whether the amygdala is necessary for the acquisition or development of normal social behavior. Existing developmental literature suggested that this was the case. For example, nursery-reared infants (i.e., infants raised with peers rather than their mothers) that received amygdala damage around 2 months of age were more "fearful" and less social than controls in social settings at approximately 1 year of age (Thompson, Schwartzbaum, & Harlow, 1969). "Fearful" behaviors included incidence of the silent bared teeth display, freezing, screeching, and rocking, whereas social behaviors included social grooming and being in physical contact with another animal. When these same animals were evaluated at 3.5 years of age, they were submissive to the neurologically intact control animals with whom they were paired (Thompson & Towfighi, 1976). Similarly, early lesions that involved the amygdala, hippocampus, and adjacent cortices in peer-reared infant monkeys reduced sociability, the propensity to explore the environment, and emotional expressivity at ages 2 and 6 months, resulting in animals that not only were socially withdrawn but also actively shunned social contact (Bachevalier, 1994). These animals also had heightened propensities for abnormal behaviors such as stereotypies (Bachevalier, 1994). These effects were so robust that Bachevalier concluded that early damage to medial temporal structures was a model for autism.

Caveats Associated with Previous
Developmental Studies

The early studies by Bachevalier and those that predated her work raised a number of questions. First, what would be the effect of *selective* amygdala damage in very young animals—that is, damage to the amygdala only that occurred before animals developed their repertoire of species-typical social behaviors? Second, would the patterns of behavior be the same in neonates with neural damage who were raised with their mothers? Existing evidence suggested that animals raised without their mothers developed abnormal behavior (e.g., Champoux, Metz, & Suomi, 1991); rearing without mother could therefore potentially alter or exacerbate the effects of early brain damage. There is actually substantial evidence from several primate centers that maternal deprivation and nursery rearing are risk factors for increased stereotypies and other forms of pathological behavior (Bellanca & Crockett, 2002; Lutz, Well, & Novak, 2003). Finally, since we had not found impairment of social behavior in adults with bilateral amygdala lesions, we wondered whether the effects of neonatal selective bilateral amygdalectomy would be more deleterious. We decided to answer these developmental questions by selectively and neurotoxically creating bilateral amygdala damage in infants who were too young to have learned a social behavior repertoire.

Of note, we are not the only team to question the impact of damaging fibers of passage and of rearing conditions on social and affective behavior following early amygdala damage. Following the start of our study (in 2001), Bachevalier and colleagues began a similar study in 2009. They produced similar early amygdala lesions using ibotenic acid in 3- to 4-week-old infants, returned them to their mothers, then housed them in large social groups. See Bachevalier, Sanchez, Raper, Stephens, and Wallen (Chapter 7, this volume) for a detailed history of that project.

A Short Primer on the Development of Rhesus Monkeys' Social Behavior

Macaque development occurs approximately four times faster than human development (for a review, see Machado, 2013; Suomi, 1999). Indeed, much of this development occurs inside the womb, such that newborn monkeys have brains approximately 60% the size of an adult monkey brain, whereas newborn humans are much more altricial and have brains only about 25% the size of an adult human brain. Although many comparisons of specific behaviors are inappropriate (e.g., monkeys are born able to walk), in general this means that between birth and their first birthday, rhesus monkeys traverse the equivalent developmental milestones that human children traverse between birth and going off to school (at 4–5 years of age). Rhesus infants spend the majority of time during their first month of life with their mothers, typically on their chests (what is referred to in primatology as "ventral–ventral contact," see Figure 6.1; Berman, 1980; Hinde & Spencer-Booth, 1967; for review, see Machado, 2013; Bauman & Amaral, 2008). Infants' social lives literally revolve around the mother during this time. During the first month of life, mothers initiate social interactions (e.g., grooming) with infants (Hinde, Rowell, & Spencer-Booth, 1964), search for mutual gaze, and generate faces such as the "lipsmack" (an affiliative signal) directed toward their infants (Ferrari, Paukner, Ionica, & Suomi, 2009; see Figure 6.1). Infants may generate lipsmacks directed toward their mothers as young as 3 days of age but typically do not begin grooming their mothers until 2 months of age (Ferrari et al., 2009) or later (Hinde & Spencer-Booth, 1967). In the period from birth to 2 months of age, mutual gaze between infants and their mothers increases (Ferrari et al., 2009). While they are readily mobile, possessing the ability to cling to their mothers as early as the day they are born, infant monkeys' time away from mother typically occurs in short bursts that increase in duration with age (Hinde et al., 1964; Hinde & Spencer-Booth, 1967). By the second month of life, however, infants begin to spend time physically outside of their mothers' reach (Ferarri et al., 2009).

The transition to weaning begins around 3 months of age and is accompanied by greater independence from mother. During the 3- to 6-month developmental window, rhesus monkeys spend increasing lengths of time away from their mothers and, as a result, begin to develop social relationships of their own with peers and kin. Play emerges at around 4 months of age (Suomi, 1984) and serves as a means by which relationships are both developed and maintained. In service of these social relationships, social communication (e.g., the appropriate use of facial displays and vocal signals) develops rapidly during the 3- to 6-month window as well (Suomi, 1984). The communication repertoire of healthy rhesus infants includes the silent bared teeth (or "fear" grimace) display (see Figure 6.1) by 3 months of age (Suomi, 1984), although there may be variability relative to when that facial display appears (Hinde et al., 1964). The threat facial display appears to come online later (Hinde et al., 1964). The complexity of social signaling continues to develop rapidly through 6 months of age (Suomi, 1984). For example, presenting rump—a communicative body posture that occurs both in sexual and nonsexual contexts—begins to appear prior to 6 months of age in females and shortly after 6 months of age in males (Hinde & Spencer-Booth, 1967). Infants are typically weaned by the mother at around 6 months of age, and the process is complete by the birth of their next sibling (Fooden, 2000).

Between 6 months and 1 year of age, rhesus monkeys spend more and more time away from their mothers and develop stronger bonds

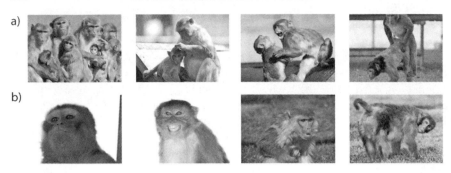

FIGURE 6.1. Examples of species-typical social and affective behaviors. (a) Social behaviors from left to right: mother–infant ventral–ventral contact; grooming; play; mounting. (b) Communicative affective behaviors from left to right: lips-mack, silent bared teeth, threat, and present rump. Photographs courtesy of Kathy West at the CNPRC.

with peers and kin. Grooming and play (see Figure 6.1) become critically important for both developing and maintaining social relationships. Play varies between "rough-and-tumble" and acting-out sexual behavior (e.g., taking turns mounting each other; see Figure 6.1), without actually having sex. Aggressive behavior emerges at around 6–7 months (Suomi, 1984). Around a monkey's first birthday, it is likely that his or her mother will have given birth to a new infant. This further reduces individuals' contact with their mothers. Macaques between 1 and 3–4 years of age typically stay integrated with their family unit, although sex differences emerge in this family integration as they approach sexual maturity (around 3 years of age for females and around 4 years of age for males; Rawlins & Kessler, 1986). Females typically remain with their natal group for the duration of their lives, resulting in families that are structured based on maternal kin (called "matrilines") (Fooden, 2000; Melnick, Pearl, & Richard, 1984). In contrast, males typically migrate from the natal group at around 4 years of age, when they reach sexual maturity, in order to join another troop (Melnick et al., 1984).

Creation of the UC Davis Cohort of Neonatally Lesioned Animals

In 2001, as the birth season unfolded at the CNPRC, we selected the animals that would become our subjects as they were born. We chose male and female infants born to mothers that had given birth to and reared healthy infants before. Our initial study group was 24 infants—eight with amygdala lesions (three males, five females), eight with hippocampus lesions (three males, five females), and eight sham-operated controls (four males, four females) that underwent only anesthesia and opening of the scalp. One methodological concern associated with our goal to mother-rear infants was that their mothers would not take them back after surgery. To address this, we exposed mothers to the smell of Betadine and ethanol to habituate them to what their infants would smell like after surgery. On postnatal days 4, 8, and 11, infants were removed from their mothers, had their heads shaved, had their heads scrubbed with Betadine and 70% ethanol, then were returned to their mothers. In the end, we had 100% success returning operated infants to their mothers after their surgery.

Presurgical Magnetic Resonance Imaging

Surgery occurred when infants were between 12 and 16 days of age. On the morning of neurosurgery, mothers were sedated and their infants removed. Infants were transported to the UC Davis Veterinary Medicine Teaching Hospital to undergo magnetic resonance imaging (MRI). The MRI was used as an individualized stereotactic atlas for plotting the location of injection sites for the ibotenic acid.

Surgery

After neuroimaging, infants were transported back to the CNPRC in the stereotaxic apparatus. At this age, the ear canals are very poorly formed and positioning the animal in the stereotaxic apparatus was much more difficult than with adult animals. Preliminary studies indicated that the best success for accurate placement of injections occurred by keeping the animal in the stereotaxic apparatus from the time it received its MRI until the surgery was completed. Surgeries occurred at the CNPRC under aseptic conditions with isoflurane and fentanyl anesthesia.

Prior to injecting the neurotoxin, we performed electrophysiological recordings to confirm the depth of the injection sites. We recorded from a location that was at the midpoint of all calculated injection sites (i.e., in the middle of both the rostrocaudal and mediolateral coordinates). Injection locations were adjusted on the basis of the electrophysiological assessment. Once coordinates had been confirmed or adjusted, injection of the neurotoxin occurred. Bilateral injections of ibotenic acid (10 mg/ml in 0.1 M phosphate-buffered solution [Biosearch Technologies, Novato, CA]; rate = 0.2 µl/minute) were made into the targeted neural issue. Amygdala lesions required 7–12 µl of ibotentic acid. Sham-operated controls received an incision to expose the scalp, had their fascia and scalp closed in two separate layers, and were maintained under anesthesia for the average duration of the neurotoxic surgeries.

Housing and Socialization

Social housing conditions are detailed in Figure 6.2. Our goal was to provide the lesioned animals with maternal and peer interaction that was as normal as possible, while maintaining experimental control of the animals for observational studies.

Subjects were returned to their mothers within 24 hours postoperatively, when they were awake and alert. Infants were housed with their mothers in standard primate caging in indoor rooms. Once infants had recovered from their surgeries, they were socialized with their mothers and other infant–mother pairs in large chain-link indoor enclosures for 3 hours, 5 days per week. Each social group included two subjects from each experimental condition, their mothers, and a novel adult male. Groups were monitored by an observer for the first five 3-hour meetings to ensure social compatibility. According to standard husbandry practices at the CNPRC, subjects were weaned from their mothers at 6 months of age and singly housed but were socialized in their groups without their mothers for 3 hours each day. The infants and adult male in each social group remained the same, and a novel adult female was added to each group. Subjects were permanently housed with their social groups in large enclosures beginning at 1 year of age.

At 3 years of age, each social group was moved to a large outdoor enclosure for 1 year. After a year, subjects were then moved into standard indoor caging and paired with compatible social partners for at least 5 hours/day, 5 days per week. At 4 years of age, females were moved to large outdoor enclosures, into groups that comprised one female from each lesion condition and one novel adult male (for further details, see Moadab, Bliss-Moreau, Bauman, & Amaral, submitted). Males were moved into smaller outdoor enclosures and paired with another male

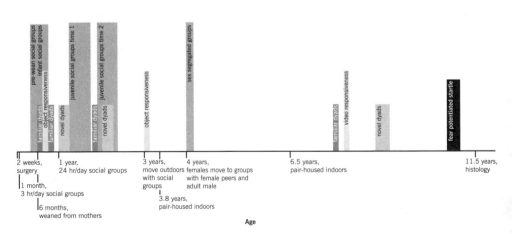

FIGURE 6.2. Time line of subject social housing and experiments.

from the project. At 6.5 years of age, animals were relocated indoors and placed into male–female pairs with either other subjects, adult males who had been members of the social groups (described earlier), or animals from the CNPRC colony.

One of the original amygdala-lesioned males died of natural causes at approximately 1 year of age (Bauman, Lavenex, Mason, Capitanio, & Amaral, 2004a). At that time, this animal was replaced with another male amygdala-lesioned animal that underwent surgery at the same time as the other animals but was raised by his mother alone for the first year of life. He was pair-housed with an age-matched female after being separated from his mother at 1 year and introduced to his social group at 1 year and 3 months. One female amygdala-lesioned subject died at approximately 5 years of age and a second died at 9 years of age. Neither were replaced as subjects.

Lesion Analysis

Lesion placement was confirmed via T2-weighted MRIs acquired 10 days after surgery (see Bauman et al., 2004a) and by T1-weighted images acquired when the animals were approximately 4 years of age (Machado, Snyder, Cherry, Lavenex, & Amaral, 2008). Histological confirmation of the lesions has now been completed and an example of one of the experimental cases is presented in Figure 6.3; the extent of amygdala sparing is detailed in Table 6.1.

Assessment of Early Damage to the Amygdala on Social and Affective Behavior

Across their lifetimes, the neonatally lesioned subjects completed two types of tasks—social behavior assessments (in groups or pairs, i.e., "dyads") and assessments with affectively potent stimuli in nonsocial settings (e.g., while being tested alone in a cage, i.e., "responsiveness" testing). Testing occurred at various developmental time points when subjects were housed in various social configurations. We detail these two features of the experiment in Figure 6.1. Below we detail the patterns of results across their lives.

The Development of Social Behavior

We evaluated social behavior using standard focal sampling techniques (Altmann, 1974) while subjects interacted with familiar and novel peers in a variety of social settings. "Focal sampling" entails watching a specific subject as he or she behaves. Behaviors generated by the subject are recorded and, in most cases, information about their interaction partners

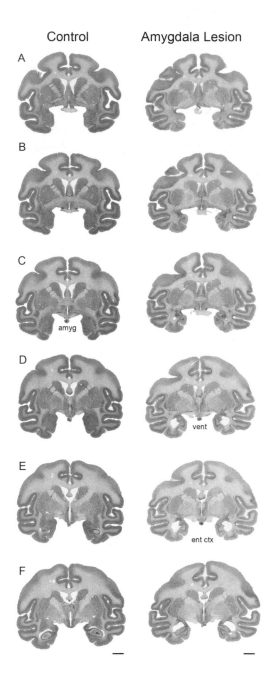

FIGURE 6.3. Six slices (A–F) illustrating the complete amygdala of one representative control animal and selective amygdala damage in one representative amygdala lesion case. Sections are arranged from rostral (A) through caudal (F). The control animal's intact amygdala (amyg) is labeled in C. Note that no tissue is present in the amygdala lesion case at the same positions. The amygdala-lesioned animal's enlarged ventricles (vent), visible in C, D, E, and F, is labeled in D. The amygdala-lesioned animal's intact entorhinal cortex (ent ctx) is labeled in E. The scale bar represents 1 cm.

is recorded as well. We recorded behaviors as indicated in a catalog of species-typical social behaviors (termed "behavioral ethograms" in the behavioral biology and anthropology literatures). These catalogs of observed behaviors evolved over the course of the study and were tailored to the particular experiments. In all cases, the behavior generated by the focal animal was recorded. We recorded both the frequency of behaviors and the duration of a subset of behaviors for which duration is meaningful ("state" behaviors, e.g., proximity with another animal, grooming bouts). Observation durations varied by experiment, lasting between 5 and 20 minutes per sample. Multiple observations were made for each subject in each experiment.

TABLE 6.1. Lesion Extent

	Volume of left amygdala	Volume of right amygdala	Percent atrophy, left amygdala	Percent atrophy, right amygdala
Control animals				
Males				
Case A	187.31	188.69	—	—
Case B	247.50	246.94	—	—
Case C	252.70	244.86	—	—
Male control average	*229.17*	*226.83*		
Females				
Case D	199.15	197.70	—	—
Case E	189.34	190.17	—	—
Case F	202.38	195.31	—	—
Case G	193.02	187.69	—	—
Female control average	*195.97*	*192.72*		
Amygdala-lesioned animals				
Males				
Case H	13.77	19.55	94.01	91.38
Case I	9.73	4.15	95.76	98.17
Case J	6.43	13.56	97.19	94.02
Average	*9.96*	*12.42*	*95.65*	*94.52*
Females				
Case K	17.00	22.01	91.32	88.58
Case L	7.29	13.38	96.28	93.06
Case M	14.21	4.85	92.75	97.49
Average	*12.84*	*13.42*	*93.45*	*93.04*

Note. Volumes are in cubic millimeters. Percent atrophy was calculated by sex and by hemisphere: (average volume for control animals – volume of each individual amygdala lesioned animal)/average volume for control animals. Calculations were computed in cubic microns and converted to cubic millimeters, then rounded to two decimal places.

Social Behavior in Social Groups

Prior to weaning, at 4.5–6.0 months of age, subjects' social behavior was evaluated while the animals were in their social groups with their mothers (Bauman et al., 2004a). Amygdala-lesioned animals, compared to control animals, spent more time in contact with their mothers, although their interactions with their mothers in social groups were comparable to those of controls. Once subjects were weaned at 6 months (Bauman, Lavenex, Mason, Capitanio, & Amaral, 2004b), social behavior was evaluated in the same social groups without the mothers present but with the adult male and novel female that were part of the group. Contrary to predictions, amygdala-lesioned animals were able to generate all social behaviors. In fact, they generated *more* communicative social signals than the unoperated controls. Interestingly, they generated more "fear" and submission signals, as well as more affiliation signals. This was despite receiving fewer affiliative gestures (e.g., lipsmack, present groom, present mount, contact, proximity) from control monkeys. While amygdala-lesioned animals did groom their peers, they did so less than control animals. When animals were tested to evaluate whether they had a preference for their mother, amygdala-lesioned animals were less distressed than controls when initially separated from their mothers and did not evidence a clear preference for their mothers (Bauman et al., 2004b). While they generally approached the mother first, before the novel female, they did not spend significantly more time with the mother. Our interpretation of this outcome was not that the infants had failed to develop an attachment for their mothers but rather that the novel environment was not perceived to be as threatening for the amygdala-lesioned neonates and they therefore did not seek the comfort of their mothers. Evidence for this came from the fact that amygdala-lesioned infants emitted fewer coos and other anxiety-related vocalizations. Taken together, these results suggest that the social behavior repertoire was largely intact following early damage to the amygdala, although the regulation of some social behaviors appeared to be subtly altered.

At 1.5–2.0 years of age, we evaluated the animals' social behaviors in their groups, both with and without the adult male and female (Bliss-Moreau, Moadab, Bauman, & Amaral, 2013; Bauman, Toscano, Mason, Lavenex, & Amaral, 2006). Again, amygdala-lesioned animals generated the same species-typical social behaviors as control animals. At this time point, we observed subtle differences in regulation of social behaviors. For example, when in the social group with the adult males and females, amygdala-lesioned animals still groomed others less frequently (Bliss-Moreau et al., 2013). Additionally, they spent less time sitting near and interacting with other monkeys than did controls (Bliss-Moreau et al., 2013). Amygdala-lesioned animals also initiated aggressive behaviors less frequently than controls (Bliss-Moreau et al., 2013). When the adult animals were temporarily removed from the social groups in order to evaluate the subjects' dominance hierarchy (Bauman et al., 2006), amygdala-lesioned animals displaced animals less frequently, were less agonistic, and generated more submission signals. These observed behaviors, in concert with behaviors observed on a food access task, led to the conclusion that as a group, amygdala-lesioned animals were lowest ranking (Bauman et al., 2006).

At 4 years of age, the female subjects were relocated outdoors into groups with novel female peers (i.e., not the animals from their social groups) and a single adult male (Moadab, Bliss-Moreau, Bauman, & Amaral, submitted). Amygdala-lesioned animals spent less time in close social interactions with the male, including less contact time and grooming, and directed fewer affiliative signals toward him. As in previous reports, they generated fewer agonistic behaviors with their female peers. Behaviors directed by the male and female peers toward the amygdala-lesioned animals also differed from those directed toward the controls. Males generated fewer affiliative signals and fewer consortship behaviors toward the amygdala-lesioned animals. Peers directed more agonistic behaviors toward them.

Our choice to house the female subjects with an adult, nonrelated male was made largely with an eye toward eventually being able to study how early damage to the amygdala might influence maternal behavior. We were particularly interested in the idea that early amygdala damage might disrupt maternal behavior, because previous experimental testing had demonstrated that the amygdala-lesioned subjects were significantly less interested in other females' babies than were control animals (Toscano, Bauman, Mason, & Amaral, 2009). As is typical for first-time pregnancies, there were many complications, and we were unable to carry out the full experiment. But we did observe that amygdala-lesioned animals became pregnant significantly later than did their peers (Moadab et al., submitted). It is likely that the altered behavior with the male and the late conception dates of the amygdala-lesioned females were driven by variation in hormonal cycling and/or the amygdala-lesioned animals' dominance status (as suggested by Wallen, 1990; see Bachevalier et al., Chapter 7, this volume). This raised the possibility that early damage to the amygdala had a direct effect on hormonal cycling and the timing of sexual maturity, which in turn influenced behavior with the male.

Taken together, these effects suggest that early amygdala damage does not eliminate the social behavior repertoire but does subtly compromise the regulation of social behavior in a few domains. Some behavioral differences remained stable over time. Across contexts with familiar social interaction partners, amygdala-lesioned animals were generally less social, although only in terms of grooming. They were less agonistic which was likely related to their low social ranks. Other behavioral patterns changed over time. Early in development, amygdala-lesioned animals, compared to controls, generated more frequent social signals than controls, but later in development they generated less frequent social signals. One possible explanation is that since the amygdala-lesioned animals' heightened early social signaling was not reciprocated by their peers, it was extinguished as they matured. At the very least, it appears that the motivation to generate social signals decreased as the animals aged.

Social Behavior with Familiar Interaction Partners, One-on-One

In addition to evaluating the subjects' social behavior while with a group of familiar animals, we also evaluated their social behavior while interacting with one other familiar animal (i.e., in a "dyad"). Again, as in the observations with social groups, amygdala-lesioned animals' social behavior repertoires were essentially intact in this setting. At 6 and 9 months (Bauman et al., 2004b) amygdala-lesioned animals generated significantly more social signals than controls when tested in dyads with familiar peers. This included signals indicative of both affiliation (e.g., cooing, grunting, following) and those indicative of "fear" or submission (e.g., silent bared teeth, screaming, fleeing). Their frequency and duration of physical contact was less frequent at 9 months despite this increased social signaling. At 2.5 years of age (Bliss-Moreau et al., 2013), the heightened affiliative signaling persisted, but there was no evidence of continued heightened "fear" or submission signaling. Consistent with the evaluation at 9 months suggesting that amygdala-lesioned animals spent less time in close social interactions (i.e., in contact), subjects spent more time in close social interactions when paired with control animals as compared to amygdala-lesioned animals.

These subtle, lesion-based differences in the amount of time spent in close social states persisted into adulthood (Moadab, Bliss-Moreau, & Amaral, 2015). We evaluated subjects' social behavior with monkeys with whom they lived in standard-size primate caging when they were approximately 7 years of age. Amygdala-lesioned animals groomed their partners for shorter durations of time. Despite these being their primary social relationships, amygdala-lesioned animals had significantly more frequent occurrences of stress-related behaviors such as yawning and scratching.

On the whole, amygdala-lesioned animals' behavior changed across development when interacting with familiar social partners in a one-on-one setting. Across their entire lives, amygdala-lesioned animals were able to generate species-typical social behavior. Early in development, amygdala-lesioned animals generated more social signals than controls of both the affiliative and submissive varieties. As they aged, these effects dissipated, such that there were no differences in either affiliative or submissive signaling as adults. Heighted "fear" or submission signaling stabilized first, with heightened affiliative signaling persisting through the 2.5-year evaluation. One consistent pattern of effects across all time points is that amygdala-lesioned animals physically explored their environments less frequently than did controls.

Social Behavior with Unfamiliar Interaction Partners, One-on-One

We evaluated subjects' social behavior with unfamiliar interaction partners in one-on-one settings at three time points: 1 year, 2.5 years, and 8.5 years. Evidence of amygdala-lesioned animals' intact social behavior repertoires was evident in these interaction contexts as well. Again, subtle differences in the execution of some classes of behavior were observed at the early time point. At 1 year (Bauman et al., 2004b) and 2.5 years of age (Bliss-Moreau et al., 2013), subjects interacted with other subjects that they did not know. At 1 year of age (Bauman et al., 2004b), amygdala-lesioned animals were groomed for longer durations of time than controls, although they themselves did not initiate longer social interactions than their peers. As in other contexts at a similar developmental time point, amygdala-lesioned animals had heightened affiliative signaling and heightened "fear" or submission signaling and were less agonistic compared to controls.

By 2.5 years of age (Bliss-Moreau et al., 2013) patterns of behaviors had changed. At this developmental time point, when interacting with other novel peers, amygdala-lesioned animals spent more time out of social states and disengaged from their environments than did controls. There were no differences in affiliative or submissive signaling, as observed at earlier time points. The only other behavioral difference that persisted is that amygdala-lesioned animals generated fewer agonistic behaviors than did controls.

Our final social evaluation of this group occurred when they were, on average, 8.5 years of age (Bliss-Moreau, Moadab, Santistevan, & Amaral, submitted). In this experiment, subjects met other monkeys, one-on-one. The other monkeys were two female and two male novel, age-matched animals from the CNPRC colony. Meetings occurred in two conditions—when animals were separated by a metal grill and when they were free to interact physically with each other. At the onset of this series of experiments, we had predicted that the social behavior of the neonatally lesioned animals would be far more impaired than that of animals lesioned as adults. But actually we observed very few notable, lesion-based differences. When separated by a metal grill, amygdala-lesioned males spent more time engaging in nonsocial behaviors than did control males. In the same experimental condition, amygdala-lesioned females generated more agonistic behaviors with male interaction partners than did control females. When allowed to interact freely, rates and durations of social behavior generated by the subjects did not differ between amygdala-lesioned and control animals. The only lesion-based differences related to the sequencing of behaviors. When subjects initiated agonistic behaviors toward their interaction partners, amygdala-lesioned animals, compared to controls, more frequently initiated avoidant behaviors or stereotypies. Similarly, when interaction partners instigated agonistic behaviors toward subjects, amygdala-lesioned animals were equally likely to respond with avoidant, engaging, or stereotypic behaviors, while control animals were more likely to respond with engaging behaviors.

The findings across three social behavioral evaluations with novel partners suggest that lesion-related differences in social behavior change over time but are fairly subtle. Early in development, amygdala-lesioned animals had heightened affiliative and submission signaling and were less agonistic. Differences in agonistic behavior persisted until 2.5 years but not beyond that point. No other social behavior differences were consistent across time. In adulthood, evaluation of the frequency and duration of social behaviors indicated that there were essentially no gross-level behavioral differences. That being said, when the sequencing of behaviors was considered, amygdala-lesioned animals did differ subtly from controls. The one lesion-based behavioral difference that was consistent across time (and contexts) is that amygdala-lesioned animals physically explored their environments significantly less frequently than did controls.

Consistency across Development or Context?

As a whole, our findings suggest that early damage to the amygdala does not alter an animal's social behavior repertoire per se (i.e., the ability to generate species-typical social behaviors), but it may alter its regulation in subtle ways. Few lesion-based differences were consistent across contexts within developmental time points, and very few lesion-based differences remained consistent across developmental time. For example, amygdala-lesioned animals generated more affiliative and submissive signals than control animals when meeting familiar and unfamiliar social interaction partners around 1 year of age (although not when tested in social groups). This propensity for increased signaling was not maintained into adulthood. In fact, in adulthood, when considering the rates and durations of social behaviors individually, there were essentially no lesion-based differences. The only difference between groups was in the sequencing of behaviors. Arguably, the most consistent finding was that amygdala-lesioned animals physically explored their environments less frequently than did control animals, though the reason for this was not clear.

The Development of Stimulus-Driven and Directed Affective Behavior

One of the now "classic" findings is that adult animals with amygdala damage do not respond to novelty and threat in the same way that neurologically intact animals do. While controls are wary of novel stimuli and stimuli representing potential threat, animals with amygdala lesions have no such wariness (Aggleton & Passingham, 1981; Zola-Morgan, Squire, Alverez-Royo, & Clower, 1991; Meunier et al., 1999; Stefanacci, Clark, & Zola, 2003; Izquierdo, Suda, & Murray, 2005; Mason et al., 2006; Machado, Kazama, & Bachevalier, 2009; Chudasama, Izquierdo, & Murray, 2009). They readily approach and interact with such objects and retrieve food from their proximity. Findings like these have led many to conclude that the amygdala plays a central role in determining the threat potential of a stimulus. In this view, novel objects have the potential to be threatening because they are unknown. In the prototypical "object responsiveness" task, objects are placed either in the animal's cage or on a platform in front of the animal (sometimes testing is carried out in a Wisconsin General Testing Apparatus) and typically co-presented with a desired food item. The rate and speed with which the food item is retrieved is thought to index the affective potency of the object—if food is retrieved quickly then the object is not so salient or potent. If food is retrieved slowly, then the object is thought to be potent because its presence deters normal food retrieval behavior.

Over the course of their lives, we tested animals in our cohort three times on a standard object responsiveness task (e.g., one that includes objects such as toy snakes)—at 9, 18, and 36 months of age. Additionally, we had two other test points at which we evaluated their responsivity to other varieties of affective stimuli. Animals were tested at ~8 years of age on their responsiveness to videos with affective content. At ~10 years of age, we evaluated their responses to potent sensory stimuli (e.g., startle tone; air puff to the cheek) during an associative learning task. Results were remarkably consistent across test points—amygdala-lesioned animals' responses to the stimuli were blunted compared to those of control animals.

At 9 and 18 months of age, amygdala-lesioned and control animals completed an object responsiveness task with two phases (Bliss-Moreau, Toscano, Bauman, Mason, & Amaral, 2010). During the first phase, animals were given 60 seconds to interact with a series of novel objects presented one at a time. No food was presented with the object. At both time points, amygdala-lesioned animals physically explored the novel objects by touching them the most. At 9 months of age, amygdala-lesioned animals were fastest to explore novel objects and explored them more frequently and for longer periods than did control animals. At 18 months of age, amygdala-lesioned animals explored objects significantly faster and for significantly longer durations than did control animals.

At 9, 18, and 36 months (Bliss-Moreau et al., 2010; Bliss-Moreau, Toscano, Bauman, Mason, & Amaral, 2011), we tested the neonatally lesioned animals with salient objects and concurrently presented food. These trials were 30 seconds in length. We used different objects at the three time points, but all time points included objects thought to engender threat responding (including toy snakes). In most cases, objects were presented in forms that varied in physical complexity—at one extreme, "complex" objects were presented in their normal form (e.g., a green toy snake, a brown stuffed bear), and at the other extreme, "simple" objects mimicked the shape and color of the complex object but were simplified either as solid wooden blocks or by masking features of the complex object. Animals were presented with stationary objects at all three time points; the 18-month evaluation included moving objects as well. A desired food treat was presented in front of the object. Food retrieval behavior and the propensity for animals physically to explore the objects were recorded. At all time points, amygdala-lesioned animals explored objects more frequently, earlier, and for longer durations than did controls animals. There were no lesion-based food retrieval differences at 9 months of age, but differences did emerge across development. At 18 months of age, there were no lesion-based food retrieval differences when food was presented with stationary objects. Amygdala-lesioned animals tended to retrieve food faster than controls in the presence of moving objects, suggesting that they were less perturbed by the moving objects than were controls. At 36 months of age, amygdala-lesioned animals retrieved food faster and more frequently in the presence of salient objects than did controls.

Patterns of behavior after early amygdala damage (Bliss-Moreau et al., 2010; Bliss-Moreau et al., 2011) were essentially the same as those reported in the adult amygdala lesion literature (Aggleton & Passingham, 1981; Zola-Morgan et al., 1991; Meunier et al., 1999; Stefanacci et al., 2003; Izquierdo et al., 2005; Mason et al., 2006; Machado et al., 2009; Chudasama et al., 2009). Early damage to the amygdala, like damage that occurs later in development, appears to disrupt the ability to assess the value of potent object stimuli. These effects extend beyond objects typically thought to engender threat (e.g., toy snakes) to both novel and moving objects. Across all three time points, the propensity to explore objects differed significantly between controls and amygdala-lesioned animals. As development proceeded, the propensity to retrieve concurrently presented food also was indicative of lesions.

Testing with salient objects left open two questions about the effect of early amygdala damage on responding to important environmental stimuli. Affective stimuli fall along a continuum that ranges from those that act directly on the nervous system in the absence of prior learning (e.g., very loud sounds, bright lights, noxious fumes; typically used as unconditioned stimuli [US] in learning experiments) and those that require learning to have value (typically used as conditioned stimuli [CS] in learning experiments). The stimuli used in classic object responsiveness tasks (e.g., snakes, spiders) arguably fall somewhere in the middle of that continuum. While some thinkers have argued that primates innately are biologically hardwired to respond robustly to snakes (Isbell, 2009), others have argued that it is not the response to snakes itself that is hardwired but rather the potential for quick learning about snakes (and other stimuli that represent potential threat; i.e., "prepared" stimuli) (Öhman, 2001; Mineka & Öhman, 2002). Our three-object responsiveness tests demonstrated that early amygdala damage perturbed responding to these sorts of stimuli. But what of the stimuli at either extreme? What of stimuli whose value must be learned or have their meaning constructed? For example, the meaning of social displays are thought to be learned (or constructed) through experience. Animals reared without social access do not generate or execute social behaviors in context-appropriate ways, which indicates that they do not know their normative meanings (Harlow, Dodsworth, & Harlow, 1965; Harlow & Suomi, 1971; Suomi & Harlow, 1972). On the other extreme, stimuli typically used as unconditioned stimuli generate responses in animals without any prior experience with them. Would early damage to the amygdala blunt responding to these types of stimuli as well?

When the animals were on average 7¾ years of age, we evaluated their behavioral responses to video clips of stimuli with constructed meaning (Bliss-Moreau, Bauman, & Amaral, 2011). Animals watched a series of videos that varied in affective and social content. Videos varied by affective content insofar as they depicted content thought to be indicative of negative, positive, and neutral valence. Control videos showed no social content (no other monkeys), whereas both classes of social videos showed other monkeys. In the first class of social videos, which we refer to as "socially nonengaging," monkeys were depicted interacting with other monkeys at a distance. These included videos of monkeys fighting (negative affective content), monkeys grooming (positive affective content) and monkeys sitting together (neutral affective content). In the second class of social videos, which we refer to as "socially engaging," monkeys were depicted making social displays to the video camera, so that it looked like they were trying to engage the subject. Videos were presented concurrently with a food reward, as in object responsiveness tasks.

Food retrieval did not differentiate lesion groups. All animals retrieved food fastest and most frequently on the control videos and slowest and least frequently on the socially engaging videos across all types of affective content. This is consistent with findings presented previously that the neonatally lesioned animals remain keenly attuned to social stimuli. Amygdala-lesioned and control animals did, however, differ in their behavioral response to the videos. Specifically, the number of socioaffective signals that subjects generated during videos varied significantly between lesion groups. We counted as socioaffective signals those that serve a social communication or affective expression purpose, including facial displays (e.g., lipsmack, silent bared teeth), vocalizations (e.g., coo, grunt) and communicative body postures (e.g., "present rump"). There were no lesion-based differences in the generation of any single socioaffective signal. However, there were differences when all socioaffective signals were considered together. Compared to control animals, amygdala-lesioned animals generated fewer socioaffective signals across all categories compared to controls. This blunted affective responsivity was driven by amygdala-lesioned animals' particularly compromised responding to videos with positive and negative content. In other words, early amygdala damage compromises responsivity to not only threat-related and novel objects but also to stimuli with constructed meaning (e.g., social signals, catcher's net). Of note, amygdala-lesioned animals, like controls, were most responsive to the most potent stimuli, indicating that although the magnitude of their response was blunted, their ability to detect which stimuli were most potent was not.

Our final test of the experimental group was an associative learning experiment (discussed in greater detail below; Bliss-Moreau & Amaral, submitted). As part of the experiment, animals were exposed to two types of stimuli that should engender responding in the absence of learning: loud bursts of white noise startle probes at different volumes and a 100-pounds-per square-inch (psi) air puff to the neck. Measuring startle magnitude during the presentation of these stimuli allowed us to evaluate whether early amygdala damage might blunt responsivity to potent stimuli that do not require learning to generate a response. Amygdala-lesioned animals had significantly smaller magnitude startles across all startle probes ranging from 80 to 115 decibels. Both amygdala-lesioned and control animals startled more in response to louder noises, indicating that their responses were calibrated to the magnitude of the stimuli. Similarly, amygdala-lesioned animals startled to the air puff to the neck significantly less than did controls. This effect was particularly robust early in testing—control animals became less responsive to the US over 8 days of testing, while amygdala-lesioned animals' level of responding was consistent across the test days. Consistent with previous findings, amygdala-lesioned animals showed blunted responsivity to the US. As in the video responsiveness task (discussed earlier), amygdala-lesioned animals, like controls, were most responsive to the most potent stimuli.

Two themes emerge from the discrete affective stimulus testing that we performed across the subjects' developmental trajectories. Amygdala-lesioned animals consistently showed blunted responding to affective stimuli. In some cases this took the form of increased behavior (more exploration of objects); in other cases, this took the form of reduced behavior (fewer socioaffective signals). In some, but not all cases, food retrieval was an indicator of altered responsivity. All of these responses are consistent with decreased detection or response to a threatening stimulus. Across all experiments, we were also able to evaluate whether early amygdala damage influenced response calibration to stimulus magnitude. In the object responsiveness tasks, stimuli were presented in forms ranging from simple to complex. At 9 and 18 months of age, all animals were slower to retrieve food during complex as compared to simple objects, suggesting that they were processing the difference in stimulus complexity and therefore potency. At 36 months of age, control animals showed a complexity effect, but amygdala-lesioned animals did not. They retrieved food at the same speed and rate across objects. Testing in adulthood supported the idea that amygdala-lesioned animals' calibration was based on stimulus intensity. In the video task, all animals were significantly more responsive to the most potent stimuli (the socially engaging stimuli) compared to other stimuli. Furthermore, all animals startled more to the loudest noises than to the softest ones, even though amygdala-lesioned animals were substantially blunted.

Consistent across Development or Context?

Taken together, these data suggest that early damage to the amygdala blunts responding to a whole host of affective stimuli—prepared stimuli, socially constructed stimuli, and those stimuli that act on the nervous system without any prior learning. These findings mirror those from the adult nonhuman animal literature, which consistently demonstrates that amygdala-lesioned animals have blunted responding. These findings suggest that the amygdala plays a putative role in affective perceiving and/or generating behavioral responses to potent affective stimuli—one that cannot be compensated for during neural development via plasticity mechanisms.

Associative Learning

Decades of research in nonhuman animals and humans have demonstrated a role for the amygdala in associative learning (often called "classical" or "fear conditioning"; for reviews, see Gallagher & Holland, 1994; Maren, 2001). Associative learning occurs when a neutral stimulus (CS) acquires affective meaning by being presented in proximity (either temporal or spatial) with an affectively potent stimulus (US). By being presented together, the CS comes to predict the occurrence of the US and itself acquires the ability to generate an affective response. In that way, the CS is said to acquire affective meaning. Although learning occurs via co-occurrence of neutral and potent stimuli, methods to measure learning vary. One method capitalizes on a phenomenon known as "potentiated startle." Previous research has demonstrated that if an affective stimulus is presented immediately prior to a startle stimulus, startle magnitude will be greater than if the startle stimulus was presented alone (for a review, see Davis, 1989). This effect is commonly referred to as "fear"-potentiated startle, because the experience of fear is thought to prepare the individual to act, thus potentiating behavior, such as startle, that leads to escape (Davis, 1989; Lang, Bradley, & Cuthbert, 1990; but see Yartz & Hawk, 2002). Whereas negative stimuli *potentiate* or increase startle, positive stimuli are thought either to have no effect or actually to reduce startle (Lang et al., 1990). The ability for an affective stimulus to increase startle magnitude is referred to as "potentiated startle." In the context of learning experiments, the CS's ability to potentiate startle should be greater after learning has occurred than before it has occurred. The extent to which the CS can potentiate startle after learning is an index of the magnitude of learning.

Decades of research in rodent models demonstrated that the amygdala is required for associative learning to occur and to be measured via potentiated startle (see Maren, 2001, for a review). In a series of studies with rhesus macaques with damage to the amygdala that occurred during adulthood, we demonstrated that this was true in nonhuman primates as well. Rhesus monkeys who sustained damage to the amygdala as adults were unable to learn via associative means (Antoniadis, Winslow, Davis, & Amaral, 2007). Whereas control monkeys demonstrated potentiated startle after a learning phase that paired the CS (a light or tone) with a US (a 100-psi air puff to the neck), amygdala-lesioned animals' startle was not potentiated, which indicates that learning did not occur (Antoniadis et al., 2007). Interestingly, whereas amygdala damage prevented learning, it did not prevent expression of learning; that is, animals that completed the learning phase prior to receiving amygdala lesions still demonstrated potentiated startle (Antoniadis et al., 2007) but were unable to learn new CS–US associations (Antoniadis, Winslow, Davis, & Amaral, 2009). Given the robustness of these amygdala-related learning effects, we reasoned that affective learning would be a good litmus test of amygdala-related functions in animals that received early damage.

Around 10 years of age, the neonatally amygdala-lesioned animals and control animals underwent potentiated startle testing (Bliss-Moreau & Amaral, submitted). The testing included three phases (as in Antoniadis et al., 2007). During the first phase, animals were presented with 40 millisecond bursts of white noise (startle probes) at five different volumes. Animals then completed a second phase during which the CS (a light presented overhead) was presented before a startle probe on multiple trials. This allowed us to index the CS's ability to potentiate startle prior to learning. In a third phase, the CS was paired on a number of occasions with a 100-psi air puff to the neck. The CS was also presented prior to the startle stimulus (CS + startle trials), allowing us to index the CS's ability to potentiate startle following learning. If early amygdala damage prevented learning as we expected, then the amygdala-lesioned animals' magnitude of startle would be the same on CS + startle trials prior to and following learning, whereas the control animals would have a greater startle on the CS + startle trials following learning than prior to learning.

As expected, control animals demonstrated learning. Their startle magnitude was significantly greater on CS + startle trials following learning than prior to learning. Surprisingly, the pattern of response was identical for the amygdala-lesioned animals. Their startle magnitude was significantly greater on CS + startle trials following learning as compared with those that preceded learning. In other words, early amygdala damage did not prevent associative learning or the expression of that learning. In the context of evidence collected with animals with amygdala-damage in adulthood, these findings suggest that neural development and brain plasticity were able to shift a putative function of the amygdala to another neural structure. Similar plasticity had previously been observed in our group relative to the function of the hippocampus. While adult animals with hippocampus damage were unable to use spatial relational cues to navigate their physical environments (Banta Lavenex, Amaral, & Lavenex, 2006), animals with early hippocampus damage were able to use such cues to navigate just as well as control animals (Lavenex, Banta Lavenex, & Amaral, 2007).

Behavioral Abnormalities

Over the 12 years of the project, the amygdala-lesioned animals gained a reputation around the CNPRC for being a bit odd. We believe that oddness was related to a few core features: low social behavior with their pair mates (discussed earlier; Moadab et al., 2015); low interest in delicious treats (e.g., the juice and fruit popsicles given out as part of standard enrichment at the CNPRC; blunted responsivity to these treats inspired Bliss-Moreau, Bauman, & Amaral, 2011); and higher levels of behavioral stereotypies (as in Bauman, Toscano, Babineau, Mason, & Amaral, 2008; Bliss-Moreau et al., 2014; Moadab et al., 2015).

Over the course of their lives, many of the experimental animals developed behavioral stereotypies. These included both whole-body stereotypies (e.g., pacing) and self-directed stereotypies (e.g., self-biting) (see Novak, 2003, for a review of stereotypy types). Stereotypies began to emerge between 1 and 2.5 years of age (Bauman, Toscano, et al., 2008). Compared to controls, amygdala-lesioned animals produced more frequent stereotypies. The number of animals that engaged in stereotypic behavior and the rates of these stereotypies increased with time (as in Moadab et al., 2013, submitted; Bliss-Moreau et al., submitted). When controls produced stereotypic behaviors, they were largely whole-body stereotypies, which are thought to be behavioral adaptations that replace species-typical motoric behaviors when animals live in small spaces (Novak, 2003). Amygdala-lesioned animals, however, engaged in more frequent self-directed stereotypies. The development of self-directed stereotypies is particularly problematic, because animals that engage in high levels of self-directed stereotypies are at risk for developing self-injurious behavior and subsequent wounding (Lutz et al., 2003). These self-directed and self-injurious behaviors are thought to be maladaptive means of down-regulating physiological arousal (Novak, 2003).

Supporting the idea that the amygdala-lesioned animals had maladaptive regulation of arousal are a number of anecdotal observations. First, two of the amygdala-lesioned animals (one female and one male) developed emesis (vomiting) in adulthood (around 7–8 years of age). Exhaustive diagnostic testing revealed no medical cause of the vomiting, suggesting a central nervous system mechanism. We treated the first animal, a female with fairly frequent episodes of vomiting, with Cerenia (maripoitant citrate; Pfizer, New York, NY), which was successful at preventing frequent emesis. Ultimately, however, we elected to euthanize this animal because of complicating medical factors. When the second animal developed less frequent emesis soon thereafter, we immediately began treatment with Cerenia and were able to maintain his health, and eliminate his vomiting, for the duration of the project.

Individual amygdala-lesioned animals also had other odd potentially arousal-related behaviors. One female had periods during adulthood during which she appeared to be narcoleptic. She was frequently observed to fall asleep in the middle of grooming her pair mate—her hands still positioned on his back—only to wake a few seconds or minutes later and pick up where she had left off. While in social group housing, she was often observed to play with a single stick or rock for hours, generating the same repetitive motion over and over again. Another female could execute the appropriate motion required for grooming but would often groom the air a few centimeters off of her pair mate's back (her adaptive pair mate would simply move backwards a bit so that she would actually groom him). This same animal would often stick her fingers in her caging, pretending to be stuck, potentially a self-stimulating behavior.

Taken together, the documented stereotypies and the anecdotal behavioral abnormalities point to the amygdala-lesioned animals being different from the controls. While each individual behavior itself might not be striking, the combination of behaviors was. Many of our monkey-naive trainees were able to determine accurately what animal had an early amygdala-lesion based on limited observations of them. When asked how they identified the animals, they would indicate that the amygdala-lesioned animals were just "different." These anecdotal observations suggest that the formal experimental observations we made throughout the lifespans of this group of animals may not have been adequately sensitive to identify more subtle personality or behavioral alterations. Of course, it is also true that there are substantial individual differences in nonhuman primate behavior. Thus, behavioral observations are complicated by the confound of lesion-induced alterations on different genetic backgrounds.

Plasticity and the Interpretation of Amygdala Lesions

When the neonatal lesion study was initiated in 2001, there was already substantial neurobiological evidence for functional brain plasticity. Somatosensory maps were shown to be reconfigurable based on increased use of digits or digit amputation in nonhuman primates even in adult animals (Jenkins, Merzenich, & Recanzone, 1990; Merzenich et al., 1984). The groundbreaking research of Hubel and Weisel demonstrated that there is a competitive process in early development of the primary visual cortex that depends on appropriate inputs from the left and right eyes (LeVay, Wiesel, & Hubel, 1980). Removing input from one eye led to a morphological alteration of the inputs from the opposite eye into the visual cortex. And, plasticity of this type was not limited to nonhuman animals. A large literature emerged that humans born with the loss of one sensation had cortical maps that saw the colonization of unused cortex by intact sensory modalities (Neville & Bavelier, 2002). While the extent of structural reorganization following insult to the nervous system is still a matter of debate and research (Perederiy & Westbrook, 2013; Starkey & Schwab, 2014), it is clear that the injured brain attempts to establish a compensatory pattern of connectivity and improvises a modified nervous system that interacts as effectively as possible with the environment in which it finds itself.

When we initiated the neonatal lesion study, we hypothesized that animals devoid of an amygdala from near birth would be far more impaired in socioemotional behavior as adults than an animal that received an amygdala lesion as an adult. But, as we have documented here, many of the behavioral alterations in the neonatally lesioned animals were actually more subtle than those observed in the animals with lesions in adulthood.

Our speculation now is that a lifetime of experience has sculpted the nervous system of the neonatally lesioned animals to respond as appropriately as possible to the environment in which they lived. An early positron emission tomography study (Machado et al., 2008b) demonstrated that, relative to controls, amygdala-lesioned animals displayed hypometabolism in three frontal lobe regions, as well as in the neostriatum and hippocampus. Hypermetabolism was also evident in the cerebellum of amygdala-lesioned animals. We are currently analyzing high-resolution magnetic resonance images of the brains of the neonatally lesioned animals acquired prior to the end of the study, as well as evaluating histological preparations. All point to the same conclusion that the early lesion has led to substantial reorganization of the nervous system of these animals. Thus, it is not surprising that the behavioral alterations observed in these animals changed during development. It is interesting that some behavioral alterations, such as responses to objects, persisted throughout life, whereas other "amygdala-based" behavioral functions, such as associative learning, were preserved.

Conclusions

With the long view on our developmental study, we identify a few take-home messages. First, early amygdala damage does not eliminate social behavior or even dramatically alter it. Animals with early amygdala damage were able to execute species-typical behaviors from the earliest point of evaluation. Although there were subtle differences that emerged over the course of development, by the final evaluation point, amygdala-lesioned animals behaved essentially like controls during formal observations. This stands in stark contrast to the pattern of results observed with adult animals with amygdala damage that occurred during adulthood. Second, early amygdala damage does alter responding to affective stimuli, much in the way we would expect based on the adult literature. These findings largely parallel those from a study by Bachevalier and colleagues (Chapter 7, this volume), in which animals with early damage to the amygdala were raised in large, seminaturalistic social groups.

A third point of note is that the context in which behaviors are evaluated matters. One of the consistent findings across developmental time points was that animals with early amygdala damage were less exploratory in social contexts but more exploratory in tests with affective stimuli. We interpret the decreased exploration during social experiences to be the result largely of the animals "tuning out" during social evaluations, perhaps suggesting altered attentional processing. In contrast, the heightened exploration during testing with affective stimuli can be interpreted as failure to evaluate or attend properly or accurately to the significance of the stimuli with which they were presented. Fourth, neurodevelopment and inherent neural plasticity allow for recovery of some, but not all, functions of the amygdala. While the social behavior of animals with early amygdala damage normalized over development (became more like that of control animals over time) and early damage did not preclude associative learning, early amygdala damage permanently blunted responding to affective stimuli such as threat-engendering objects and social videos. This suggests that there has been a selective redistribution of functions to other brain structures. It is our hope that ongoing histological analyses will help us to identify candidate neural regions that were altered as a result of development following early damage, thus spurring future study. Related to this point, a fifth matter of note is that the impact of early neural damage changes over development. At early time points, amygdala-lesioned animals' behavior was objectively different from age-matched control animals. At later time points, the differences in frequencies and durations of social behaviors between amygdala-lesioned and control animals all but disappeared. Without a decade of study, we would not have seen this pattern of effects.

The fact that we were able to create early amygdala damage and study the same cohort of animals over a period of more than a decade speaks to the incredible potential power of nonhuman primate models. Preliminary neuroanatomical analyses suggest that early damage to the amygdala causes changes to cortical structures that are either absent or underdeveloped in mice and rats. These findings point to the importance of nonhuman primate models for understanding human brain function. The use of nonhuman primates in biobehavioral and neuroscience research has dramatically increased our knowledge of how primate systems function and develop in ways that would be untenable if we were to study only humans (Phillips et al., 2014). A fundamental goal of studies such as these is that they contribute to an understanding of the extent of brain plasticity leading to recovery of function. Once understood, our hope is that these forces can be controlled and enhanced in order to promote a better quality of life for individuals with neurodevelopmental disorders.

ACKNOWLEDGMENTS

This research was supported by funding from the National Institute of Mental Health (Grant No. R37MH57502 to David G. Amaral), and by the base grant of the CNPRC (No. RR00169). Eliza Bliss-Moreau was supported by Grant No. K99MH10138 during preparation of this chapter. This work was also supported through the Early Experience and Brain Development Network of the MacArthur Foundation. We thank the veterinary and husbandry staff of the CNPRC for excellent care of the animal subjects. We thank Dr. Pierre Lavenex, Jeffrey Bennett, and Pamela Tennant for assistance with surgical procedures.

REFERENCES

Aggleton, J. P., & Passingham, R. E. (1981). Syndrome produced by lesions of the amygdala in monkeys (*Macaca mulatta*). *Journal of Comparative and Physiological Psychology, 95*, 961–977.

Altmann, J. (1974). Observational study of behavior: Sampling methods. *Behavior, 49*, 227–267.

Amaral, D. G., & Price, J. L. (1984). Amygdalo-cortical projections in the monkey (*Macaca fascicularis*). *Journal of Comparative Neurology, 230*, 465–496.

Amaral, D. G., Price, J. L., Pitkänen, A., & Carmichael, S. T. (1992). Anatomical organization of teh primate amygdaloid complex. In J. Aggleton (Ed.), *The amygdala: Neurobiological aspects of emotion, memory and mental dysfunction* (pp. 1–66). Wilmington, DE: Wiley-Liss.

Antoniadis, E. A., Winslow, J. T., Davis, M., & Amaral D. G. (2007). Role of the primate amygdala in fear-potentiated startle: Effects of chronic lesions in the rhesus monkey. *Journal of Neuroscience, 27*, 7386–7396.

Antoniadis, E. A., Winslow, J. T., Davis, M., & Amaral D. G. (2009). The nonhuman primate amygdala is necessary for the acquisition but not the retention of fear-potentiated startle. *Biological Psychiatry, 65*, 241–248.

Bachevalier, J. (1994). Medial temporal lobe structures and autism: A review of clinical and experimental findings. *Neuropsychologia, 32*, 627–648.

Banta Lavenex, P., Amaral, D. G., & Lavenex, P. (2006). Hippocampal lesion prevents spatial relational learning in adult macaque monkeys. *Journal of Neuroscience, 26*, 4546–4558.

Bauman, M. D., & Amaral, D. G. (2008). Nonhuman primate models of autism. In D. Amaral, D. Dawson, & G. Geschwind (Eds.), *Autism spectrum disorders* (pp. 963–980). New York: Oxford University Press.

Bauman, M. D., Lavenex, P., Mason, W. A., Capitanio, J. P., & Amaral, D. G. (2004a). The development of mother–infant interactions after neonatal amygdala lesions in rhesus monkeys. *Journal of Neuroscience, 24*, 711–721.

Bauman, M. D., Lavenex, P., Mason, W. A., Capitanio, J. P., & Amaral, D. G. (2004b). The development of social behavior following neonatal amygdala lesions in rhesus monkeys. *Journal of Cognitive Neuroscience, 16*, 1388–1411.

Bauman, M. D., Toscano, J. E., Mason, W. A., Lavenex, P., & Amaral, D. G. (2006). The expression of social dominance following neonatal lesions of the amygdala or hippocampus in rhesus Monkeys (*Macaca mulatta*). *Behavioral Neuroscience, 120*, 749–760.

Bauman, M. D., Toscano, J. E., Babineau, B. A., Mason, W. A., & Amaral, D. G. (2008). Emergence of stereotypies in juvenile monkeys (*Macaca mulatta*) with neonatal amygdala or hippocampus lesions. *Behavioral Neuroscience, 122*, 1005–1015.

Bellanca, R. U., & Crockett, C. M. (2002). Factors predicting increased incidence of abnormal behavior in male pigtailed macaques. *American Journal of Primatology, 58*, 57–69.

Berman, C. I. (1980). Mother–infant relationships among free-ranging rhesus monkeys on Cayo Santiago: A comparison with captive pairs. *Animal Behaviour, 28*, 860–873.

Bliss-Moreau, E., & Amaral, D. G. (2014). *Associative affective learning persists following early amygdala damage in nonhuman primates.* Manuscript in preparation.

Bliss-Moreau, E., Bauman, M. D., & Amaral, D. G. (2011). Neonatal amygdala lesions result in globally blunted adult affect in adult rhesus macaques. *Behavioral Neuroscience, 125,* 848–858.

Bliss-Moreau, E., Moadab, G., Bauman, M. D., & Amaral, D. G. (2013). The impact of early amygdala damage on juvenile rhesus macaque social behavior. *Journal of Cognitive Neuroscience, 25,* 2124–2140.

Bliss-Moreau, E., Moadab, G., Stanstitevan, A. C., & Amaral, D. G. (2014). *Adult social behavior with novel partners following neonatal amygdala or hippocampus damage.* Manuscript in preparation.

Bliss-Moreau, E., Toscano, J. E., Bauman, M. D., Mason, W. A., & Amaral, D. G. (2010). Neonatal amygdala or hippocampus lesions influence responsiveness to objects. *Developmental Psychobiology, 52,* 487–503.

Bliss-Moreau, E., Toscano, J. E., Bauman, M. D., Mason, W. A., & Amaral, D. G. (2011). Neonatal amygdala lesions alter responsiveness to objects in juvenile rhesus macaques. *Neuroscience, 178,* 132–132.

Brothers, L. (1990). The social brain: A project for integrating primate behavioral and neurophysiology in a new domain. *Concepts in Neuroscience, 1,* 27–51.

Capitanio, J. P., Mendoza, S. P., Mason, W. A., Maninger, N. (2005). Rearing environment and hypothalamic–pituitary–adrenal regulation in young rhesus monkeys (*Macaca mulatta*). *Developmental Psychobiology, 46,* 318–330.

Champoux, M., Metz, B., & Suomi, S. J. (1991). Behavior of nursery/peer-reared and mother-reared rhesus monkeys from birth through 2 years. *Primates, 32,* 509–514.

Chudasama, Y., Izquierdo, A., & Murray, E. A. (2009). Distinct contributions of the amygdala and hippocampus to fear expression. *European Journal of Neuroscience, 30,* 2327–2337.

Davis, M. (1989). Neural systems involved in fear-potentiated startle. *Annals of the New York Academy of Sciences, 563,* 165–183.

Dicks, D., Myers, R. E., & Kling, A. (1969). Uncus and amygdala lesions: Effects on social behavior in the free-ranging rhesus monkey. *Science, 165,* 69–71.

Dukelow, W. R., & Whitehair, L. A. (1995). A brief history of the Regional Primate Centers. *Comparative Pathology Bulletin, 27,* 1–2.

Dunbar, R. I. M. (1998). The social brain hypothesis. *Evolutionary Anthropology, 6,* 178–190.

Emery, N. J., Capitanio, J. P., Mason, W. A., Machado, C. J., Mendoza, S. P., & Amaral, D. G. (2001). The effects of bilateral lesions of the amygdala on dyadic social interactions in rhesus monkeys (*Macaca mulatta*). *Behavioral Neuroscience, 115,* 515–544.

Ferrari, P. F., Paukner, A., Ionica, C., & Suomi, S. J. (2009). Reciprocal face-to-face communication between rhesus macaque mothers and their newborn infants. *Current Biology, 19,* 1768–1772.

Fooden, J. (2000). Systematic review of the rhesus macaque, *Macaca mulatta* (Zimmermann, 1780). *Fieldiana Zoology, 96,* 1–180.

Gallagher, M., & Holland, P. C. (1994). The amygdala complex: Multiple roles in associative learning and attention. *Proceedings of the National Academies of Sciences USA, 25,* 11771–11776.

Golub, M. S., Hogrefe, C. E., Widaman, K. F., & Capitanio, J. P. (2009). Iron deficiency anemia and affective response in rhesus monkey infants. *Developmental Psychobiology, 51,* 47–59.

Harlow, H. F., Dodsworth, R. O., & Harlow, M. K. (1965). Total social isolation in monkeys. *Proceedings of the National Academies of Sciences USA, 54,* 90–97.

Harlow, H. F., & Suomi, S. J. (1971). Social recovery by isolation-reared monkeys. *Proceedings of the National Academies of Sciences USA, 68,* 1534–1538.

Hinde, R. A., Rowell, T. E., & Spencer-Booth, Y. (1964). Behavior of socially living rhesus monkeys in their first six months. *Proceedings of the Zoological Society London, 143,* 609–649.

Hinde, R. A., & Spencer-Booth, Y. (1967). The behaviour of socially living rhesus monkeys in their first two and a half years. *Animal Behaviour, 15,* 169–196.

Isbell, L. A. (2009). *The fruit, the tree, and the serpent: Why we see so well.* Cambridge, MA: Harvard University Press.

Izquierdo, A., Suda, R. K., & Murray, E. A. (2005). Comparison of the effects of bilateral orbital prefrontal cortex lesions and amygdala lesions on emotional responses in rhesus monkeys. *Journal of Neuroscience, 25,* 8534–8542.

Jarrard, L. E.(1989). On the use of ibotenic acid to lesion selectively different components of the hippocampal formation. *Journal of Neuroscience Methods, 29,* 251–259.

Jenkins, W. M., Merzenich, M. M., & Recanzone, G. (1990). Neocortical representational dynamics in adult primates: Implications for neuropsychology. *Neuropsychologia, 28,* 573–584.

Kling, A. (1974). Differential effects of amygdalectomy in male and female non-human primates. *Archives of Sexual Behavior, 3,* 129–134.

Kling, A., & Cornell, R. (1971). Amygdalectomy and social behavior in the caged stump-tailed macaque (*Macaca speciosa*). *Folia Primatologica, 14,* 190–208.

Klüver, H., & Bucy, P. C. (1939). Preliminary analysis of functions of the temporal loves in monkeys. *Archives of Neurology and Psychiatry, 42,* 979–1000.

Lang, P. J., Bradley, M. M., & Cuthbert, B. N. (1990). Emotion, attention, and the startle reflex. *Psychological Review, 97,* 377–395.

Lavenex, P., Banta Lavenex, P., & Amaral, D. G. (2007). Spatial relational learning persists following neonatal lesions in macaque monkeys. *Nature Neuroscience, 10,* 234–239.

LeVay, S., Wiesel, T. N., & Hubel, D. H. (1980). The development of ocular dominance columns in normal and visually deprived monkeys. *Journal of Comparative Neurology, 191,* 1–51.

Lutz, C., Well, A., & Novak, M. (2003). Stereotypic and self-injurious behavior in rhesus macaques: A survey and retrospective analysis of environment and early experience. *American Journal of Primatology, 60,* 1–15.

Machado, C. J. (2013). Maternal influences on social and neural development in macaque monkeys. In K. B. H. Clancy, K. Hinde, & J. N. Rutherford (Eds.), *Building babies: Primate development in proximate and ultimate perspective* (pp. 259–279). New York: Springer.

Machado, C. J., Emery, N. J., Capitanio, J. P., Mason, W. A., Mendoza, S. P., & Amaral, D. G. (2008a). Bilateral neurotoxic amygdala lesions in Rhesus monkeys (*Macaca mulatta*): Consistent pattern of behavior across different social contexts. *Behavioral Neuroscience, 22*, 251–266.

Machado, C. J., Kazama, A. M., & Bachevalier, J. (2009). Impact of amygdala, orbital frontal, or hippocampal lesions on threat avoidance and emotional reactivity in nonhuman primates. *Emotion, 9*, 147–163.

Machado, C. J., Snyder, A. Z., Cherry, S. R., Lavenex, P., & Amaral, D. G. (2008b). Effects of neonatal amygdala or hippocampus lesions on resting brain metabolism in the macaque monkey: A microPET imagining study. *NeuroImage, 15*, 832–846.

Maren, S. (2001). Neurobiology of Pavlovian fear conditioning. *Annual Review of Neuroscience, 24*, 897–931.

Mason, W. A., Capitanio, J. P., Machado, C. J., Mendoza, S. P., & Amaral, D. G. (2006). Amygdalectomy and responsiveness to novelty in Rhesus monkeys (*Macaca mulatta*): Generality and individual consistency of effects. *Emotion, 6*, 73–81.

Melnick, D. J., Pearl, M. C., & Richard, A. F. (1984). Male migration and inbreeding avoidance in wild rhesus monkeys. *American Journal of Primatology, 7*, 229–243.

Merzenich, M. M., Nelson, R. J., Stryker, M. P., Cynader, M. S., Schoppmann, A., & Zook, J. M. (1984). Somatosensory cortical map changes following digit amputation in adult monkeys. *Journal of Comparative Neurology, 224*, 591–605.

Meunier, M., Bachevalier, J., Murray, E. A., Malkova, L., & Mishkin, M. (1999). Effects of aspiration versus neurotoxic lesions of the amygdala on emotional responses in monkeys. *European Journal of Neuroscience, 11*, 4403–4418.

Mineka S., & Öhman, A. (2002). Phobias and preparedness: the selective, automatic, and encapsulated nature of fear. *Biological Psychiatry, 52*, 927–937.

Mirsky, A. F. (1960). Studies of the effects of brain lesions on social behavior in *Macaca mulatta:* Methodological and theoretical considerations. *Annals of the New York Academy of Sciences, 85*, 785–794.

Moadab, G., Bliss-Moreau, E., & Amaral, D. G. (2015). Adult social behavior with familiar partners following neonatal amygdala or hippocampus damage. *Behavioral Neuroscience, 129*(3), 339–350.

Moadab, G., Bliss-Moreau, E., Bauman, M. D., & Amaral, D. G. (2013). *Female sex and sociability following early amygdala damage in Macaca mulatta.* Manuscript under review.

Myers, R. E., & Swett, C., Jr. (1970). Social behavior deficits of free-ranging monkeys after anterior temporal cortex removal: A preliminary report. *Brain Research, 18*, 548–551.

Neville, H., & Bavelier, D. (2002). Human brain plasticity: Evidence from sensory deprivation and altered language experience. *Progress in Brain Research, 138*, 177–188.

Novak, M. A. (2003). Self-injurious behavior in rhesus monkeys: New insights into its etiology, physiology, and treatment. *American Journal of Primatology, 59*, 3–19.

Öhman, A., & Mineka, S. (2001). Fears, phobias, and preparedness: Toward an evolved module of fear and fear learning. *Psychological Review, 108*, 483–522.

Phillips, K. A., Bales, K. L., Capitanio, J. P., Conley, A., Czoty, P. W., 't Hart, B.

A., et al. (2014). Why primate models matter. *American Journal of Primatology, 76*(9), 801–827.

Perederiy, J. V., & Westbrook G. L. (2013). Structural plasticity in the dentate gyrus—Revisiting a classic injury model. *Frontiers in Neural Circuits, 7,* 17.

Pitkänen, A., & Amaral, D. G. (1998). Organization of the intrinsic connections of the monkey amygdaloid complex: Projections originating in the lateral nucleus. *Journal of Comparative Neurology, 398,* 431–458.

Powell, D. A. (2010). A framework for introduction and Socialization Processes for Mammals. In D. G. Kleiman, K. V. Thompson, & C. K. Baer (Eds.), *Wild mammals in captivity: Principles and techniques for zoo management* (pp 49–61). Chicago: University of Chicago Press.

Price, J. L., & Amaral, D. G. (1981). An autoradiographic study of the projections of the central nucleus of the monkey amygdala. *Journal of Neuroscience, 1,* 1242–1259.

Rawlins, R. G., & Kessler, M. J. (1986). *The Cayo Santiago macaques: History, behavior, and biology.* New York: State University of New York Press.

Rosvold, H. E., Mirsky, A. F., & Pribram, K. H. (1954). Influence of amygdalectomy on social behavior in monkeys. *Journal of Comparative and Physiological Psychology, 47,* 173–178.

Starkey, M. L., & Schwab, M. E. (2014). How plastic is the brain after a stroke? *The Neuroscientist, 20,* 359–371.

Stefanacci, L., & Amaral, D. G. (2000). Topographic organization of cortical inputs to the lateral nucleus of the macaque monkey amygdala: A retrograde tracing study. *Journal of Comparative Neurology, 421,* 52–79.

Stefanacci, L., Clark, R. E., & Zola, S. M. (2003). Selective neurotoxic amygdala lesions in monkeys disrupt reactivity to food and object stimuli and have limited effects on memory. *Behavioral Neuroscience, 117,* 1029–1043.

Stefanacci, L., Suzuki, W. A., & Amaral, D. G. (1996). Organization of connections between the amygdaloid complex and the perirhinal and parahippocampal cortices in macaque monkeys. *Journal of Comparative Neuroscience, 25,* 552–582.

Suomi, S. J. (1984). The development of affect in rhesus monkeys. In N. Fox & R. J. Davidson (Eds.), *Affective development: A psychobiological perspective* (pp. 119–159). Hillsdale, NJ: Erlbaum.

Suomi, S. J. (1999). Attachment in rhesus monkeys. In J. Cassidy & P. R. Shaver (Eds.), *Handbook of attachment: Theory, research, and clinical applications* (pp. 181–197). New York: Guilford Press.

Suomi, S. J., & Harlow, H. F. (1972). Depressive behavior in young monkeys subjected to vertical chamber confinement. *Journal of Comparative and Physiological Psychology, 80,* 11–18.

Thompson, C. I., Schwartzbaum, J. S., & Harlow, H. F. (1969). Development of social fear after amygdalectomy in infant rhesus monkeys. *Physiology and Behavior, 4,* 249–254.

Thompson, C. I., & Towfighi, J. T. (1976). Social behavior of juvenile rhesus monkeys after amygdalectomy in infancy. *Physiology and Behavior, 17,* 831–836.

Toscano, J. E., Bauman, M. D., Mason, W. A., & Amaral, D. G. (2009). Interest in infants by female rhesus monkeys with neonatal lesions to the amygdala or hippocampus. *Neuroscience, 162*, 8881–8891.

Wallen K. (1990). Desire and ability: Hormones and the regulation of female sexual behavior. *Neuroscience and Biobehavioral Reviews, 14*, 223–241.

Weiskrantz, L. (1956). Behavioral changes associated with ablation of the amygdaloid complex in monkeys. *Journal of Comparative and Physiological Psychology, 49*, 381–391.

Yartz, A. R., & Hawk, L. W. (2002). Addressing the specificity of affective startle modulation: Fear versus disgust. *Biological Psychology, 59*, 55–68.

Zola-Morgan, S., Squire, L. R., Alverez-Royo, P., & Clower, R. P. (1991). Independence of memory functions and emotional behavior: Separate contributions of the hippocampal formation and the amygdala. *Hippocampus, 1*, 207–220.

CHAPTER 7

The Effects of Neonatal Amygdala Lesions in Rhesus Monkeys Living in a Species-Typical Social Environment

Jocelyne Bachevalier
Mar Sanchez
Jessica Raper
Shannon B. Z. Stephens
Kim Wallen

The chapter summarizes the behavioral development of infant monkeys with neonatal amygdala lesions and living in large social groups with a species-typical social structure. The impacts of the neonatal lesions on infant social development were at best mild and transitory, and indistinguishable from their controls in adolescence. Thus, adolescent amygdalectomized males (2–2.5 years of age) were able to recognize hierarchical status signals and to form stable social hierarchies, and pubertal amygdala-operated females (2.5–3.5 years of age) showed normal levels of female-initiated behavior toward the males. The results demonstrated nonetheless an interesting sex-dependent role of the amygdala in the early development of social skills. Despite the moderate impact on social behavior, neonatal amygdala lesions had robust effects on emotional regulation and stress physiology, including elevated basal secretion of stress hormones and increased reactivity to threatening stimuli. Thus, some of the subtle emotional changes observed in the group setting became more apparent when emotional reactivity of the animals was assessed in response to novelty and in a more controlled experimental context. The neonatal amygdala lesions reduced the magnitude of the expression of emotional behaviors and in some cases reduced the contextual modulation of these behaviors. These changes in emotional reactivity became more pronounced as the animals matured and were associated with increased cortisol stress responses in juvenile monkeys, suggesting that the absence of a functional amygdala may be more detrimental to the development of emotional and neuroendocrine functions due to critical amygdala interactions with subcortical centers, such as the hypothalamus, required for emotional and stress regulatory mechanisms. The results of this longitudinal study share many similarities to, and also extend, those previously reported (Bliss-Moreau, Modab, & Amaral, Chapter 6, this volume) and are in line with those found in human patients with bilateral amygdala damage (for review, see Buchanan, Tranel, & Adolphs, 2009).

Klüver and Bucy's (1939) cornerstone studies imprinted very early the idea of a link between the primate amygdala and socioemotional cognition. Studies by Rosvold, Mirsky, and Pribram (1954) and Mirsky (1960) indicated that amygdalectomized monkeys, when tested in their individual cages, were less fearful of the experimenter offering food but fell from top to bottom in the hierarchy when socially grouped in a large enclosure. Since these original reports, several other studies have substantiated the marked changes in social interactions that follow amygdalectomy in monkeys. Thus, aspiration lesions of the anterior temporal cortex, which includes the amygdala, yielded marked decrements in aggression and dominance in squirrel monkeys placed in small laboratory cage groups (Plotnik 1968). In rhesus monkeys observed in free-ranging social groups, these changes resulted in complete social isolation of the operated animals from the social groups (Kling & Brothers 1992). The role of the amygdala in social interactions has also been demonstrated by electrophysiological recording studies in monkeys. Radiotelemetry recordings of the activity of neurons in the amygdala during social interactions showed the highest responses to ambiguous or threatening situations, such as threat face display, and the lowest responses to tension-lowering behaviors, such as grooming and huddling (Kling, Steklis, & Deutsch, 1979).

Although these earlier reports demonstrated that the amygdala contributes significantly to affiliative behaviors, several factors appear to influence the effects of amygdala lesions on social and emotional responses. Aside from the extent of amygdala lesions, including or not the adjacent cortical areas and fibers of passage, these factors comprise species-specific behaviors, sex of the subjects, age at the time of surgery, and amount of preoperative social experience with conspecifics in a social group. Thus, bilateral amygdalectomy appears to have less disruptive effects in species that display intense positive social behaviors of grooming and embracing, such as in *Macaca speciosa*, than in *Macaca mulatta* and *Macaca ira* (Kling & Cornell, 1971). Furthermore, male amygdalectomized monkeys showed less aggressive behaviors than did female monkeys and, more often than females, fell in social rank (Rosvold et al., 1954; Kling, 1974). In adult monkeys, the deleterious effects of amygdala lesions are present when the animals are placed in small laboratory groups and in free-ranging social groups, whereas in juvenile operated monkeys, these effects emerged only when the social groups increased in complexity (Dicks, Myers, & Kling, 1969; Kling, 1972). Last, changes in social interactions following amygdalectomy depend on the length of time the social relationships had preoperatively existed, with greater and more rapid changes in operated animals being associated with less preoperative experience in a social group (Rosvold et al., 1954).

Given the crucial role of the amygdala for social cognition in adult subjects, it has been proposed that this structure should likewise play a critical role in the development of social cognition. The first observations of the effects of early amygdalectomy were made by Kling and Green (1967) and Kling (1972), who followed over a period of 2 years the development of four monkeys amygdalectomized during infancy. They noted that when returned to their mothers, the amygdalectomized infant monkeys could successfully be raised maternally. They displayed normal nipple orientation, sucking, and grasping, with a somatic and affective development grossly in the normal range. In addition, following repeated presentations of inedible objects, these operated animals did not display the typical compulsive oral behavior seen in amygdalectomized adult monkeys. This lack of effects of neonatal amygdalectomy in monkeys parallels results indicating that the behavioral effects of brain damage are minimized when the injury occurs early in life and can be accounted for by an incomplete maturation of the brain at the time of the insult (Goldman, 1971). Alternatively, the normal behavioral responses after early amygdala lesions could have resulted from the lack of specific quantification of behavioral responses and from the limited aspects of amygdala functions investigated. Indeed, more systematic and detailed investigations of the effects of neonatal amygdala lesions in rhesus monkeys reared in small peer groups (for review, see Thompson, 1981; Bachevalier, 1994) or reared with their mothers in small social groups (for review, see Bliss-Moreau et al., Chapter 6, this volume) clearly showed that bilateral amygdalectomy does not leave the subject unaltered, even when the surgery is performed during infancy. Thus, bilateral aspiration or neurotoxic lesions of the amygdaloid complex in the first months of life significantly altered social affiliation. However, in none of these developmental studies were the infants reared by their mothers in large multimatrilineal, species-typical, social groups (Sade, 1967). Given the earlier observations that the effects of amygdala lesions on social interactions in juvenile monkeys emerge only when the social groups increased in complexity (Dicks et al., 1969; Kling, 1972), we reinvestigated the effects of neonatal neurotoxic amygdala lesions on behavioral development of infant monkeys raised with their mothers in large social groups at the Field Station of the Yerkes National Primate Research Center, Lawrenceville (Georgia). Although procedures used to produce the neonatal lesions and return the infants to their mothers and to small social groups have already been described (Bauman, Lavenex, Mason, Capitanio, & Amaral, 2004), in this chapter we first describe the methods used to return the mother–infant pairs to their large species-typical social groups, because this procedure may be relevant to many other researchers interested in following the development of behavioral and cognitive processes, and their neural bases in nonhuman primates raised in a species-typical social troop. We then summarize the findings collected on the maturation of their social skills and abilities to regulate emotional and stress neuroendocrine responses when observed in their natural social group or tested in more standardized experimental settings.

Animal Handling Procedures for Neonatal Brain Lesions

The animals lived in large, outdoor compounds (38 m × 39 m) with attached, climate-controlled indoor areas at the Yerkes National Primate Research Center (YNPRC) Field Station (Lawrenceville, Georgia) of Emory University (Figure 7.1). Each outdoor compound also had an elevated observation tower, with unobstructed visual access, and electricity for computers used for behavioral observations. Experimental subjects were an integral part of these groups, which duplicate the social context and structure of wild rhesus monkey groups (e.g., sex ratios, age demographics, and social structure) and served as the outdoor laboratory in which social behavior, cognitive function, emotion, and neuroendocrine function could be investigated.

Our groups have lived together for more than 15 years and consist of multiple matrilines organized in a rhesus-typical social hierarchy. The groups are age-graded with members of all age classes. Offspring are routinely cropped to maintain a manageable group size and for other research, but cropping is done so that an appropriate matrilineal balance is maintained. Two to five adult males are part of each group and are routinely replaced every 2 to 5 years, as occurs naturally in native groups. Females live their whole lives within their natal group, becoming integrated into the matriarchal power structure. Males develop relatively more independently, eventually emigrating to a new social group between ages 3 and 5 years (Berard, 1989). Thus, males and females, even in the same social group, experience markedly different social rearing contexts (Lovejoy & Wallen, 1988; Wallen & Tannebaum, 1997; Wallen 2005). Therefore, our nonhuman primate groups preserve critical social aspects of native rhesus monkey groups, while allowing experimental control typical of less complex social conditions. In addition, during 30 years of working with large, complex social groups of rhesus monkeys, we have also developed animal training and handling procedures and techniques that allow us to enter the groups and select individuals, using a pointing

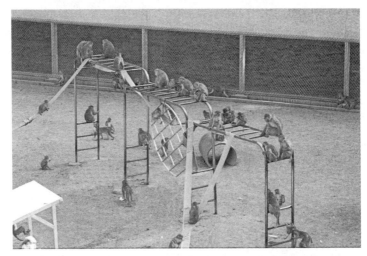

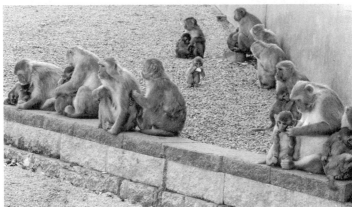

FIGURE 7.1. Upper photo: An aerial view from the observation tower of a large species-specific social group at the YNPRC Field Station (Lawrenceville, Georgia); photograph by Dr. Janice Vick and Amy Henry. Lower photo: A close-up view of mother–infant pairs interacting in a large species-typical social group; photograph by Dr. Kim Wallen.

procedure, to enter an indoor area with specialized caging that facilitates transfer of subjects to cages designed for collecting physiological samples and formal behavioral testing. We have used these animal handling procedures on monkeys at all stages of life, from mother–infant pairs to individual adults, to routinely access subjects daily.

Thus, as compared to previous studies on the effects of neonatal amygdala lesions on socioemotional behavior (Thompson, 1981; Bachevalier 1994), including the most recent studies from Bliss-Moreau et al. (Chapter 6, this volume), our research facility offered us the unique advantage of longitudinally following the development of infants with neonatal amygdala lesions, while maintaining the animals with their mothers in the large and species-typical challenging social groups, and at the same time allowing us to access animals individually to study their behavior in laboratory emotional tests with more experimental control, as well as collect blood samples to examine the effects of the neonatal amygdala lesions on stress neuroendocrine function. Finally, given that males and females in the same social group experience markedly different social rearing contexts, the environment at the Yerkes Field Station allowed us to investigate the influence of rearing contexts on the effects of neonatal amygdala damage in males and females separately. Thus, our study included a total of 12 sham-operated animals (six males, six females) and 15 animals with neonatal amygdala lesions (nine males, six females) and allowed us to measure gender differences in the effects of neonatal lesions.

At this unique facility, we used two social groups that comprised 80–100 animals with known matrilineal relations and selected our subjects over two successive breeding seasons, such that two cohorts of mother–infant pairs were used over 2 years. Pregnant females that had already successfully reared at least one infant were monitored during the birth season, and their infants (males or females) were randomly assigned to either the amygdala-operated or sham-operated groups. Infants from the highest- and lowest-ranking matrilines were not enrolled to make the social context across subjects as similar as possible. Upon selection, when the infants were 22–26 days of age, mothers and their infants were removed from their social group and transported and housed in individual cages at the YNPRC Main Station, where the lesions were performed. After 24 hours, infants were removed from their mother using standard animal procedures, then received either an amygdala lesion or a sham surgery (see details in Raper, Bachevalier, Wallen, & Sanchez, 2013a). For the amygdala lesions, animals received first a neuroimaging procedure to acquire high-resolution T1 structural images to select the injection sites for each monkey. Following surgery, infants were kept in a temperature-controlled isolette, where they were monitored hourly and bottle-fed to document that the infants were capable of nursing. Within 24 hours postsurgery, infants were reunited with their mothers by bringing the infant inside a transfer box to its mother's cage, attaching the transfer box to the mother's cage, and opening a sliding door, allowing the mother access to her infant. Three of our first four postsurgery reunions experienced difficulties, such that the mothers retrieved their infants initially but rejected them after a few minutes. In these three cases, repeated reunion attempts were made and in one case the reunion was successful after 5 days, whereas in the other two cases, reunions with the mother were never successful but the infants were adopted by another mother in the infant's natal group that already had an infant in the study. The difficulty in these initial reunions of mothers and babies likely resulted from the use of cyanoacrylate adhesive on the sutures to prevent the mothers from removing them. This glue has a pungent odor and our first three mothers initially retrieved their babies, sniffed the sutures, and rejected their babies. After these initial problems, we ceased using cyanoacrylate glue, instituted a trial separation prior to surgery, applied Betadine solution to the infant's shaved head, as would be done in surgery, and reunited the infant with its mother. We also monitored all mother–infant pairs during postsurgery reunions via Internet cameras allowing around-the-clock monitoring. After instituting these procedures, only one reunion of the next 39 failed, and this infant was successfully cross-fostered to a mother in its natal group that had recently lost her infant.

Mother–infant pairs were kept in the YNPRC Main Station for 1 week, at which time the amygdala-operated infants underwent a second magnetic resonance imaging (MRI; FLAIR = fluid-attenuated inversion recovery) to identify hypersignals indicative of cell death in the amygdala that were used to measure the extent of damage. Sham-operated controls did not experience this second episode of anesthesia but were separated from the mother for the same amount of time as the amygdalectomized animals. Following the second MRI, mothers and infants were reunited and, in all cases, the mothers immediately retrieved their infants. Upon return to the YNPRC Field Station, mother–infant pairs were kept in a separate area visible to their groups and were released into the group 12 hours later. All mother–infant pairs immediately reintegrated into the group.

Because of the large number of subjects created in the 3-month birth season, we substituted some surgical shams for behavioral shams. Behavioral-sham infants were separated from their mothers and their heads were shaved and cleaned with betadine as with the operated animals, and were then reunited with their mothers. They received a second separation 1 week later to simulate the postoperative MRI and separation that operated animals received, after which they were reunited with their mothers and returned to their social groups using the same procedures as used for the other subjects. Behavioral measures were taken either while the animals were actively interacting with their mothers or other group members, or when they were temporarily removed from their social groups for no more than 4 hours to be tested on behavioral tasks or to collect cerebrospinal fluid or blood samples. Given that the two types of control animals (surgical shams and behavioral shams) did not differ for the behavioral measures reported below, they were combined into a single control group (Neo-C, 11 females and 12 males) for comparisons with those with neonatal amygdala lesions (Neo-A, 6 females and 9 males).

Development of Social Relationships from Infancy through Adolescence

The effects of neonatal amygdala lesions on the development of social skills were investigated after the 1-month-old amygdalectomized rhesus monkeys and their controls were returned with their mothers to their species-typical social groups.

Mother Preference

Infant primates of either sex become attached to their mothers and show a preference for them compared to other familiar adult females (Ainsworth & Bell, 1970; Mason & Mendoza, 1998). This preference, expressed very early in development, continues throughout the juvenile period and even into adulthood for females remaining in their natal group as adults. We investigated whether amygdalectomy at 1 month of age affected the development and expression of mother preference at 3 and 6 months of age when infant monkeys maintained close proximity with their mothers.

Using a large enclosure described in detail elsewhere (Goursaud, Wallen, & Bachevalier, 2014), infants were given the opportunity to approach and interact with either their caged mother or a caged familiar female not part of the infant's matriline. The mother–infant pair and the familiar female were separated from their group. The two adult females were kept in separate cages attached to one wall of the enclosure and positioned approximately 3 meters apart. The infant was sequestered in a small animal handling box, attached on the opposite wall of the enclosure and positioned about 3 meters away from and equidistant to the adult females' cages. Upon release from the handling box, the infant's position, vocalizations, and interactions with the females were video-recorded for 10 minutes using three cameras covering different angles of the testing environment.

At both 3 and 6 months, amygdala-operated and control subjects significantly preferred their mother (see Figure 7.2). However, at 6 months, when in proximity of their mothers, Neo-A infants reached out to their

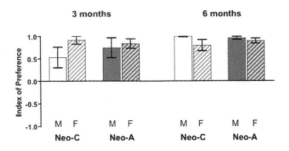

FIGURE 7.2. Average index of preference (IP; mean ± *SEM*) for males (M) and females (F) in groups Neo-C (surgical and behavioral controls) and Neo-A (animals with neonatal amygdala lesions) at both 3 and 6 months of age. IP = (duration of proximity with mother/duration of proximity with familiar female)/ (total duration of proximity with both stimuli). This IP value expressed the ability of the animal to discriminate between the two stimuli and choose one of them (IP > 0, preference for the mother; IP < 0, preference for the familiar female; and IP = 0, no preference). Based on Goursaud et al. (2014).

mothers significantly less than did control animals (mean ± *SEM* [standard error of the mean], Neo-A = 7.33 ± 1.47, control: 15.33 ± 1.59, $t(19)$ = 3.66, p = .002, Cohen's d = 1.62). Thus, although amygdalectomized infants displayed a clear mother preference, they did not attempt to reach their mothers as much as did control subjects. Whether this change reflects reduced secure-base behavior (alterations in attachment?) in amygdalectomized subjects or reduced anxiety triggered by being separated from their mothers needs to be investigated further. It is, however, clear that, even in the absence of a functional amygdala, monkeys form essential social relationships (e.g., maternal bond) in a manner that is hard to distinguish from infants with intact amygdalae. Thus, the findings confirmed the predictions enunciated in an earlier report (Bauman et al., 2004; see also Bliss-Moreau et al., Chapter 6, this volume).

Mother–Infant Social Behavior

Infant male and female rhesus monkeys differ in the age at which they venture away from their mothers' protective zone and strike out on their own (Hinde, Rowell, & Spencer-Booth, 1964; Jensen, Bobbit, & Gordon, 1968). Development of independence typically occurs earlier in males than it does in females (Jensen et al., 1968), but after 6 months of age, there is little difference in independence status. Behavioral data were collected for each subject starting from their return to the social group after surgery (approximately 30 days old) through 12 months of age. Subjects were focally observed twice per week (for 30 minutes each time) in their social group's outdoor compound, from a tower above one corner of the compound, and were clearly identified by a distinctive dye-mark on their bodies. Neonatal amygdalectomy produced subtle changes in mother–infant interactions, such that Neo-A female infants showed earlier independence from their mothers, spending less time in contact and proximity with them at 4 months of age and signficantly more time 3 meters away from them as compared to Neo-C female infants, and did not differ from Neo-C males (Raper, Stephens, Sanchez, Bachevalier, & Wallen, 2014b). By contrast, Neo-A males showed a nonsignificant delay in independence, compared to Neo-C males, but were not different from Neo-C females. Interestingly, both Neo-A male and female infants produced more emotional vocalizations (coos and screams) than did Neo-C subjects at this early age.

Mothers' behavior toward their infants varied with the sex of the infant and whether it had an intact amygdala or not (Raper et al., 2014b). Rhesus monkey mothers cradle their infants for a substantial time whether they are male or female. However, mothers of Neo-A males cradled their infants significantly longer than did mothers of either Neo-A females or Neo-C males, but not of Neo-C females. Thus, for both independence and maternal cradling, Neo-A females looked more like Neo-C males, whereas Neo-A males looked more like Neo-C females. The reasons for this sex role reversal are not known but suggest that the social and emotional impact of amygdala damage differs between males and females, with amygdalectomized females experiencing a greater reduction in fearfulness than did males.

Composite behavioral measures during infancy (time in contact, time away, coo vocalizations, and amount of grooming received from the mother) accounted for 78% of the variance and accurately classifying 94% of the female infants by lesion status (Press's $Q = 13.24$, df [degrees of freedom] = 1, $p < .001$), whereas this classification was not found for the males (Raper et al., 2014b). Thus, there was a clear sex difference in the ability of infant behavioral measures to distinguish amygdala-operated from control subjects, further supporting that the effects of amygdalectomy were more pronounced in females than in males. Interestingly, during this early developmental period, these results highlighted the presence of sexual dimorphism in mother–infant relations after neonatal amygdalectomy that had not been noticed in the earlier study of Bauman and colleagues (2004).

After 6 months of age, lesion status did not predict any behavioral differences either from the mothers toward the juveniles or by the juveniles themselves, with the exception that Neo-A juveniles of both sexes followed their mothers less frequently than did Neo-C juveniles (Raper et al., 2014b). In addition, the behavioral measures that successfully discriminated Neo-A female infants from Neo-C female infants no longer did so.

Thus, when our subjects reached the juvenile period, it was not possible to distinguish males from females or amygdala-operated from control subjects based on their interactions with their mothers. The lack of changes after 6 months of age may reflect the final expression of independence at this time period, or that the effects of amygdalectomy are subtle and transitory during the first year of life, thus echoing the lack of changes in social interactions described earlier (Bauman et al., 2004).

Social Status Achievement

Male rhesus monkeys do not spend their lives in their natal group but emigrate to a new, typically unfamiliar group, where they become socially integrated for 5 or so years, after which they emigrate again to a new group (Berard, 1989). Prior to integration in a new group, males spend time in all-male bands living on the periphery of heterosexual groups. Entering all-male bands requires that males achieve social rank without maternal aid. Male integration provides a unique opportunity to explore social status achievement and its relationship to neural function. We modeled male emigration by removing the Neo-A (n = 9) and Neo-C (n = 9) males (between 2 and 2.5 years of age) from their natal group and forming three age-matched, six-member all-male groups, including both familiar and unfamiliar males in each group. Group hierarchy formation was followed for 10 months, with weekly behavioral observations. All three groups formed stable social hierarchies, with the average social rank not differing between Neo-A and Neo-C males. Neonatally operated males did not assume low social status, unlike those in previous studies (Bauman, Toscano, Babineau, Mason, & Amaral, 2006; Rosvold et al., 1954), a finding similar to that reported by Machado and Bachevalier (2006) after adult-onset amygdala lesions in males. Neonatally amygdalectomized males appeared to recognize hierarchical status signals and to form stable social hierarchies. In addition, amygdala-operated males were not socially withdrawn, as has been previously suggested under quite different social and observational conditions (Bliss-Moreau, Moadab, Bauman, & Amaral, 2013; Dicks et al., 1969).

Adolescent Sexual Behavior (Pair Tests)

Social context influences the relationship between ovarian hormones and female sexual behavior (Wallen, 1990, 2001), but the brain region(s) integrating social context and mediating these effects on female sexual behavior are unknown. The amygdala is involved in social recognition and in producing species-typical behavioral responses (Bennett, Greco, Blasberg, & Blaustein, 2002; Kling & Cornell, 1971; Spiteri et al., 2010; Thompson, Schwartzbaum, & Harlow, 1969). It also has projections to the ventromedial hypothalamus, an area that is critical for the expression of sexual behavior (Amaral, Price, Pitkänen, & Carmichael, 1992; Mathews & Edwards, 1977; Mathews, Donovan, Hollingsworth, Hutson, & Overstreet, 1983; Oomura, Aou, Koyama, Fujita, & Yoshimatsu, 1988). Thus, the amygdala appears well positioned to facilitate the integration of social context and the relationship between estradiol and sexual behavior.

We examined the effects of neonatal amygdala lesions on female sexual behavior during pair tests with an adult male in pubertal rhesus macaques (2.5–3.5 years of age). Female sexual receptivity, measured by the rate of mounting by the male, as well as female-initiated behaviors, such as initiating proximity to the male (within arm's reach), approaching the male, following the male, sexual solicitations, and presentation of hindquarters to the male (present), were measured. We predicted that female-initiated behaviors would be displayed less by Neo-A females, but that male-initiated behavior would not differ between Neo-A and Neo-C females.

Testing occurred between September and January, the breeding season in rhesus macaques (Wilson, Gordon, & Collins, 1986; Wilson & Gordon, 1989), once all females reached menarche. Females were tested once or twice a week, with increased testing when estradiol levels were expected to be elevated. On testing days, females were removed from their social group and transferred to an outdoor behavioral testing facility (4.9 m × 4.9 m × 2.4 m), where they received two separate 30-minute tests (60 minutes, if any mating was observed) with each of two adult males not from their natal group. Subjects were habituated to the testing procedure and to the adult males prior to collecting sexual behavior data. Vaginal swabs and blood samples were collected at least three times a week to determine the timing of menstrual cycles and estradiol levels, respectively.

Only tests in which estradiol was > 5 pg (picograms)/ml were analyzed (Neo-C: 46 tests; Neo-A: 22 tests) and estradiol levels did not significantly differ between Neo-A ($M = 64.19 \pm 14.5$ pg/ml) and Neo-C ($M = 72.51 \pm 12.89$ pg/ml) female pair tests. Means ($\pm$ *SEM*) for each behavioral rate are presented in Table 7.1, which also shows the regression of estradiol levels followed by neonatal treatment (Neo-A vs. Neo-C) as predictor variables. Given that these data have not been published yet, a more complete description of the results is given below.

Unlike adult-onset amygdala lesions, which decreased female-initiated proximity (Spies et al., 1976), neonatal lesions did not account for any additional variance to that accounted for by estradiol levels in the frequency of female-initiated proximity to the male, $\beta = .06$, $t(65) = 0.52$, $p = .602$, or the duration of proximity to the male, $\beta = -.04$, $t(65) = -0.35$, $p = .73$. Though there were no differences in the frequency or duration of initiating proximity, amygdala-operated females approached to within 1 meter of the male more frequently ($\beta = .46$, $t(65) = 4.32$, $p < .001$; $R^2 =$

TABLE 7.1. Mean ± *SEM* and Regression Statistics for Female- and Male-Initiated Behaviors during Pair Tests

Behavior	Statistics	Measure	Neo-A	Neo-C
Frequency of female proximity initiation	$\beta = .06$, $t(65) = 0.52$, $p = .602$; $R^2 = .12$, $F(2,67) = 4.39$, $p = .016$	Mean frequency/hr	4.784 ± 1.40	4.01 ± 1.43
Duration of time in proximity	$\beta = .04$, $t(65) = 0.35$, $p = .730$; $R^2 = .06$, $F(2,67) = 2.20$, $p = .119$	Mean duration min/hr	1.82 ± 0.38	2.20 ± 0.58
Frequency of female initiation within 1 meter	$\beta = .46$, $t(65) = 4.32$, $p <.001$***; $R^2 = .25$, $F(2,67) = 10.54$, $p <.001$	Mean frequency/hr	15.42 ± 2.39	5.71 ± 1.14
Duration of time at 1 meter	$\beta = .38$, $t(65) = 3.30$, $p <.002$*; $R^2 = .16$, $F(2,67) = 6.15$, $p <.001$	Mean duration min/hr	4.92 ± 0.94	2.06 ± 0.38
Frequency of following the male	$\beta = .34$, $t(65) = 2.94$, $p <.005$**; $R^2 = .12$, $F(2,67) = 4.35$, $p <.017$	Mean frequency/hr	8.43 ± 2.56	2.20 ± 0.75
Duration of time following the male	$\beta = .30$, $t(65) = 2.58$, $p <.012$*; $R^2 = .09$, $F(2,67) = 3.35$, $p <.041$*	Mean duration min/hr	0.66 ± 0.23	0.16 ± 0.07
Mount frequency	$\beta = .15$, $t(65) = -1.28$, $p = .205$; $R^2 = .16$, $F(2,67) = 6.09$, $p = .004$	Mean frequency/hr	0.00 ± 0.00	2.92 ± 1.49
Sexual solicit frequency	$\beta = .11$, $t(65) = 0.90$, $p = .372$; $R^2 = .06$, $F(2,67) = 2,11$, $p = .129$	Mean frequency/hr	0.63 ± 0.37	3.26 ± 1.87
Present frequency	$\beta = .25$, $t(65) = 2.05$, $p = .045$*; $R^2 = .06$, $F(2,67) = 2,09$, $p = .132$	Mean frequency/hr	3.87 ± 1.98	0.95 ± 0.29
Threats received frequency	$\beta = .26$, $t(65) = 2.12$, $p = .038$*; $R^2 = .07$, $F(2,67) = 2,26$, $p = .112$	Mean frequency/hr	3.58 ± 0.93	1.72 ± 0.41
Submissive gestures frequency/hr	$\beta = .04$, $t(65) = 0.29$, $p = .776$; $R^2 = .004$, $F(2,67) = 0.12$, $p = .88$	Mean frequency/hr	24.08 ± 3.68	25.85 ± 4.20
Scratch frequency	$\beta = .44$, $t(65) = 3.87$, $p = .001$***; $R^2 = .21$, $F(2,67) = 8.39$, $p = .001$***	Mean frequency/hr	2.65 ± 0.75	0.48 ± 0.15

*p < .05; ** p < .01; *** p < .001; *** p < .001 when neonatal treatment was a significant predictor in the regression model.

.25, $F(2, 67) = 10.54$, $p < .001$) and spent more time within 1 meter of the male ($\beta = .38$, $t(65) = 3.30$, $p = .002$; $R^2 = .16$, $F(2, 67) = 6.15$, $p = .004$) than did control females. Neonatal amygdala-operated females also followed the male (an indicator of sexual interest) more frequently ($\beta = .34$, $t(65) = 2.94$, $p = .005$; $R^2 = .12$, $F(2, 67) = 4.35$, $p = .017$) and for longer durations ($\beta = .30$, $t(65) = 2.58$, $p = .012$; $R^2 = .09$, $F(2, 67) = 3.35$, $p = .041$) than did control females. Thus, amygdala-operated females spent more time near the male than did control females.

Frequency of presents and sexual solicits did not differ between adult amygdala-operated females and control females (Spies et al., 1976); similarly, we found that neonatal lesions did not account for any additional variance in the frequency of sexual solicits ($\beta = -.11$, $t(65) = -0.90$, $p = .372$; $R^2 = .06$, $F(2, 67) = 2.11$, $p = .129$). In contrast to sexual solicits, female present frequency was significantly predicted by neonatal treatment ($\beta = .25$, $t(65) = 2.05$, $p = .045$), with Neo-A females displaying more presents to the male than did Neo-C females. However, the regression model for female presents, including estradiol levels and neonatal treatment, was not statistically significant ($R^2 = .06$, $F(2, 67) = 2.09$, $p = .132$).

Neonatal treatment did not significantly account for any additional variance in mount rate ($\beta = -.15$, $t(65) = -1.28$, $p = .205$). However, amygdala-operated females were never mounted; thus, it was not possible to assess receptivity. The lack of mounting of Neo-A females may reflect their adolescent status and small size compared to the adult males that may not have regarded these females as potential sexual partners.

Amygdala-operated females received more threatening gestures from the male in comparison to control females ($\beta = .26$, $t(65) = 2.123$, $p = .038$), but despite receiving more threats by the male, Neo-A females did not display more submissive gestures than did Neo-C females ($\beta = -.04$, $t(65) = -0.29$, $p = .776$).

Self-scratching, a measure of anxiety, was displayed more by Neo-A females than by Neo-C females ($\beta = .44$, $t(63) = 3.87$, $p < .001$), with estradiol levels and neonatal treatment accounting for 21% of the variation in scratching ($R^2 = .21$, $F(2, 65) = 8.39$, $p = .001$). The cause of this heightened anxiety in amygdalectomized females is unclear, but it demonstrates that even without a functional amygdala, females are capable of displaying anxious behaviors. In summary, when sexual behavior was examined in a pair test, neonatal amygdala-operated females did not show decreased levels of female-initiated behavior towards the males, and, if any neonatal treatment difference existed, Neo-A females displayed more of that behavior than did Neo-C females. Thus, contrary to findings reported by Moadab, Bliss-Moreau, and Amaral (2015), when raised in a large social group, females with neonatal amygdala lesions exhibited apparently normal social interactions with unfamiliar males when there was no competition for access to adult males.

Emotional Reactivity to Threatening Social Stimuli

From the review we just presented, it is clear that animals living without a functional amygdala in a large social group displayed little or no severe changes in their interactions with their mothers or other group members. Remarkably, these animals remained undetected by others in the group according to animal caretakers or casual observers. Yet, the limited effects of neonatal amygdala lesions on social interactions contrasts with the robust effects on the emotional and stress reactivity that we found in the same animals when tested in a more controlled experimental setting.

A critical role of the amygdala in the modulation of behavioral and physiological responses to social signals has been well documented after either electrical amygdala stimulation in humans (Fish, Gloor, Quesney, & Olivier, 1993; Lanteaume et al., 2007; Stevens, Mark, Erwin, Pacheco, & Suematsu, 1969) and monkeys (Delgado, Rivera, & Mir, 1971; Jurgens & Richter, 1986) or amygdala lesion in adult primates (Kalin, Shelton, & Davidson, 2004; Machado & Bachevalier, 2008; Mason, Capitanio, Machado, Mendoza, & Amaral, 2006; Meunier, Bachevalier, Murray, Malkova, & Mishkin, 1999). A few developmental studies in monkeys have also shown that neonatal amygdala lesions yield abnormal threat detection and inappropriate reactivity toward objects and social partners in animals either surrogate peer-reared (Raper, Wilson, Sanchez, Machado, & Bachevalier, 2013c; Thompson et al., 1969; Thompson, Bergland, & Towfighi, 1977; Thompson, 1981) or mother-reared in small social groups (Bauman et al., 2004; Bliss-Moreau, Toscano, Bauman, Mason, & Amaral, 2010; Bliss-Moreau, Toscano, Bauman, Mason, & Amaral, 2011b; Bliss-Moreau, Bauman, & Amaral, 2011a; Bliss-Moreau et al., 2013; Prather et al., 2001). These studies showed that early amygdala damage left intact species-typical emotional behaviors (i.e., fear grimaces, freezing, hostility), but impaired the animal's ability to modulate appropriately those behaviors based on the level of threat in the environment. Therefore, we tested whether similar outcomes were observed in rhesus monkeys with neonatal amygdala lesions living in large, species-typical social groups.

The human intruder paradigm (see Figure 7.3A) assesses emotional responses toward different levels of social threat and has proven to be a robust and precise experimental tool for measuring modulation of emotional responses in monkeys (Kalin & Shelton, 1989; Kalin, Shelton, & Takahashi, 1991). In the Alone condition, when monkeys are separated from their social groups and placed in a novel environment, they typically emit coo vocalizations and exploratory behavior in an attempt to reunite with their social group (Kalin, Shelton, Fox, Oakes, & Davidson, 2005). In the Profile condition (also termed "No Eye Contact" in other publications), when an unfamiliar human enters the room, avoiding eye contact and presenting their profile to the animal (mild threat), monkeys

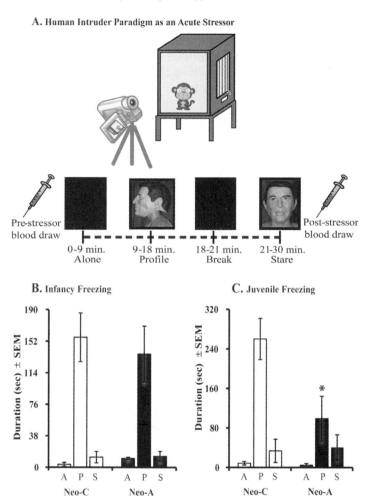

FIGURE 7.3. Schematic representation of the human intruder paradigm used as an acute stressor (A). After a habituation period of 9 minutes to the experimental room (Alone condition), the animal is faced with the presence of an unfamiliar human presenting his or her profile for 9 minutes (Profile condition). Animal is then left alone in the room for a 3-minute period, after which the human intruder reappears, this time staring at the animal (Stare condition) for 9 minutes. Blood samples were collected immediately before and after the task to measure neuro-endocrine responses (ACTH, cortisol) to the social stressor. Mean (± *SEM*) freezing behavior during the Alone (A), Profile (P), and Stare (S) conditions of the human intruder paradigm during infancy (B: 2.5 months) and juvenile (C: 12 months) periods. Control animals (Neo-C, open bars) and animals with neonatal amygdala lesions (Neo-A, black bars). * indicates a group difference of *p* < .05. Graphs in B and C are reprinted with modifications from Raper et al. (2013a) with permission from Elsevier.

emit fearful defensive or antipredator detection behaviors, such as ceasing vocalization and freezing. Last, in the Stare condition, when the unfamiliar human makes direct eye contact with the animal (salient threat), monkeys now emit hostile and anxious behaviors. Animals with neonatal amygdala lesions and their controls were tested on this task at the ages of 2, 4, and 12 months of age.

Neonatal amygdala lesions did not disrupt the animals' ability to exhibit species-typical defensive and emotional behaviors, but they did impact the magnitude and modulation of emotional responses depending on the context (Raper et al., 2013b). During infancy, there was no difference in the level of freezing or hostility between amygdala-operated and control animals; however, when the animals were retested as juveniles, neonatal amygdala-operated animals exhibited lower levels of freezing and hostility compared to controls that showed higher reactivity with age (see Figure 7.3B and 7.3C; Raper et al., 2013b). These findings replicate those of a previous study demonstrating similar protracted changes in emotional reactivity to threat signals in animals reared in a more restricted environment (Raper et al., 2013c). In addition to providing additional support to earlier observations of blunted emotional reactivity after neonatal amygdalectomy (see review in Bliss-Moreau et al., Chapter 6, this volume), our findings demonstrate that the emotional changes were not present in the first few months of life, but they emerged as the animals reached early adolescence. This protracted development in the modulation of freezing behaviors parallels the increase in amygdala morphology and volume from birth through 2 years of age (Chareyron, Banta Lavenex, Amaral, & Lavenex, 2012; Payne, Machado, Bliwise, & Bachevalier, 2010), which suggests that, unlike control animals that are able to refine their emotional behavior as the amygdala reaches functional maturity, those with neonatal amygdala lesions are not able to do so.

Not all animals' emotional behaviors exhibited these same maturational alterations after neonatal amygdalectomy. For example, coo vocalizations were expressed more among animals with early amygdala lesions as compared to controls during both infancy and the juvenile periods (Raper et al., 2013b). This finding is similar to increased coo vocalizations reported after adult-onset amygdala lesions in monkeys (Kalin et al., 2004), suggesting that the expression of some emotional behaviors is controlled by the amygdala early in life, as well as later in development. The increased cooing is also in line with the role of the amygdala in detecting dangers in the environment and adapting an appropriate behavioral response according to the level of threat presented (Davis & Whalen, 2001). The fact that animals with neonatal amygdala lesions are willing to emit coos regardless of the presence of gaze direction of the human intruder suggests that they have difficulty discerning the difference in threat level between conditions or in modulating their emotional responses to these conditions. Other changes in emotional behavior responses were also sex-dependent. For example, in the case of scream vocalizations, infant females with neonatal amygdala lesions emitted more screams in the Alone condition compared to control females. Sex differences in screaming vocalizations have been previously reported, with females giving longer, more complex vocalizations in response to maternal separation than males (Jiang, Kanthaswamy, & Capitanio, 2013; Tomaszycki, Davis, Gouzoules, & Wallen, 2001). These vocalizations can be masculinized in females whose mothers were exposed to elevated testosterone during pregnancy, raising the possibility that the sex differences in emotional vocalizations may reflect sexual differentiation of the amygdala under prenatal androgen exposure.

Last, during the juvenile period only, but not in infancy, discriminant function analyses based on emotional responses (coo vocalizations, freezing, hostility, and anxious behaviors) correctly classified individual animals with and without an intact amygdala (Raper et al., 2013b). Interestingly, although reduced freezing is the most common finding across studies examining the effects of amygdala lesions (Meunier et al., 1999; Kalin et al., 2004; Machado & Bachevalier, 2008; Raper et al., 2013c), in our study, freezing was only moderately predictive of whether an animal had amygdala damage, whereas hostility and anxiety expression were stronger predictors. Overall, the discriminant analyses further support the idea that the impact of early amygdala damage on emotional reactivity worsens and becomes more apparent with age. Therefore, it became critical to investigate whether these emotional reactivity changes were related to, or at least paralleled, significant changes in hypothalamic–pituitary–adrenal (HPA) axis functioning.

Stress Physiology

The HPA axis plays a critical role in both the neuroendocrine stress response and homeostasis, with a basal circadian secretory rhythm characterized by a peak in cortisol secretion upon awakening and a decline across the day, with a trough at night (Weitzman et al., 1971; Keller-Wood & Dallman, 1984). The amygdala plays a crucial role in coordinating behavioral, autonomic, and neuroendocrine stress responses, via mostly excitatory influences on the hypothalamus and brainstem (Aggleton, 2000). The amygdala's main stimulatory role in HPA axis stress reactivity is mediated through indirect projections to the hypothalamic paraventricular nucleus (PVN) that involve disinhibition of gamma-aminobutyric acid (GABA)ergic projections (Amaral et al., 1992; Beaulieu, Di Paolo, & Barden, 1986; Ehle, Mason, & Pennington, 1977; Feldman, Conforti, & Saphier, 1990; Feldman, Conforti, Itzik, & Weidenfeld, 1994; Feldman,

Conforti, & Weidenfeld, 1995; Freese & Amaral, 2009; Herman et al., 2003; Herman, Ostrander, Mueller, & Figueiredo, 2005; Kalin et al., 2004; Machado & Bachevalier, 2008; Mason, 1959; Pitkänen, 2000; Price & Amaral, 1981; Redgate & Fahringer, 1973). In response to a psychogenic threat, this PVN disinhibition provokes the release of corticotropin-releasing factor (CRF) to the median eminence portal blood system for transport to the anterior pituitary, where it stimulates the release of adrenocorticotropic hormone (ACTH) into systemic circulation. ACTH then stimulates the synthesis and release of glucocorticoids (GCs) by the adrenal cortex (cortisol in primates or corticosterone in rodents; Herman, et al., 2003; Myers, McKlveen, & Herman, 2012; Ulrich-Lai & Herman, 2009). In addition to their role as highly catabolic stress hormones, these circulating GCs also play a critical negative-feedback role by acting back on the pituitary, hypothalamus, and extrahypothalamic areas to shut down this stress-induced HPA axis mediated by binding to glucocorticoid receptors (GRs). A few rodent studies have also indicated that the amygdala plays a stimulatory role on basal HPA axis activity (Allen & Allen, 1975; Furay, Bruestle, & Herman, 2008; Regev, Tsoory, Gil, & Chen, 2012), but this role is less clear.

The HPA axis exhibits a progressive postnatal maturation in human and nonhuman primates, such that the basal HPA secretory diurnal rhythm does not emerge until human infants are 8–12 weeks of age (for review, see Tarullo & Gunnar 2006), and in macaques, the basal HPA secretory activity is either stable or slightly decreases between 2 and 24 weeks of age (Champoux, Coe, Schanberg, Kuhn, & Suomi, 1989; Clarke, 1993; Higley, Suomi, & Linnoila, 1992), with an adult-like diurnal pattern of cortisol secretion reported by 1 year of age (Barrett et al., 2009; Sanchez et al., 2005). The study of the impact of amygdala lesions during infancy on HPA axis functioning (Goursaud, Mendoza, & Capitanio, 2006; Norman & Spies, 1981; Raper et al., 2013c) has so far yielded inconsistent results. Similarly, the two studies that have investigated the impact of neonatal amygdala lesions on the HPA axis-reactive stress response (Goursaud et al., 2006; Raper et al., 2013c) have also led to inconsistent results. Thus, we examined whether the emotional alterations described in the previous section were associated (or at least paralleled) with developmental alterations in the HPA axis function after the neonatal amygdalectomy. Using the same cohorts of neonatally amygdalectomized monkeys and their controls, HPA axis basal secretory rhythm and its reactivity to stress were thoroughly studied at different developmental time points (Raper et al., 2013a, 2013b, 2014a). For this, baseline blood samples were collected following a very quick access of the subjects from their home cages during the infant and juvenile periods, followed (or not) by exposure to the human intruder stress task described earlier for measurement of basal or stress-induced plasma cortisol and ACTH levels.

Diurnal HPA Axis Rhythm

At 2.5 months of age, control infants exhibited sexually dimorphic difference in basal cortisol levels (i.e., higher cortisol levels in control males than in females), but this sex-difference was not apparent at 5 months. This sex difference coincided with the transient period of elevated testosterone (T) levels normally seen from birth until approximately 4 months of age in male infant rhesus monkeys (Mann, Gould, Collins, & Wallen, 1989; Robinson & Bridson 1978). In fact, a positive correlation was found between cortisol levels and T levels in males at 2.5 months (i.e., at the time of T surge), but not at 5 months, when the postnatal T surge had ended. This sex difference in cortisol secretion at 2.5 months was eliminated by neonatal amygdalectomy as Neo-A male infants had basal cortisol levels similar to those of females, and lower than those of control males. Although the amygdala lesions eliminated sex differences in basal cortisol seen at this age, they did not affect the postnatal T surge. Therefore, the amygdala's effect on HPA axis development and sexual dimorphism does not seem to be due to a direct effect on T secretion, but potentially is mediated by a stimulatory effect of T on basal cortisol release. Although the underlying mechanisms of this relationship are unknown, one potential substrate could be the high expression of androgen receptors (ARs) found in the amygdala (Choate, Slayden, & Resko, 1998), particularly in males (Pomerantz, & Sholl, 1987). Although neonatal amygdala lesions could affect normal T binding to amygdala ARs, there are other mechanisms by which the lesions could influence the hypothalamic–pituitary–gonadal (HPG)–HPA interactions.

At later ages (5 months), neither the sex difference in cortisol nor its correlation with T levels were apparent any longer in control animals. At 5 months, the diurnal cortisol rhythm was present but not fully mature in control animals, characterized by high cortisol levels in the morning, a nonsignificant decline in cortisol from morning to afternoon, and a steep cortisol decline from afternoon to evening (Figure 7.4A). This immature rhythm has also been reported in human infants and toddlers (Larson, White, Chochran, Donzella, & Gunnar, 1998; Watamura, Donzella, Kertes, & Gunnar, 2004). Neonatal amygdalectomy resulted in a blunted cortisol decline from afternoon to evening, driven by increased cortisol levels in the evening compared to controls. This finding is consistent with adult rodent studies demonstrating that CRF knockdown in the central nucleus of the amygdala (CeA) leads to increased basal corticosterone close to the sleep phase of the diurnal rhythm (Regev et al., 2012) or that GR knockdown in the basolateral amygdala (BLA) complex increases basal corticosterone secretion (Furay et al., 2008). These effects of neonatal amygdala lesions on diurnal cortisol rhythm became more prominent with age, leading to higher cortisol secretion throughout the day during

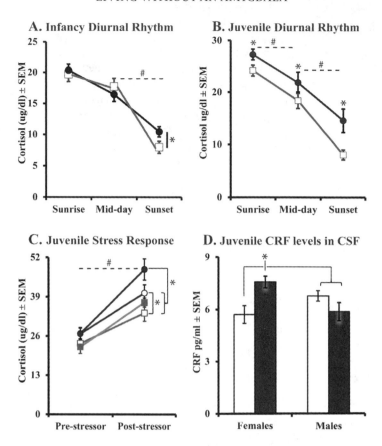

FIGURE 7.4. HPA axis functioning during infancy and juvenile periods. Mean (± *SEM*) diurnal plasma cortisol levels during infancy (5 months shown in A), juvenile (12 months shown in B), and pre- and post-human intruder stressor during juvenile (12 months shown in C). Corticotropin-releasing factor levels in cerebrospinal fluid during the juvenile period are shown in D. Control animals (Neo-C; open bars or open symbols) and animals with neonatal amygdala lesions (Neo-A; black bars or filled symbols). In C, Neo-C females are represented with black squares and Neo-C males with open squares, and Neo-A females are represented with open circles and Neo-A males with black circles.# indicates a significant change in cortisol across time, and * indicates significant group difference of *p* < .05. A and C are reprinted with modifications from Raper et al. (2013a, 2013b) with permission from Elsevier. B and D are reprinted with modifications from Raper et al. (2014b) with permission from the Society for Neuroscience.

the juvenile macaque period (see Figure 7.4B; Raper et al., 2014a). Interestingly, the higher basal HPA axis activity observed in Neo-A animals during the juvenile period could be a consequence of higher central levels of the stress neuropeptide CRF detected in amygdalectomized animals in that study, at least in females.

In short, the results summarized here suggest that the amygdala is essential for the expression of sexually dimorphic HPA axis basal functioning in early infancy and for the establishment of the typical diurnal rhythm by the HPA axis during the juvenile period. However, our findings of elevated baseline HPA axis activity in the juvenile period suggest that the amygdala may have an opposite role during development on HPA axis activity (inhibitory) than that reported in adults (excitatory).

HPA Axis Stress Reactivity

The impact of neonatal amygdala lesions on the stress reactivity was investigated when the animals were juveniles, at 12 months of age (Raper et al., 2013b). The human intruder paradigm was used as a psychogenic stressor, because it has been shown to activate the HPA axis significantly, resulting in rapid increases in ACTH and cortisol in blood (Jahn et al., 2010; Raper et al., 2013c). Amygdalectomized juvenile monkeys exhibited greater cortisol secretions after the social stressor as compared to controls, and this increase in cortisol secretion was greater in Neo-A females than in all other animals (see Figure 7.4C). The results contrast with those of our previous studies reporting blunted HPA axis stress-induced activations in adult monkeys with neonatal amygdala lesions (Raper et al., 2013c). These different outcomes of neonatal amygdala lesions on HPA axis stress reactivity may be related to the developmental period used to assess HPA axis reactivity. Thus, our previous studies examined the HPA axis stress response in adulthood, after the animals had already undergone puberty, whereas the current study has focused on prepubertal animals, a developmental period during which the neural pathways regulating the HPA axis stress response are not fully developed (Andersen, 2003; Lidow, Goldman-Rakic, & Rakic, 1991; Perlman, Webster, Herman, Kleinman, & Weickert, 2007; Pryce, 2008; Sinclair, Webster, Wong, & Weickert, 2011). Prepubertal rodents and monkeys exhibit an exaggerated stress response compared to adults (Clarke, 1993; Davenport et al., 2003; Romeo, Lee, Chhua, McPherson, & McEwen, 2004a; Romeo, Lee, & McEwen, 2004b; Romeo & McEwen, 2006; Sanchez et al., 2005). Thus, the increased cortisol stress response observed in Neo-A animals suggests that the early lesions could have impacted this normative HPA axis development, including the typical developmental changes in corticosteroid receptor systems (Perlman et al., 2007; Pryce, 2008; Sinclair et al., 2011). Indeed, and as described earlier, we also recently demonstrated that the increase in basal HPA axis activity during the juvenile period may involve increased central CRF activity (See Figure 7.3D; Raper et al., 2014a).

In summary, although the amygdala plays an important stimulatory role in adult HPA axis activity, particularly in its response to stress, our findings suggest that during development, the primate amygdala may instead have an inhibitory role on HPA axis maturation. These differences in the effects of neonatal versus adult amygdala lesions are very provocative and may indicate a regulatory role of the amygdala on the development of other brain regions that control the HPA axis, including the medial prefrontal cortex.

Conclusions

Our longitudinal developmental study of the effects of neonatal amygdala lesions in monkeys living in large social groups with a species-typical social structure has yielded important new findings. First, the impacts of the neonatal lesions on infant social development were at best mild and transitory, and upon reaching adolescence, animals with neonatal amygdalectomy were indistinguishable from their controls. Yet, in early infancy, there was a clear but transient amygdalectomy × sex effect in the infant relationship to their mothers, with Neo-A animals spending less time in contact or proximity to their mothers, with the effects of amygdalectomy being slightly, but significantly, more pronounced in females than in males. Upon reaching adolescence, neonatally amygdalectomized males were able to recognize hierarchical status signals and to form stable social hierarchies, and when paired with an adult male, pubertal neonatally amygdala-operated females (2.5–3.5 years of age) showed normal levels of female-initiated behavior toward the males.

These findings contrast with earlier studies that have reported more severe changes in behavioral and social responses in animals with neonatal amygdala lesions. In these earlier reports (Bachevalier, 1994; Thompson, 1981), neonatal aspiration lesions of the amygdala in peer-reared infant monkeys yielded changes in socioemotional behaviors that became increasingly evident when the monkeys reached adulthood. Our data are more consistent with those reported in a series of studies that followed in greater details the long-term effects of neonatal damage of the amygdala in monkeys reared by their biological mother until the age of 6 months and placed in small social groups thereafter (for review, see Bliss-Moreau et al., Chapter 6, this volume). However, notable differences were still evident between these later studies and ours. For example, unlike animals in Bliss-Moreau and colleagues' study, males and females with damage to the amygdala did not display a reduction in exploratory behaviors in social contexts, and in no instances did we observe abnormal behaviors (stereotypies) in our animals. Thus, it appears that the severity of the effects of neonatal amygdala lesions on social behavior largely depends on the complexity of the social contexts in which the animals navigate, with less impact when animals are raised in large social groups than when raised in more restricted groups. The combination of the immaturity of the neural structures, and especially the cortical areas at the time of the neonatal lesions, with the beneficial effects of a socially enriched environment on brain development (see for review Lewis, 2004; Will, Galani, Kelche, & Rosenzweig, 2004) may explain such different impacts of neonatal amygdala damage. The rich social environment could have promoted greater anatomical and functional plasticity in brain structures normally implicated in the regulation of social behaviors and intimately connected with the amygdala, such as the orbitofrontal and anterior cingulate cortex.

Despite the subtle effects of neonatal amygdala lesions on social interactions, the results demonstrated significant changes in emotional and stress neuroendocrine reactivity. Thus, although neonatal amygdala lesions spared the basic expression of emotional or defensive behaviors, they reduced the magnitude of the expression of emotional behaviors, and in some cases reduced the contextual modulation of these behaviors depending on the presence and gaze direction of a social intruder. These emotional changes became more pronounced as the animals matured, and were associated with increased cortisol basal and stress-induced responses in juvenile monkeys, suggesting a developmental trajectory in which the consequences of neonatal amygdala damage became magnified with age or social experience. Thus, in contrast to social behaviors, the absence of a functional amygdala may be more detrimental to the development of emotional and stress neuroendocrine functions due to critical amygdala interactions with subcortical centers, such as the hypothalamus, required for emotional and stress regulatory mechanisms.

Altogether, the effects of neonatal amygdala lesions in monkeys that have been raised with their mothers in a large social group are in line with those reported in human patients with bilateral amygdala damage, such as patients S. M. and A. P. (for review, see Buchanan et al., 2009). Both of these patients present with an almost intact social life, except for being very open and forthcoming in their social interactions. In addition, as for the monkeys, despite normal social behaviors, these subjects demonstrated clear changes in reactivity to fearful stimuli, in recognizing intensity of fear from facial expressions, and in rating truthfulness when viewing face stimuli. The nonhuman and human data now converge, with a revised view of the role of the amygdala on social cognition by Adolphs and Spezio (2006), who posits that in the absence of a functional amygdala, subjects "retain their ability to display the full range of basic social behavior while being impaired in the appropriate context-dependent deployment of these behaviors and of more complex social behaviors" (pp. 364–365).

ACKNOWLEDGMENTS

The study was supported by the National Institute of Mental Health (Grant No. MH050268) and by the National Center for Research Resources to the Yerkes National Research Center (Grant No. P51 RR00165; YNRC base grant), which is currently supported by the Office of Research Infrastructure Programs/OD P51OD11132.

REFERENCES

Adolphs, R., & Spezio, M. (2006). Role of the amygdala in processing visual social stimuli. *Progress in Brain Research, 156,* 363–378.

Aggleton, J. P. (2000). *The amygdala: A functional analysis* (2nd ed.). New York: Oxford University Press.

Ainsworth, M. D. S., & Bell, S. M. (1970). Attachment, exploration, and separation: Illustrated by the behavior of one-year-olds in a strange situation. *Child Development, 41,* 49–67.

Allen, J. P., & Allen, C. F. (1975). Amygdalar participation in tonic ACTH section in the rat. *Neuroendocrinology, 19,* 115–125.

Amaral, D. G., Price, J. L., Pitkänen, A., & Carmichael, S. T. (1992). Anatomical organization of the primate amygdaloid complex. In J. P. Aggleton (Ed.), *The amygdala: Neurobiological aspects of emotion, memory, and mental dysfunction* (1st ed., pp. 1–66). New York: Wiley-Liss.

Andersen, S. L. (2003). Trajectories of brain development: Point of vulnerability or window of opportunity? *Neuroscience and Biobehavioral Review, 27,* 3–18.

Bachevalier, J. (1994). Medial temporal lobe structures and autism: A review of clinical and experimental findings. *Neuropsychologia, 32,* 627–648.

Barrett, C. E., Noble, P., Hanson, E., Pine, D. S., Winslow, J. T., & Nelson, E. E. (2009). Early adverse rearing experiences alter sleep–wake patterns and plasma cortisol levels in juvenile rhesus monkeys. *Psychoneuroendocrinology, 34,* 1029–1040.

Bauman, M. D., Lavenex, P., Mason, W. A., Capitanio, J. P., & Amaral, D. G. (2004). The development of social behavior following neonatal amygdala lesions in rhesus monkeys. *Journal of Cognitive Neuroscience, 16,* 1388–1411.

Bauman, M. D., Toscano, J. E., Babineau, B. A., Mason, W. A., & Amaral, D. G. (2006). The expression of social dominance following neonatal lesions of the amygdala and hippocampus in rhesus monkeys (*Macaca mulatta*). *Behavioral Neuroscience, 120,* 749–760.

Beaulieu, S., Di Paolo, T., & Barden, N. (1986). Control of ACTH secretion by the central nucleus of the amygdala: Implication of the serotoninergic system and its relevance to the glucocorticoid delayed negative feedback mechanism. *Neuroendocrinology, 44,* 247–254.

Bennett, A. L., Greco, B., Blasberg, M. E., & Blaustein, J. D. (2002). Response to male odours in progestin receptor- and oestrogen receptor-containing cells in female rat brain. *Journal of Neuroendocrinology, 14*, 442–449.

Berard, J. (1989). Male life histories. *Puerto Rico Health Sciences Journal, 8*, 47–58.

Bliss-Moreau, E., Bauman, M. D., & Amaral, D. G. (2011a). Neonatal amygdala lesions result in globally blunted affect in adult rhesus macaques. *Behavioral Neuroscience, 125*, 848–858.

Bliss-Moreau, E., Moadab, G., Bauman, M. D., & Amaral, D. G. (2013). The impact of early amygdala damage on juvenile rhesus macaque social behavior. *Journal of Cognitive Neuroscience, 25*, 2124–2140.

Bliss-Moreau, E., Toscano, J. E., Bauman, M. D., Mason, W. A., & Amaral, D. G. (2010). Neonatal amygdala or hippocampus lesions influence responsiveness to objects. *Developmental Psychobiology, 52*, 487–503.

Bliss-Moreau, E., Toscano, J. E., Bauman, M. D., Mason, W. A., & Amaral, D. G. (2011b). Neonatal amygdala lesions alter responsiveness to objects in juvenile macaques. *Neuroscience, 178*, 123–132.

Buchanan, T. W., Tranel, D., & Adolphs, R. (2009). The human amygdala in social function. In P. J. Whalen & E. A. Phelps (Eds.), *The human amygdala* (pp. 289–320). New York: Guilford Press.

Chareyron, L. J., Banta Lavenex, P., Amaral, D. G., & Lavenex, P. (2012). Postnatal development of the amygdala: A sterological study in macaque monkeys. *Journal of Comparative Neurology, 520*, 1965–1984.

Champoux, M., Coe, C. L., Schanberg, S. M., Kuhn, C. M., & Suomi, S. J. (1989). Hormonal effects of early rearing conditions in the infant rhesus monkey. *American Journal of Primatology, 19*, 111–117.

Choate, J. V., Slayden, O. D., & Resko, J. A. (1998). Immunocytochemical localization of androgen receptors in brains of developing and adult male rhesus monkeys. *Endocrine, 8*, 51–60.

Clarke, A. S. (1993). Social rearing effects on HPA axis activity over early development and in response to stress in rhesus monkeys. *Developmental Psychobiology, 26*, 433–446.

Davenport, M. D., Novak, M. A., Meyer, J. S., Tiefenbacher, S., Higley, J. D., & Lindell, S. G. (2003). Continuity and change in emotional reactivity in rhesus monkeys throughout the perpubertal period. *Motivation and Emotion, 27*, 57–76.

Davis, M., &Whalen, P. J. (2001). The amygdala: Vigilance and emotion. *Molecular Psychiatry, 6*, 13–34.

Delgado, J. M., Rivera, M. L., & Mir, D. (1971). Repeated stimulation of amygdala in awake monkeys. *Brain Research, 27*, 111–131.

Dicks, D., Myers, R. E., & Kling, A. (1969). Uncus and amygdala lesions: Effects on social behavior in the free-ranging rhesus monkey. *Science, 165*, 69–71.

Ehle, A. L., Mason, J. W., & Pennington, L. L. (1977). Plasma growth hormone and cortisol changes following limbic stimulation in conscious monkeys. *Neuroendocrinology, 23*, 52–60.

Feldman, S., Conforti, N., Itzik, A., & Weidenfeld, J. (1994). Differential effect of amygdaloid lesions on CRF-41, ACTH, and corticosterone response following neural stimuli. *Brain Research, 658*, 21–26.

Feldman, S., Conforti, N., & Saphier, D. (1990). The preoptic area and bed nucleus of the stria terminalis are involved in the effects of the amygdala on adrenocortical secretion. *Neuroscience, 37,* 775–779.

Feldman, S., Conforti, N., & Weidenfeld, J. (1995). Limbic pathways and hypothalamic neurotransmitters mediating adrenocortical responses to neural stimuli. *Neuroscience and Biobehavioral Review, 19,* 235–240.

Fish, D. R., Gloor, P., Quesney, F. L., & Olivier, A. (1993). Clinical responses to electrical brain stimulation of the temporal and frontal lobes in patients with epilepsy: Pathophysiological implications. *Brain, 116,* 397–414.

Freese, J. L., & Amaral, D. G. (2009). Neuroanatomy of the primate amygdala. In P. J. Whalen & E. A. Phelps (Eds.), *The human amygdala* (pp. 1–42). New York: Gilford Press.

Furay, A. R., Bruestle, A. E., & Herman, J. P. (2008). The role of the forebrain glucocorticoid receptor in acute and chronic stress. *Endocrinology, 149,* 5482–5490.

Goldman, P. S. (1971). Functional development of the prefrontal cortex in early life and the problem of neuronal plasticity. *Experimental Neurology, 32,* 640–650.

Goursaud, A.-P. S., Mendoza, S. P., & Capitanio, J. P. (2006). Do neonatal bilateral ibotenic acid lesions of the hippocampal formation or of the amygdala impair HPA axis responsiveness and regulation in infant rhesus macaques (*Macaca mulatta*)? *Brain Research, 1071,* 97–104.

Goursaud, A.-P. S., Wallen, K., & Bachevalier, J. (2014). Mother recognition and preference after neonatal amygdala lesions in rhesus macaques (*Macaca mulatta*) raised in a semi-naturalistic environment (Special issue). *Developmental Psychobiology, 56*(8), 1723–1734.

Herman, J. P., Figueiredo, H., Mueller, N. K., Ulrich-Lai, Y., Ostrander, M. M., Choi, D. C., et al. (2003). Central mechanisms of stress integration: Hierarchical circuitry controlling hypothalamo–pituitary–adrenocortical responsiveness. *Frontiers in Neuroendocrinology, 24,* 151–180.

Herman, J. P., Ostrander, M. M., Mueller, N. K., & Figueiredo, H. (2005). Limbic system mechanisms of stress regulation: Hypothalmo–pituitary–adrenocortical axis. *Progress in Neuropsychopharmacology and Biological Psychiatry, 29,* 1201–1213.

Higley, J. D., Suomi, S. J., & Linnoila, M. (1992). A longitudinal assessment of CSF monoamine metabolite and plasma cortisol concentrations in young rhesus monkeys. *Biological Psychiatry, 32,* 127–145.

Hinde, R. A., Rowell, T. E., Spencer-Booth, Y. (1964). Behavior of socially living rhesus monkey in their first six months. *Proceedings of the Zoological Society London, 143,* 609–649.

Jahn, A. L., Fox, A. S., Abercrombie, H. C., Shelton, S. E., Oakes, T. R., Davidson, R. J., et al. (2010). Subgenual prefrontal cortex activity predicts individual differences in hypothalamic–pituitary–adrenal activity across different contexts. *Biological Psychiatry, 67,* 175–181.

Jensen, G. D., Bobbitt, R. A., & Gordon, B. N. (1968). Sex difference in the development of independence of infant monkeys. *Behaviour, 30,* 1–14.

Jiang, J., Kanthaswamy, S., & Capitanio, J. P. (2013). Degree of Chinese ancestry affects behavioral characteristics of infant rhesus macaques (*Macaca mulatta*). *Journal of Medical Primatology, 42,* 20–27.

Jurgens, U., & Richter, K. (1986). Glutamate-induced vocalization in the squirrel monkey. *Brain Research, 373*, 349–358.

Kalin, N., & Shelton, S. E. (1989). Defensive behaviors in infant rhesus monkeys: Environmental cues and neurochemical regulation. *Science, 243*, 1718–1721.

Kalin, N., Shelton, S. E., & Davidson, R. J. (2004). The role of the central nucleus of the amygdala in mediating fear and anxiety in primate. *Journal of Neuroscience, 24*, 5506–5515.

Kalin, N., Shelton, S. E., & Takahashi, L. K. (1991). Defensive behaviors in infant rhesus monkeys: ontogeny and context-dependent selective expression. *Child Development, 62*, 1175–1183.

Kalin, N. H., Shelton, S. E., Fox, A. S., Oakes, T. R., & Davidson, R. J. (2005). Brain regions associated with the expression and contextual regulation of anxiety in primates. *Biological Psychiatry, 58*, 796–804.

Keller-Wood, M. E., & Dallman, M. F. (1984). Corticosteroid inhibition of ACTH secretion. *Endocrine Review, 5*, 1–24.

Kling, A., & Cornell, R. (1971). Amygdalectomy and social behavior in the caged stump-tailed (*M. speciosa*). *Folia Primatology, 14*, 91–103.

Kling, A., & Green, P. C. (1967). Effects of neonatal amygdalectomy in the maternally reared and maternally deprived macaque. *Nature, 213*, 742–743.

Kling, A. S. (1972). Effects of amygdalectomy on social-affective behavior in non-human primates. In B. E. Eleftheriou (Ed.), *The neurobiology of the amygdala* (pp. 511–536). New York, Plenum.

Kling, A. S. (1974). Differential effects of amygdalectomy in male and female nonhuman primates. *Archives of Sexual Behavior, 3*, 129–134.

Kling, A. S., & Brothers, L. (1992). The amygdala and social behavior. In J. P. Aggleton (Ed.), *The amygdala: Neurobiological aspects of emotion, memory, and mental dysfunction* (pp. 353–377). New York: Wiley-Liss.

Kling, A. S., Steklis, H. D., & Deutsch, S. (1979). Radiotelemetered activity from the amygdala during social interactions in the monkeys. *Experimental Neurology, 66*, 88–96.

Klüver, H., & Bucy, P. (1939). Preliminary analysis of functioning of the temporal lobes in monkeys. *Archives of Neurology and Psychiatry, 42*, 979–1000.

Lanteaume, L., Khalfa, S., Regis, J., Marquis, P., Chauvel, P., & Bartolomei, F. (2007). Emotion induction after direct intracerebral stimulations of human amygdala. *Cerebral Cortex, 17*, 1307–1313.

Larson, M. C., White, B. P., Chochran, A., Donzella, B., & Gunnar, M. (1998). Dampening of the cortisol response to handling at 3 months in human infants and its relation to sleep, circadian cortisol activity, and behavioral distress. *Developmental Psychobiology, 33*, 327–337.

Lewis, M. H. (2004). Environmental complexity and central nervous system development and function. *Mental Retardation and Developmental Disabilities Research Reviews, 10*, 91–95.

Lidow, M. S., Goldman-Rakic, P. S., & Rakic, P. (1991). Synchronized overproduction of neurotransmitter receptors in diverse regions of the primate cerebral cortex. *Proceedings of the National Academy of Sciences USA, 88*, 10218–10221.

Lindberg, D. G. (1971). The rhesus monkey in Northern India: An ecological and behavioral study. In L. A. Rosenblum (Ed.), *Primate behavior* (Vol. 2, pp. 1–106). New York: Academic Press.

Lovejoy, J., & Wallen, K. (1988). Sexually dimorphic behavior in group-housed rhesus monkeys (*Macaca Mulatta*) at 1 year of age. *Psychobiology, 16*, 348–356.

Machado, C. J., & Bachevalier, J. (2006). The impact of selective amygdala, orbital frontal cortex or hippocampal formation lesions on established social relationships in monkeys. *Behavioral Neuroscience, 120*, 761–786.

Machado, C. J., Bachevalier, J. (2008). Behavioral and hormonal reactivity to threat: Effects of selective amygdala, hippocampal, or orbital frontal lesions in monkeys. *Psychoneuroendocrinology, 33*, 926–941.

Mann, D. R., Gould, K. G., Collins, D. C., & Wallen, K. (1989). Blockade of neonatal activation of the pituitary–testicular axis: Effect on perpubertal luteinizing hormone and testosterone secretion and on testicular development in male monkeys. *Journal of Clinical Endocrinology and Metabolism, 68*, 600–607.

Mason, J. W. (1959). Plasma 17-hydroxycorticosteroid levels during electrical stimulation of the amygdaloid complex in conscious monkeys. *American Journal of Physiology, 196*, 44–48.

Mason, W. A., Capitanio, J. P., Machado, C. J., Mendoza, S. P., & Amaral, D. G. (2006). Amygdalectomy and responsiveness to novelty in rhesus monkeys (*Macaca mulatta*): Generality and individual consistency of effects. *Emotion, 6*, 73–81.

Mason, W. A., & Mendoza, S. P. (1998). Generic aspects of primate attachments: Parents, offspring and mates. *Psychoneuroendocrinology, 23*, 765–778.

Mathews, D., Donovan, K. M., Hollingsworth, E. M., Hutson, V. B., & Overstreet, C. T. (1983). Permanent deficits in lordosis behavior in female rats with lesions of the ventromedial nucleus of the hypothalamus. *Experimental Neurology, 79*, 714–719.

Mathews, D., & Edwards, D. A. (1977). Involvement of the ventromedial and anterior hypothalamic nuclei in the hormonal induction of receptivity in the female rat. *Physiology and Behavior, 19*, 319–326.

Meunier, M., Bachevalier, J., Murray, E. A., Malkova, L., & Mishkin, M. (1999). Effects of aspiration versus neurotoxic lesions of the amygdala on emotional responses in monkeys. *European Journal of Neurosciemce, 11*, 4403–4418.

Mirsky, A. F. (1960). Studies of the effects of brain lesions on social behaviors in *Macaca mulatta*: Methodological and theoretical considerations. *Annals of the New York Academy of Sciences, 85*, 785–794.

Moadab, G. Bliss-Moreau, E., & Amaral, D. G. (2015). Adult social behavior with familiar partners following neonatal amygdala or hippocampus damage. *Behavioral Neuroscience, 129*(3), 339–350.

Myers, B., McKleen, J. M., & Herman, J. P. (2012). Neural regulation of the stress response: The many faces of feedback. *Cellular and Molecular Neurobiology*. [Epub ahead of print].

Norman, R. L., & Spies, H. G. (1981). Brain lesions in infant female rhesus monkeys: Effects on menarche and first ovulation and on diurnal rhythms of prolactin and cortisol. *Endocrinology, 108*, 1723–1729.

Oomura, Y., Aou, S., Koyama, Y., Fujita, I., & Yoshimatsu, H. (1988). Central control of sexual behavior. *Brain Research Bulletin, 20*, 863–870.

Payne, C., Machado, C. J., Bliwise, N. G., & Bachevalier, J. (2010). Maturation of the hippocampal formation and amygdala in *Macaca mulatta*: A volumetric magnetic resonance imaging study. *Hippocampus, 20*, 922–935.

Perlman, W. R., Webster, M. J., Herman, M. M., Kleinman, J. E., & Weickert, C. S. (2007). Age related differences in glucocorticoid receptor mRNA levels in the human brain. *Neurobiology of Aging, 28*, 447–458.

Pitkänen, A. (2000). Connectivity of the rat amygdaloid complex. In J. P. Aggelton (Ed.), *The amygdala: A functional analysis* (pp. 31–115). New York: Oxford University Press.

Plotnik, R. (1968). Changes in social behavior of squirrel monkeys after anterior temporal lobectomy. *Journal of Comparative Physiological Psychiatry, 66*, 369–372.

Pomerantz, S. M., & Sholl, S. A. (1987). Analysis of sex and regional differences in androgen receptors in fetal rhesus monkey brain. *Developmental Brain Research, 36*, 151–154.

Prather, M. D., Lavenex, P., Mauldin-Jourdain, M. L., Mason, W. A., Capitanio, J. P., Mendoza, S. P., et al. (2001). Increased social fear and decreased fear of objects in monkeys with neonatal amygdala lesions. *Neuroscience, 106*, 653–658.

Price, J. L., & Amaral, D. G. (1981). An autoradiography study of the projections of the central nucleus of the monkey amygdala. *Journal of Neuroscience, 1*, 1242–1259.

Pryce, C. R. (2008). Postnatal ontogeny of expression of the corticosteroid receptor genes in mammalian brains: Inter-species and intra-species differences. *Brain Research Review, 57*, 596–605.

Raper, J., Bachevalier, J., Wallen, K., & Sanchez, M. (2013a). Neonatal amygdala lesions alter basal cortisol levels in infant rhesus monkeys. *Psychoneuroendocrinology, 38*, 818–829.

Raper, J., Stephens, S., Henry, A., Villareal, T., Bachevalier, J., Wallen, K., et al. (2014a). Neonatal amygdala lesions lead to increased activity of brain CRF systems and hypothalamic–pituitary–adrenal axis of juvenile rhesus monkeys. *Journal of Neuroscience, 34*, 11452–11460.

Raper, J., Stephens, S. B. Z., Sanchez, M., Bachevalier, J., & Wallen, K. (2014b). Neonatal amygdala lesions alter mother–infant interactions in rhesus monkeys living in a species-typical social environment (Special issue). *Developmental Psychobiology, 56*(8), 1711–1722.

Raper, J., Wallen, K., Sanchez, M., Stephens, S. B. Z., Henry, A., Villareal, T., et al. (2013b). Sex-dependent role of the amygdala in the development of emotional reactivity to threatening stimuli in infant rhesus monkeys. *Hormones and Behavior, 63*, 646–658.

Raper, J., Wilson, M. E., Sanchez, M., Machado, C., & Bachevalier, J. (2013c). Pervasive alterations of emotional and neuroendocrine responses to an acute stressor after neonatal amygdala lesions in rhesus monkeys. *Psychoneuroendocrinology, 38*, 1021–1035.

Redgate, E. S., & Fahringer, E. E. (1973). A comparison of the pituitary adrenal activity elicited by electrical stimulation of preoptic, amygdaloid, and hypothalamic sites in the rat brain. *Neuroendocrinology, 12*, 334–343.

Regev, L., Tsoory, M., Gil, S., & Chen, A. (2012). Site-specific genetic manipulation of amygdala corticotropin-releasing factor reveals its imperative role in mediating behavioral response to challenge. *Biological Psychiatry, 71*, 317–326.

Robinson, J. A., & Bridson, W. E. (1978). Neonatal hormone patterns in the macaque. *Steroids and Biological Reproduction, 19,* 773–778.

Romeo, R. D., Lee, S. J., Chhua, N., McPherson, C. R., & McEwen, B. S. (2004a). Testosterone cannot activate an adult-like stress response in prepubertal male rats. *Neuroendocrinology, 79,* 125–132.

Romeo, R. D., Lee, S. J., & McEwen, B. S. (2004b). Differential stress reactivity in intact and ovariectomized prepubertal and adult female rats. *Neuroendocrinology, 80,* 387–393.

Romeo, R. D., & McEwen, B. S. (2006). Stress and the adolescent brain. *Annals of the New York Academy of Sciences, 1094,* 202–214.

Rosvold, H. E., Mirsky A. F., & Pribram K. H. (1954). Influence of amygdalectomy on social behavior in monkeys. *Journal of Comparative and Physiological Psychology, 47,* 173–178.

Sade, D. S. (1967). Determinants of dominance in a group of free-ranging rhesus monkeys. In S. Altmann (Ed.), *Social communication among primates.* Chicago: University of Chicago.

Sanchez, M. M., Noble, P. M., Lyon, C. K., Plotsky, P. M., Davis, M., Nemeroff, C. B., et al. (2005). Alterations in diurnal cortisol rhythm and acoustic startle response in nonhuman primates with adverse rearing. *Biological Psychiatry, 57,* 373–381.

Sinclair, D., Webster, M. J., Wong, J., & Weickert, C. S. (2011). Dynamic molecular and anatomical changes in the glucocorticoid receptor in human cortical development. *Molecular Psychiatry, 16,* 504–515.

Spies, H. G., Norman, R. L., Clifton, D. K., Ochsner, A., J., Jensen, J. N., & Phoenix, C. H. (1976). Effects of bilateral amygdaloid lesions on gonadal and pituitary hormones in serum and on sexual behavior female rhesus monkeys. *Physiology and Behavior, 17,* 985–992.

Spiteri, T., Musatov, S., Ogawa, S., Ribeiro, A., Pfaff, D. W., & Agmo, A. (2010). The role of the estrogen receptor α in the medial amygdala and ventromedial nucleus of the hypothalamus in social recognition, anxiety, and aggression. *Behavioural Brain Research, 210*(2), 211–220.

Stevens, J. R., Mark, V. H., Erwin, F., Pacheco, P., & Suematsu, K. (1969). Deep temporal stimulation in man: Long latency, long lasting psychological changes. *Archives of Neurology, 21,* 157–169.

Tarullo, A. R., & Gunnar, M. R. (2006). Child maltreatment and the developing HPA axis. *Hormones and Behavior, 50,* 632–639.

Thompson, C. I. (1981). Learning in rhesus monkeys after amygdalectomy in infancy or adulthood. *Behavioural Brain Research, 2,* 81–101.

Thompson, C. I., Bergland, R. M., & Towfighi, J. T. (1977). Social and nonsocial behaviors of adult rhesus monkeys after amygdalectomy in infancy and adulthood. *Journal of Comparative and Physiological Psychology, 91*(3), 533–548.

Thompson, C. I., Schwartzbaum, J. S., & Harlow, H. F. (1969). Development of social fear after amygdalectomy in infant rhesus monkeys. *Physiology and Behavior, 4,* 249–254.

Tomaszycki, M. L., Davis, J. E., Gouzoules, H., & Wallen, K. (2001). Sex differences in infant rhesus macaque separation-rejection vocalizations and effects prenatal androgens. *Hormones and Behavior, 39,* 267–276.

Ulrich-Lai, Y. M., & Herman, J. P. (2009). Neural regulation of endocrine and autonomic stress response. *Nature Reviews Neuroscience, 10*, 397–409.

Wallen, K. (1990). Desire and ability: Hormones and the regulation of female sexual behavior. *Neuroscience and Biobehavioral Reviews, 14*, 233–241.

Wallen, K. (2001). Sex and context: Hormones and primate sexual motivation. *Hormones and Behavior, 40*, 339–357.

Wallen, K. (2005). Hormonal influences on sexually differentiated behavior in nonhuman primates. *Frontiers in Neuroendocrinology, 26*, 7–26.

Wallen, K., & Tannenbaum, P. L. (1997). Hormonal modulation of sexual behavior and affiliation in rhesus monkeys. *Annals of the New York Academy of Sciences, 807*, 185–202.

Watamura, S. E., Donzella, B., Kertes, D. A., & Gunnar, M. R. (2004). Developmental changes in baseline cortisol activity in early childhood: Relations with napping and effortful control. *Developmental Psychobiology, 45*, 125–133.

Weitzman, E. D., Fukushima, D., Nogeire, C., Roffwarg, H., Gallagher, T. F., & Hellman, L. (1971). Twenty-four hour pattern of the episodic secretion of cortisol in normal subjects. *Journal of Clinical Endocrinology and Metabolism, 33*, 14–22.

Will, B., Galani, R., Kelche, C., & Rosenzweig, M. R. (2004). Recovery from brain injury in animals: Relative efficacy of environmental enrichment, physical exercise ore formal training (1990–2002). *Progress in Neurobiology, 72*, 167–182.

Wilson, M. E., & Gordon, T. P. (1989). Season determines timing of first ovulation in rhesus monkeys (*Macaca mulatta*) housed outdoors. *Journal of Reproduction and Fertility, 86*, 435–444.

Wilson, M. E., Gordon, T. P., & Collins, D. C. (1986). Ontogeny of luteinizing hormone secretion and first ovulation in seasonal breeding rhesus monkeys. *Endocrinology, 118*, 293–301.

CHAPTER 8

The Central Nucleus of the Amygdala Is a Critical Substrate for Individual Differences in Anxiety

JONATHAN A. OLER
ANDREW S. FOX
ALEXANDER J. SHACKMAN
NED H. KALIN

In this chapter we review work exploring the role of the amygdala and associated brain structures in mediating anxious temperament, which is a nonhuman primate model of the childhood risk for developing anxiety and depressive disorders. We begin with an abridged history of the scientific inquiry into the role of amygdala in emotion, and specifically in anxiety. We recount the development of our nonhuman primate model of dispositional anxiety and discuss the behavioral, neuroimaging, and molecular genetic evidence from the rhesus monkey, showing that anxious temperament is heritable and strongly related to individual differences in amygdala function. We then review mechanistic studies demonstrating that primate anxiety critically depends on the integrity of the central nucleus of the amygdala, drawing parallels to humans living without an amygdala. The implications of these findings for understanding the risk for anxiety-related psychopathology are outlined, and we highlight the potential for developing more effective early-life interventions based on data derived from the nonhuman primate model.

Research into the function of the amygdala began with experiments in rhesus monkeys, performed by Brown and Schaefer (1888) and later by Klüver and Bucy (1937, 1939). These studies led to further critical experiments in nonhuman primates that continued to specify the amygdala's role in emotion and social behavior (Weiskrantz, 1956; Kling, 1968; Kapp, Frysinger, Gallagher, & Haselton, 1979; Pribram, Reitz, McNeil, &

Spevack, 1979; Aggleton & Passingham, 1981; Rolls, 1984; Zola-Morgan, Squire, Alvarez-Royo, & Clower, 1991). The advances in lesion techniques and other invasive and noninvasive methodologies have motivated more nuanced hypotheses regarding the adaptive role of the amygdala in fear, danger detection, social behavior, vigilance, and temperament (Kalin, 2002; Whalen, 1998; LeDoux, 2000; Adolphs, 2003; Amaral, 2003). There is now great interest in understanding alterations in amygdala function in relation to psychopathology, with a particular emphasis on anxiety and affective disorders.

Understanding the role of the amygdala in anxiety and affective disorders is essential, because these disorders are among the most common psychiatric illnesses in youth and adults (33.7% lifetime incidence of any anxiety disorder; 18.3% lifetime incidence of major depressive disorder), and they are highly comorbid and often resistant to treatment (Kessler, Petukhova, Sampson, Zaslavsky, & Wittchen, 2012). Anxiety disorders frequently begin during the preadolescent years and in many cases are associated with the subsequent onset of depression during adolescence and early adulthood. Research demonstrates that very young children with extreme anxiety, as manifested by marked reactivity to novelty and/ or strangers, are at increased risk to develop anxiety and affective disorders. For example, extreme temperamental childhood anxiety is a strong predictor of the development of social anxiety disorder (Schwartz, Snidman, & Kagan, 1999; Prior, Smart, Sanson, & Oberklaid, 2000; Biederman et al., 2001; Hirshfeld-Becker et al., 2007; Chronis-Tuscano et al., 2009; Essex, Klein, Slattery, Goldsmith, & Kalin, 2010), and depressive disorders (Caspi, Moffitt, Newman, & Silva, 1996; Gladstone & Parker, 2006; Beesdo et al., 2007). A recent meta-analysis supports the contention that extreme childhood temperamental anxiety may represent the single best predictor of the development of social anxiety disorder (Clauss & Blackford, 2012). Appreciating why certain individuals are vulnerable to developing anxiety disorders requires an understanding of the neural mechanisms that influence the development of adaptive anxiety, as well as extreme temperamental anxiety (Yehuda & LeDoux, 2007; McEwen, Eiland, Hunter, & Miller, 2012; Galatzer-Levy, Bonnano, Bush, & LeDoux et al., 2013; Goswami, Rodriguez-Sierra, Cascardi, & Pare, 2013; Grupe & Nitschke, 2013; Holmes & Singewald, 2013; Shackman et al., 2013).

Our ultimate goal is to provide insight into the developmental issues related to the onset of mood and anxiety disorders. Therefore, we have focused our efforts on understanding the developmental pathophysiology of these illnesses by studying the role of the amygdala early in the life of primates as it relates to the initial manifestations of extreme anxiety. Our studies in young rhesus monkeys suggest that the central nucleus of the amygdala (Ce) and the bed nucleus of the stria terminalis (BST; part of the extended amygdala), are key substrates for trait-like differences in anxiety.

The Ce is often conceptualized as the major output structure of the amygdala for projections to the brainstem and hypothalamus, and it is thought to coordinate and gate the physiological and behavioral effects of fear (Davis, 2000; Paré, Quirk, & LeDoux, 2004; Ciocchi et al., 2010; Haubensak et al., 2010). Additional hypotheses of Ce function have been postulated to account for its role in appetitive learning and attention (Kapp, Whalen, Supple, & Pascoe, 1992; Gallagher & Holland, 1994; Gallagher, 2000; Everitt, Cardinal, Parkinson, & Robbins, 2003; Gabriel, Burhans, & Kashef, 2003). The Ce is also conceptualized as the temporal lobe component of the "central extended amygdala," a hypothesized macrostructural anatomical entity that extends into the basal forebrain (Alheid & Heimer, 1988; de Olmos & Heimer, 1999; Heimer & Van Hoesen, 2006). The basal forebrain is a complex region that has only recently become accessible to study in the living primate. Because of its strategic location and putative functions, dysfunction of the basal forebrain has been implicated in various neuropsychiatric disorders (Heimer, 2003). The major components of the basal forebrain, including the cholinergic nucleus basalis of Meynert, the ventral striatopallidal system, and the extended amygdala, are highly interdigitated, which makes it challenging to elucidate selective functions of these basal forebrain components (Zaborszky et al., 2008). The central extended amygdala concept proposed by Heimer and colleagues to describe the continuum of gamma-aminobutyric acid (GABA)ergic neurons that runs from the Ce, through the substantia innominata, to the BST and the shell of the nucleus accumbens complements the other models of Ce function mentioned earlier. In addition to being highly interconnected, the Ce and BST share many of the same efferent targets, reinforcing the idea that the Ce and BST together form a coherent functional unit (de Olmos & Heimer, 1999). Consistent with these anatomical and neurochemical findings, functional magnetic resonance imaging (fMRI) data from our laboratory demonstrate that in monkeys and humans the Ce and BST display highly significant functional connectivity at rest or under anesthesia, supporting the hypothesis that these structures form a discrete circuit (Oler et al., 2012). An alternative view, however, considers the Ce, sublenticular substantia innominata, and BST continuum as differentiated components of a striatopallidal projection system (Dong, Petrovich, & Swanson, 2001; Swanson, 2003).

Rodent studies suggest an important dissociation between subdivisions of the Ce and the BST with respect to defensive behaviors, such that the medial division of the Ce (CeM) is involved in rapid, phasic, fear-related responding, whereas the BST, via inputs from the lateral division of the Ce (CeL), is thought to mediate slower, sustained, anxiety-like responses to diffuse or ambiguous threats (Walker & Davis, 2008). More recent data, providing updates to this model, highlight the importance of the reciprocal (BST → Ce) projection in determining the functions of these central extended amygdala microcircuits (Gungor, Yamamoto, & Paré, 2015). Additionally, recent human imaging studies have associated the BST region with vigilance, threat monitoring, and anticipatory anxiety (Straube, Mentzel, & Miltner, 2007; Alvarez, Chen, Bodurka, Kaplan, & Grillon, 2011; Mobbs et al., 2010; Somerville, Whalen, & Kelley, 2010; Choi, Padmala, Spechler, & Pessoa, 2014; Grupe, Oathes, & Nitschke, 2013; Avery et al., 2014), and some evidence for a Ce and BST functional dissociation, similar to that in rodents, has been reported in humans (Davis, Walker, Miles, & Grillon, 2010).

Here we review studies from rhesus monkeys, with the aim of understanding the role of the amygdala in temperamental anxiety, and provide evidence demonstrating that the central extended amygdala plays a critical role in early-life anxiety. We first recount the development and validation of the nonhuman primate model of childhood anxiety. Next, we discuss neuroimaging and genetic evidence from the rhesus monkey, showing that the anxious phenotype, or anxious temperament, is heritable and strongly related to individual differences in Ce function. We then describe evidence from mechanistic studies demonstrating that behavioral expression of primate anxiety critically depends on the integrity of the Ce. We conclude by outlining the implications of these findings for understanding the risk for anxiety-related psychopathology, for potentially developing more effective early-life interventions, and for understanding normal variation in childhood temperament.

Developing the Human Intruder Paradigm and the Concept of Anxious Temperament

From our nonhuman primate studies, we developed the term anxious temperament to describe an individual's underlying predisposition to display extreme anxiety-related behavioral and physiological responses early in life. There is considerable evidence that the amygdala plays a critical role in normal fear and emotional processing (Adolphs et al., 2005; Whalen & Phelps, 2009; Choi & Kim, 2010; Duvarci & Paré, 2014; Wolff et al., 2014); altered amygdala function has been reported in adults with anxiety disorders (Etkin & Wager, 2007); and administration of clinically effective anxiolytics reduces amygdala activation in a dose-dependent manner (Paulus, Feinstein, Castillo, Simmons, & Stein, 2005). In addition, adults with a history of childhood anxious temperament display increased amygdala reactivity to novel or potentially fearful stimuli (Schwartz, Wrigh, Shin, Kagan, & Rauch, 2003; Blackford & Pine, 2012). However, the amygdala's contribution to early-life presentation of trait-like individual differences in childhood anxiety remains unclear. Specifying the processes within the amygdala that underlie the development of normal and abnormal anxiety will be essential for developing novel, neuroscientifically grounded interventions for treating and preventing anxiety-related psychopathology.

There are a number of standardized behavioral paradigms that measure childhood behavioral inhibition (Fox et al., 2005b). These paradigms include the introduction of a stranger to the room with a young child (Buss, Davidson, Kalin, & Goldsmith, 2004), and exposure of a child to novel objects and social situations (Kagan, Reznick, & Snidman, 1988). Individual differences in physiological responses to stress have also been examined in relation to behavioral inhibition. Many of these studies have focused on pituitary–adrenal activity and report mixed results. Initial studies demonstrated associations between cortisol and behavioral inhibition in children, or between cortisol and anxious temperament in monkeys (Kalin, Larson, Shelton, & Davidson, 1998a; Essex, Klein, Cho, & Kalin, 2002); however, later studies did not consistently replicate these findings (Shackman et al., 2013). While not as extensively studied, evidence points to an association between heart rate and right frontal electroencephalographic (EEG) asymmetry with extreme childhood behavioral inhibition and monkey anxious temperament (Davidson, Kalin, & Shelton, 1992, 1993; Kalin et al., 1998a; Fox, Henderson, Marshall, Nichols, & Ghera, 2005b).

The behavioral assay for monkeys developed by Kalin and Shelton (1989), termed the "human intruder paradigm," was conceptualized, in part, to map onto studies characterizing behavioral inhibition in human children. The human intruder paradigm consists of three different, consecutively presented conditions ("Alone," "No Eye Contact," and "Stare") that elicit different, contextually appropriate, anxiety-related defensive responses (see Figure 8.1). In the Alone condition, animals are separated from their cagemates and placed by themselves in a novel test cage. During the No Eye Contact (NEC) condition, which follows the Alone condition, a human intruder enters the room and at 2.5 meters from the cage presents his or her profile to the monkey. The critical component of this condition is the lack of eye contact between the human intruder and the test monkey. Whereas eye contact signals a direct threat, the avoidance of eye contact provides a sustained, potentially threatening context. The intruder then leaves the room for a brief period. Upon reentering, the Stare condition ensues, during which the intruder continuously stares at the monkey with a neutral facial expression (Kalin, 2002).

Our definition of "anxious temperament" parallels the construct of behavioral inhibition used by Kagan and colleagues (1988) in their description of extremely shy toddlers who were observed to become immobile and hesitant to vocalize in the face of potential threat. Freezing behavior in response to the NEC condition of the human intruder paradigm, because of its obvious similarity to human behavioral inhibition, was the initial metric used to assess threat-related anxiety in young monkeys (Kalin & Shelton, 1989, 2000, 2003; Kalin, Shelton, Fox, Oakes, & Davidson, 2005).

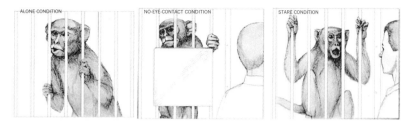

FIGURE 8.1. The three anxious temperament (AT) experimental conditions of the human intruder paradigm elicit distinct fear-related behaviors in young rhesus monkeys. When alone and separated from their cagemate (left), young monkeys actively explore the test cage and spontaneously emit "coo" calls, thought to reflect an attempt to attract help from their mothers or other conspecifics. In the next condition, a human intruder presents his or her profile, while avoiding direct eye contact with the monkey (NEC, center). In this situation, the monkeys typically orient their focus on the intruder, trying to evade discovery by remaining completely still (freezing) or hiding behind their food bin (opaque box in the center panel). In the third condition, the human intruder enters the room and stares at the animal (right). This direct threat condition often elicits aggressive behaviors (e.g., barking, threatening gestures, cage rattling). From Kalin (2002). Copyright 2002 by Scientific American, Inc. Reprinted by permission.

As a validation of its relevance to anxiety, we demonstrated that NEC-induced freezing in monkeys can be reduced by administration of the benzodiazepine, diazepam, a common pharmacological treatment for clinically significant anxiety (Kalin & Shelton, 1989; Davidson et al., 1993; Kalin, 2003), and increased with administration of β-carboline, an anxiogenic benzodiazepine inverse agonist (Kalin, Shelton, & Turner, 1992). We later expanded the assessment of monkey anxiety to move beyond just a single behavioral measure (i.e., freezing) to a composite measure by including decreases in spontaneous coo-calls (Fox et al., 2005a), as well as individual differences in threat-induced cortisol levels (Jahn et al., 2010). This was, in part, based on the observation that animals with elevated freezing in response to the NEC condition concomitantly emitted fewer vocalizations (Kalin & Shelton, 1989). Threat-induced cortisol was added to gauge individual differences in pituitary–adrenal reactivity (Kalin & Shelton, 1989; Kalin, Shelton, Rickman, & Davidson, 1998b). It is important to note that when examining the relations among the three components of anxious temperament (freezing, reduced cooing, and cortisol levels) in a large sample, individual differences in cortisol levels do not significantly correlate with either behavioral metric, whereas freezing and cooing are moderately inversely correlated (Shackman et al., 2013). The inclusion of cortisol in the composite measure of anxious temperament is intended to capture the heterogeneity in individual differences in the physiological response to fear- and anxiety-eliciting stimuli. Interestingly, the anxious temperament composite better predicts individual differences in amygdala metabolism than any one of its three components (Fox, Shelton, Oakes, Davidson, & Kalin, 2008; Shackman et al., 2013).

To be clear, we specifically use the term "anxious temperament" to operationalize the theoretical construct representing an individual's disposition to behave with reticence and respond to potential threat with extreme behavioral and physiological reactivity. Our definition of "anxious temperament" not only includes behavioral inhibition (i.e., freezing and decreased spontaneous vocalization) but also takes into account the degree of pituitary–adrenal stress-responsiveness of the individual (see Figure 8.2A).

Table 8.1 demonstrates the translational utility of anxious temperament as a model for childhood behavioral inhibition or the early childhood risk for developing social anxiety. As mentioned earlier, it is well documented that highly anxious children are at substantial risk for social anxiety disorder (SAD).

As shown in Table 8.1, the anxious temperament phenotype in young monkeys and the behaviorally inhibited phenotype in young children share a number of common features. Many of these common features are antecedents of SAD. We believe that extreme anxious temperament in children, when stable and trait-like, has the hallmarks of subthreshold SAD but is not severe enough to satisfy the functional impairment criterion. Box 8.1 lists the DSM-5 criteria for SAD diagnosis, many features of which are shared by both childhood behavioral inhibition and monkey anxious temperament.

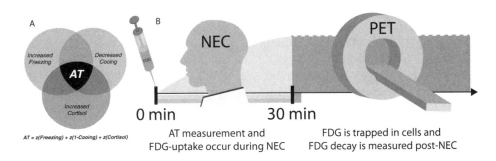

FIGURE 8.2. (A) Anxious temperament (AT) is calculated as the mean z-scores of NEC-induced freezing, coo vocalizations (reverse-scored), and plasma cortisol levels. (B) To measure NEC-induced regional brain metabolism, monkeys were injected with a radiotracer (18-FDG) immediately prior to exposure of the 30-minute NEC challenge depicted in Figure 8.1. Following NEC exposure the monkeys were anesthetized, blood was collected for cortisol, and the animals were placed in a high-resolution microPET scanner to measure FDG uptake, integrated across the 30-minute NEC challenge.

TABLE 8.1. Parallels between Monkey Anxious Temperament (AT) and Childhood Behavioral Inhibition (BI)

Phenotypic features	AT in juvenile monkeys	BI in children
Increased freezing/ reduced motor activity/ passive avoidance in the presence of adult strangers	Yes (Kalin & Shelton, 1989; Kalin et al., 1998b; Fox et al., 2008, 2012; Oler et al., 2010; Shackman et al., 2013)	Yes (Fox et al., 2005; Hirshfeld-Becker et al., 2008; Degnan et al., 2010)
Less frequent vocal communication	Yes (Kalin & Shelton, 1989; Fox et al., 2008; Oler et al., 2010; Fox et al., 2012; Shackman et al., 2013)	Yes (Fox et al., 2005b; Hirshfeld-Becker et al., 2008; Degnan et al., 2010)
Moderate stability across time and context	Yes (Fox et al., 2008, 2012; Shackman et al., 2013)	Yes (Pfeifer et al., 2002; Fox et al., 2005b; Hirshfeld-Becker et al., 2008; Degnan et al., 2010; Brooker et al., 2013)
Significant functional impairment or distress	Unknown	Variable (Fox et al., 2005b; Hirshfeld-Becker et al., 2008; Degnan et al., 2010)
Heritable	Yes (Williamson et al., 2003; Oler et al., 2010)	Yes (Rickman & Davidson, 1994; Hirshfeld-Becker et al., 2008)
Reduced by anxiolytic administration	Yes (Kalin & Shelton, 1989; Davidson et al., 1992, 1993)	Unknown
Increased pituitary–adrenal activity (cortisol)	Not consistently observed (Kalin et al., 1998b; Fox et al., 2008, 2012; Oler et al., 2010; Shackman et al., 2013)	Not consistently observed (Schmidt et al., 1997; de Haan et al., 1998; Fox et al., 2005b)
Right-lateralized frontal EEG activity	Yes (Davidson et al., 1993; Kalin et al., 1998a)	Yes (Davidson and Rickman, 1999; Buss et al., 2003; Fox et al., 2005b)
Increased or sustained amygdala activity to novelty and potential threat	Yes (Fox et al., 2008, 2012; Oler et al., 2010; Shackman et al., 2013)	Yes (some data are from retrospective studies in adults) (Schwartz et al., 2003; Blackford et al., 2011)
Altered functional connectivity between the amygdala and prefrontal cortex	Yes (Birn et al., 2014)	Yes (Hardee et al., 2013)

BOX 8.1. *Diagnostic and Statistical Manual of Mental Disorders (DSM-5) Criteria for Social Anxiety Disorder (SAD) Diagnosis*

A. Marked fear or anxiety about one or more social situations in which the individual is exposed to possible scrutiny by others. Examples include social interactions (e.g., having a conversation, *meeting unfamiliar people*), being observed (e.g., eating or drinking), and performing in front of others (e.g., giving a speech). *Note.* In children, the anxiety must occur in peer settings and not just during interactions with adults.

B. The individual fears that he or she will act in a way or show anxiety symptoms that will be negatively evaluated (i.e., will be humiliating or embarrassing; will lead to rejection of offend others).

C. The social situations almost always provoke fear or anxiety. *Note.* In children, the fear or anxiety may be expressed by crying, tantrums, *freezing*, clinging, shrinking, or *failing to speak in social situations*.

D. The social situations are avoided or endured with intense fear or anxiety.

E. The fear or anxiety is out of proportion to the actual threat posed by the social situation and to the sociocultural context.

F. The fear, anxiety, or avoidance is persistent, typically lasting for 6 months or more.

G. The fear, anxiety, or avoidance causes clinically significant distress or impairment in social, occupational, or other important areas of functioning.

H. The fear, anxiety, or avoidance is not attributable to the physiological effects of a substance (e.g., a drug of abuse, a medication) or another medical condition.

I. The fear, anxiety, or avoidance is not better explained by the symptoms of another mental disorder, such as panic disorder, body dysmorphic disorder, or autism spectrum disorder.

J. If another medical condition (e.g., Parkinson's disease, obesity, disfigurement from burns or injury) is present, the fear, anxiety, or avoidance is clearly unrelated or is excessive.

Italics added. From American Psychiatric Association (2013, pp. 202–203). Copyright 2013 by the American Psychiatric Association. Reprinted by permission.

Neuroimaging Studies Linking Individual Differences in Ce Function to Anxiety

Our initial [^{18}F] fluorodeoxyglucose (FDG)–positron emission tomography (PET) imaging studies demonstrated that monkey anxious temperament was correlated with metabolism in the amygdala and the extended amygdala (i.e., BST), as well as the anterior hippocampus, anterior temporal lobe, and periaqueductal gray (PAG) (Fox et al., 2005a, 2008; Kalin et al., 2005). FDG is a radiolabeled glucose analogue with a half-life of ~110 minutes that does not get metabolized and remains trapped in metabolically active cells (Sokoloff et al., 1977). Because the time course of FDG uptake reflects brain activity over approximately 30 minutes and remains stably detectable in the brain, it is an ideal radiotracer to study simultaneously study behavior and brain activity elicited by exposure to ethologically relevant situations (see Figure 8.2B). FDG–PET is therefore particularly useful in understanding the sustained brain responses associated with temperament, which, by definition, is a persistent and relatively context-independent emotional disposition.

We performed FDG-PET scans on animals exposed to four different conditions, two of which were stressful (NEC and Alone–separation from cagemate into a test cage), and two of which were nonstressful (in home cage without cagemate, and in homecage with cagemate). Our findings revealed consistent positive correlations between individual differences in NEC-elicited anxious temperament with metabolism in the amygdala, hippocampus, anterior temporal pole, and PAG, regardless of the stressful or nonstressful condition in which brain metabolic activity was assessed (Fox et al., 2008). Remarkably, the anxious temperament brain metabolism phenotype was discernible in the absence of provocation, when monkeys were at home with their cagemate, something that is virtually impossible to measure in humans. These results suggest that the neural correlates of anxious temperament are stable across contexts and not as context-dependent as the observable behavioral and pituitary–adrenal responses associated with anxious temperament. Similarly, we examined the stability of anxious temperament's neural substrates across time by assessing FDG–PET and anxious temperament in response to NEC in 24 animals, three times over the course of 6–18 months (Fox et al., 2012). Results demonstrated that brain metabolism within anxious temperament-related regions was stable over time, and mean brain metabolism (across the three assessments) predicted mean anxious temperament (Fox et al., 2012). Collectively, these data indicate that the trait-like nature of anxious temperament is reflected by context-independent and temporally stable neural substrates that are instantiated in the inherent activity of an individual's brain.

To explore further the neural substrate underlying anxious temperament and to elucidate the heritable basis of anxious temperament, we performed an experiment examining FDG–PET and anxious temperament in response to the NEC context in a large sample ($n = 238$) of young rhesus monkeys (Oler et al., 2010). Because of the statistical power afforded by the large sample size, we used extremely stringent statistical thresholds (Šidák correction), which increases confidence in the findings. Consistent with earlier findings, the imaging data demonstrated that metabolism in anterior temporal lobe structures, including the Ce region, anterior hippocampus, and anterior temporal cortex, predicted individual differences in anxious temperament (Figure 8.3).

At the Šidák threshold ($p = .00000005875$), large bilateral anterior temporal lobe clusters that correlated positively with anxious temperament were observed (Oler et al., 2010). The anterior temporal lobe clusters contained multiple spatial peaks, each of which correlated with anxious temperament. Therefore, we further resolved the location of the peak correlations within the anterior temporal lobe clusters by calculating the spatial confidence intervals representing volumes that with 95% certainty contained the peak correlations between metabolic activity and anxious temperament (see Oler et al., 2010, for details). To further demarcate and define the location of these peaks, we used *in vivo* chemoarchitectonic techniques to demonstrate that this functionally defined region corresponds to the Ce, a degree of precision that is difficult to achieve using conventional imaging techniques in humans. The volumes contained within the 95% confidence intervals were superimposed on a voxelwise map of serotonin transporter (5-HTT) binding created from an independent sample of rhesus monkeys assessed with [^{11}C]-3-amino-4-(2-dimethylaminomethylphenylsulfanyl)-benzonitrile (DASB) PET (Christian et al., 2009; Oler et al., 2009). This 5-HTT map (see Figure 8.4) can be used to localize the Ce and differentiate it from the anterior hippocampus, since compared to surrounding regions, CeL has the highest density of 5-HTT binding (O'Rourke & Fudge, 2006).

Demonstrating Heritability of Anxious Temperament and Initial Studies of the Genetic Basis of Anxious Temperament

To ascertain whether individual differences in anxious temperament are heritable, we took advantage of the fact that young rhesus monkeys in the study all belonged to a single multigenerational pedigree of more than 1,800 individuals. The power of the extended pedigree approach to quantitative genetic analysis stems from the many closely related, distantly

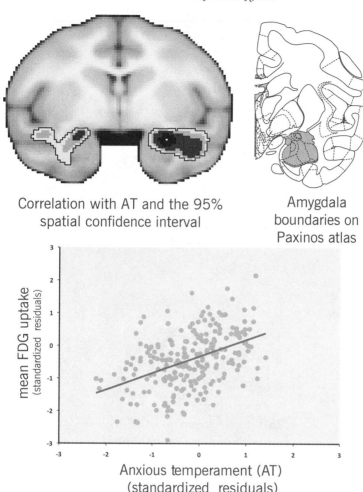

Correlation with AT and the 95% spatial confidence interval

Amygdala boundaries on Paxinos atlas

FIGURE 8.3. To understand the relation between individual differences in regional brain metabolism and anxious temperament (AT), whole-brain voxel-wise regression analysis was performed in 238 young monkeys, while researchers controlled for nuisance effects of age, sex, and voxelwise gray-matter probability. Results revealed a peak FDG–AT correlation in the region of the Ce (significance of correlations: light gray, $p < .05$; medium gray, $p < .01$; dark gray, $p < .001$, adjusted for multiple comparisons using the Šidák correction). The area in black represents the 95% spatial confidence interval of the peak FDG–AT correlation in the amygdala. Adapted with permission of Nature Publishing Group from Oler et al. (2010).

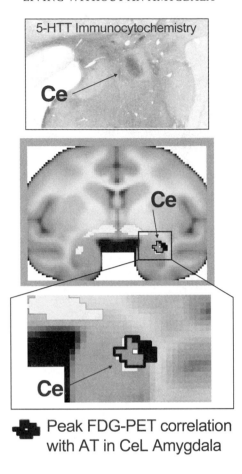

FIGURE 8.4. *In vivo* serotonin transporter (5-HTT) binding localized the dorsal amygdala cluster to the Ce. Top: A low-power photomicrograph of *ex vivo* 5-HTT immunohistochemistry showing substantial immunoreactivity in the lateral division of Ce. Adapted from O'Rourke and Fudge (2006). Copyright 2006 by Elsevier. Adapted by permission. High levels of 5-HTT are a chemoarchitectonic hallmark of the lateral subdivision of the Ce (CeL). Middle: Overlap between the amygdala 95% spatial confidence interval of the peak FDG–AT correlation (black) and *in vivo* 5-HTT availability (off white = 250 × background 5-HTT binding). High 5-HTT availability was also observed within the substantia innominata, which can be seen just below the anterior commissure, medial and dorsal to the Ce and in the region of the dorsal raphe nucleus (not shown). Bottom: Magnified coronal view of the overlap between 5-HTT binding and the FDG–PET correlation, as shown in the middle panel.

related, and unrelated pairs of individuals that all contribute information about the effects of shared genes on phenotypic similarity. Specifically, among the monkeys with phenotype data and confirmed lineage, there were three full-sibling pairs, 189 half-sibling pairs, 128 third-degree relative pairs, 372 fourth-degree relative pairs, and much larger numbers of more distantly related and unrelated pairs. Using a general variance components method (Almasy & Blangero, 1998), we estimated the heritability of anxious temperament while including covariates such as sex, age, and their interactions in the mean effects model to control for extraneous sources of variance (for methodological details, see supplemental materials from Oler et al., 2010). Consistent with previous reports in rhesus monkeys (Williamson et al., 2003; Rogers, Shelton, Shelledy, Garcia, & Kalin, 2008) and the genetic epidemiology of human anxiety disorders (Hettema, Neale, & Kendler, 2001), approximately 36% of the variability in anxious temperament was accounted for by the pairwise relationships among the animals.

We used this same quantitative genetic approach to estimate the heritability of metabolic activity at each voxel in which FDG metabolism significantly predicted differences in the anxious phenotype (see Figure 8.5). Remarkably, although glucose metabolism in the Ce and anterior hippocampal peak regions were similarly predicative of anxious temperament, these regions were differentially heritable. Unlike Ce metabolism, anterior hippocampal metabolism was significantly heritable, and this level of heritability was significantly greater than the heritability estimate for the Ce (Oler et al., 2010). We interpreted these findings cautiously, because even this large sample size is relatively modest for tests of additive genetic effects, but the results suggest that the Ce may be particularly influenced by the environment and experience, and set the stage for further experiments aimed at understanding the neurodevelopmental origins of anxious temperament. These results also highlight the important observation that it is possible to dissociate heritable from nonheritable neural substrates—something that, to our knowledge, had never been shown in prior work.

At a more specific level, we examined DNA variation in candidate genes as they relate to anxious temperament and its underlying amygdalar and hippocampal metabolism. We selected the serotonin transporter repeat length polymorphic region (5-HTTLPR), because variation in this gene was shown by numerous groups to predict fear-related behaviors and the risk for affective disorders (Hariri & Holmes, 2006). The effects of the 5-HTTLPR genotype on the risk to develop anxiety are not straightforward and may only be revealed when examining brain reactivity, for example, when comparing stressful and nonstressful conditions or, as is required in the analysis of fMRI data, a change from baseline. We

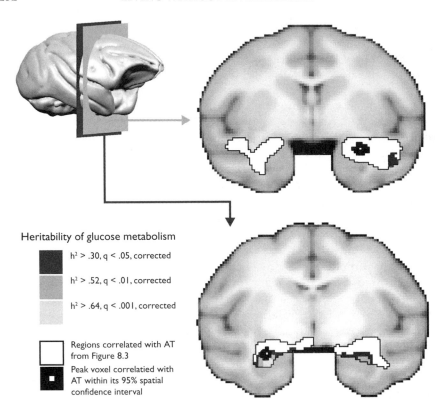

FIGURE 8.5. Overlap between regional metabolic activity predictive of anxious temperament (AT; white) and regions that are significantly heritable. No significantly heritable voxels were observed in the dorsal amygdala region (top), although within the same slice, significant heritability was detected in the superior temporal sulcus (bottom). Glucose metabolism was significantly heritable in both the right and left anterior hippocampus, where it overlaps with the left anterior hippocampal region that correlated with anxious temperament (white, regions predictive of AT; dark gray to light gray, false discovery rate: $q = .05$, $q = .01$, $q = .001$). Adapted with permission of Nature Publishing Group from Oler et al. (2010).

observed no effect of the *5-HTTLPR* on anxious temperament or anxious temperament-related glucose metabolism (Oler et al., 2010). This was not surprising considering that (1) a large imaging study using arterial spin labeling found no effect of *5-HTTLPR* genotype on baseline amygdala blood flow (Viviani et al., 2010), and (2) a previous study in a smaller sample of monkeys failed to observe *5-HTTLPR* genotype-related differences in NEC-related metabolism (Kalin et al., 2008). Kalin et al. did, however, find *5-HTTLPR* genotype-related alterations when comparing the *difference* in metabolism between the NEC condition and a "safe" condition, in which the animals were administered FDG in their home cages. In contrast to the anxious temperament findings, these data demonstrate an association between context-dependent metabolic changes and the *5-HTTLPR* genotype. Interestingly, in the same sample of monkeys, the *5-HTTLPR* genotype was not significantly associated with [^{11}C] DASB binding, a measure of 5-HT transporter availability (Christian et al., 2009). Collectively, these findings highlight the complexity of the influence that the *5-HTTLPR* and other functional polymorphisms have on behavior and the risk for psychopathology, and support the idea that neurogenetics research should focus on gene × environment interactions (Caspi, Hariri, Holmes, Uher, & Moffitt, 2010; Hyde, Bogdan, & Hariri, 2011; Bogdan, Hyde, & Hariri, 2013).

In contrast to the short and long allelic variation in the *5-HTTLPR*, single-nucleotide polymorphisms (SNPs) in the corticotropin-releasing hormone receptor 1 (*CRHR1*) gene, which has been associated with risk for the development of anxiety-related disorders (Bradley et al., 2008), were significantly associated with both anxious temperament and anxious temperament-related glucose metabolism. Specifically, SNPs in exon 6 of the rhesus *CRHR1* gene appear to confer an increased likelihood of elevated anxious temperament and greater NEC-related metabolism in the Ce and anterior hippocampus (Rogers et al., 2013). This finding is particularly interesting, because exon 6 is found primarily in anthropoid primates. Much of the human *CRHR1* genetic data report gene × environment interactions, especially interactions with early childhood trauma (Bradley et al., 2008). Thus, these findings suggest that the early-life effects of *CRHR1* genetic variation may be to support the development of a diathesis that interacts with early adversity to increase the likelihood of developing pathological anxiety.

Molecular Substrates within the Ce Relevant to Anxious Temperament

As anxiety and affective disorders can be resistant to current treatments, and many of these treatments are associated with significant adverse effects (Bystritsky, 2006; Cloos & Ferreira, 2009; Kessler et al., 2012) there is great need to identify new anxiolytic and antidepressant molecular targets. Furthermore, because of the early-life onset of anxiety, establishing novel early-life interventions aimed at preventing chronic and debilitating outcomes would be an ideal treatment approach. To develop novel interventions for anxiety disorders, it is necessary to identify potential treatment targets and to test their therapeutic feasibility in a species that expresses anxiety-related symptomatology that is similar to human psychopathology. In this regard, quantitative messenger RNA (mRNA) approaches are particularly useful, because they capture the combined impact of genetic and environmental epigenetic regulation (Jaenisch & Bird, 2003). With microarray or deep RNA sequencing data, we can identify individual differences in mRNA expression levels of specific genes that predict anxious temperament and altered metabolism within the anxious temperament neural circuit (Fox et al., 2012; Roseboom et al., 2014).

The monkey model of childhood anxious temperament allows us to dovetail the same multimodal imaging methods routinely used in humans with in-depth postmortem brain molecular analyses. Our initial approach has been to collect brain tissue punches from a subset of monkeys phenotyped for anxious temperament. Using the imaging data as a guide, from the brains of 24 male monkeys, we selectively biopsied the region of the dorsal amygdala where its metabolism was most predictive of anxious temperament (Figure 8.6). Affymetrix rhesus microarray chips were used to assess mRNA expression that was analyzed in relation to individual differences in anxious temperament and Ce metabolism (see Figure 8.6). Analyses controlling for housing differences, hemisphere sampled, and age revealed that anxious temperament was associated with a number of mRNA transcripts that had at least moderate expression levels [>log2(100)], and remained significantly correlated with anxious temperament after correcting for multiple comparisons (false discovery rate [FDR] q [adjusted p value] < .05, two-tailed; see Fox et al., 2012, for detailed methods). A gene ontology enrichment analysis of all the significant anxious temperament-related mRNAs revealed that expression levels of gene families associated with neuroplasticity and neurodevelopment significantly predicted differences in anxious temperament (Fox et al., 2012). Specifically, this transcriptome-wide analysis revealed that anxious temperament and increased Ce metabolism were associated with decreased expression levels of several genes in the NTF-3 (neurotrophin-3)–NTRK3 pathway (see Figure 8.6). NTRK3 (neurotrophic tyrosine kinase receptor-3, also termed TrkC) is of considerable interest because its activation can initiate synaptogenesis and neurogenesis (Bernd, 2008). In addition, NTRK3 genetic variation has been linked to human psychopathology (Otnaess et al., 2009), and because the NTRK3 protein is a cell surface receptor, NTRK3 may provide an accessible drug target. These unique findings in a primate species suggest that the expression and maintenance of anxious temperament and the subsequent increased risk to develop anxiety and depression may be due to early maladaptive neurodevelopmental processes (Fox et al., 2012).

The findings from the microarray experiment also demonstrated that Ce metabolism and anxious temperament were associated with altered expression of some expected candidates genes (e.g., 5HT2C and NPY1R).

Prospective longitudinal
FDG–PET imaging guided tissue
extraction for microarray

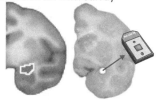

☐ Mean FDG-PET predicts mean AT (n=24)

NTRK3 mRNA levels predict
amygdala metabolism

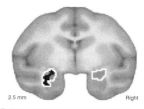

2.5 mm   Right

■ NTRK3 mRNA expression negatively predicts mean
   FDG–PET in stable AT-related regions (pink)

Decreased Ce expression of
plasticity-related genes relates to
increased AT

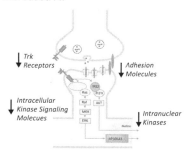

FIGURE 8.6. Microarray data demonstrated that individuals with higher levels of Ce *NTRK3* mRNA expression exhibited lower anxious temperament. Top: Ce regions predictive of dispositional anxious temperament were used to guide amygdala biopsy for analysis of anxious temperament-related RNA expression. A slice through the functionally defined amygdala region juxtaposed with a representative single-subject slab in which the dorsal amygdala was biopsied. Middle: *NTRK3* expression negatively predicts Ce metabolism. Individuals showing higher levels of *NTRK3* mRNA expression, indexed by quantitative real-time reverse transcription polymerase chain reaction (qRT-PCR), show reduced Ce metabolism *in vivo* (black) (FDR-corrected within the stable anxious temperament-related region [white]). Bottom: Portrayal of the neuroplasticity-associated *NTRK3* (neurotropic tyrosine receptor kinase [Trk]) pathway. A similar pattern in relation to anxious temperament was found for *IRS2* and *RPS6KA3*, two downstream targets of *NTRK3*. Other molecules in the *NTRK3* pathway are also depicted in light gray. Aadapted from Fox et al. (2012). Copyright 2012 by the National Academy of Sciences. Adapted by permission.

Levels of mRNAs for both of these genes were negatively correlated with anxious temperament, such that individuals with the lowest expression levels of *NPY1R* mRNA, for example, were those with the most extreme anxious temperament (Roseboom et al., 2014). *NYP1R* is of interest because of the numerous reports linking decreased neuropeptide Y (NPY) system activity to depression. While Ce *NYP1R* mRNA levels did not predict Ce metabolism, a whole-brain voxelwise analysis revealed several other regions where Ce *NYP1R* mRNA expression did predict metabolism. These regions included the dorsolateral prefrontal cortex (dlPFC) and perigenual anterior cingulate cortex, cortical regions known to be part of the circuit that regulates amygdalar activity (Davidson, 2002; Etkin, Egner, Peraza, Kandel, & Hirsch, 2006; Buhle et al., 2014; Shackman et al., 2013). These data suggest that *NPY1R* mRNA levels in the Ce may be regulated by prefrontal cortical inputs to *NPY1R*-expressing Ce neurons. Alternatively, *NPY1R*-expressing Ce neurons could modulate metabolism in these distal brain regions via direct or indirect mechanisms.

Living without an Amygdala

Lesion studies in human and nonhuman primates suggest a causal role for the amygdala in anxious temperament. Initial studies by Brown and Schafer (1888) demonstrated decreased fearfulness in monkeys with amygdala damage. Specific experimental lesions to the amygdala have been shown to decrease the reticence to act in potentially threatening situations (Kalin, Shelton, Davidson, & Kelley, 2001; Murray & Izquierdo, 2007; Machado & Bachevalier, 2008; Chudasama, Izquierdo, & Murray, 2009) and alter stress-induced cortisol release (Machado & Bachevalier, 2008). Importantly, amygdala lesions also resulted in less anxiety in social situations in which human anxious temperament is most commonly observed (Emery et al., 2001; Machado et al., 2008). We note that other studies, reviewed in other chapters in this volume, have used the human intruder paradigm to assess the effects of amygdala lesions on behavior. Also reviewed elsewhere in this volume are the seminal studies of patient S. M., a woman with calcification of the amygdala as a result of Urbach–Wiethe disease. Years of clinical and experimental assessment have revealed that S. M. is more trusting of and more likely to approach strangers (Adolphs, Tranel, & Damasio, 1998), does not recognize fear in others (Adolphs, Tranel, Damasio, & Damasio, 1994), shows a "blindness" for socially acceptable physical space (Kennedy, Glascher, Tyszka, & Adolphs, 2009), does not readily learn novel Pavlovian fear associations (Bechara et al., 1995), and does not show typical signs of anxiety (Feinstein, Adolphs, Damasio, & Tranel, 2011). Taken together, these data suggest that S. M. displays less anxiety in social and other threatening situations, and fit with data from adult rhesus monkeys with amygdalar lesions that display altered social behavior (Emery et al., 2001; Amaral, 2002; Machado et al., 2008). See also Terburg et al. (2012), and van Honk, Terburg, Thornton, Stein, and Morgan (Chapter 12, this volume) for a different interpretation of the deficits associated with human amygdala lesions resulting from Urbach–Wiethe disease.

In an initial study aimed at understanding the role of the amygdala in monkey anxious temperament, we lesioned the entire amygdala with the neurotoxin ibotenic acid (Kalin et al., 2001). Lesioned animals displayed less fear-related behavior in the presence of a live snake or novel adult conspecific. However, no reduction in freezing behavior was observed in response to the human intruder. In hindsight, we believe that this null result reflects an unintended consequence of the fact that the lesioned monkeys in this study were repeatedly exposed to the human intruder paradigm prior to surgery. Other work by our group (Fox et al., 2012) indicates that although individual differences in freezing are moderately stable, absolute levels of freezing tend to decrease with repeated exposure to the human intruder paradigm. Thus, it is possible that the apparent lack of effect of the lesions on freezing in this experiment was due to repeated exposure-associated habituation.

Alterations in sleep were also observed in the monkeys with large amygdala lesions (Benca, Obermeyer, Shelton, Droster, & Kalin, 2000). Specifically, lesioned and control monkeys were adapted to EEG recording during their nocturnal sleep period. Despite apparent adaptation, the sleep patterns of control animals were punctuated by frequent arousals. Monkeys with large bilateral lesions of the amygdala had more sleep and a higher proportion of rapid eye movement (REM) sleep compared to control animals, suggesting that the amygdala may be important in mediating the effects of stress on sleep. This is of interest considering that anxiety is the psychiatric symptom most often associated with insomnia, and the growing recognition that sleep disturbances accompany almost all forms of psychopathology (Benca, Obermeyer, Thisted, & Gillin, 1992).

In a follow-up lesion study, we focused more specifically on the Ce. In that study, the monkeys were intentionally kept naive to the human intruder paradigm and were exposed to it only once, following recovery from the lesion surgery (Kalin, Shelton, & Davidson, 2004). Small selective lesions in the Ce region were produced to examine the extent to which the Ce mediates unconditioned fear, anxious temperament-related behavioral responses, and stress-induced pituitary–adrenal activity (Figure 8.7). There were two experimental groups (bilateral lesion [$n = 9$] and unilateral [$n = 5$] Ce lesions) and an age-matched unoperated control group ($n = 16$).

The Ce lesions significantly affected coo vocalizations and freezing duration, the two behavioral components of anxious temperament. Compared with the age-matched controls, cooing was increased in the

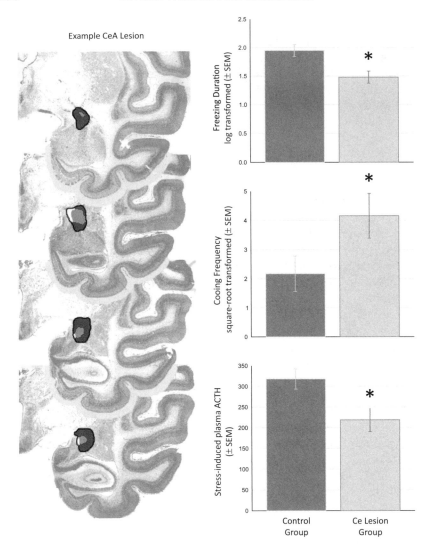

FIGURE 8.7. The effects of Ce lesions on components of anxious temperament. Left: A representative lesion is displayed on four coronal sections through the anterior–posterior (top to bottom) extent of Ce. The intact Ce is depicted in white, the area of the total lesion is displayed in black, and the lesioned Ce region is depicted by the overlap in gray. Right: Monkeys with Ce lesions displayed less freezing (top), emitted more coo calls (middle), and released less ACTH (bottom) during exposure to the human intruder paradigm. Adapted from Kalin, Shelton, and Davidson (2004). Copyright 2004 by the Society for Neuroscience. Adapted by permission.

bilateral lesion and unilateral lesion groups ($p < .04$). The bilateral lesion group showed significantly less freezing behavior compared to the other groups ($p < .023$). The animals with bilateral lesions also displayed less fear when exposed to a live snake, suggesting that these effects generalize beyond the human intruder paradigm. Decreases in adrenocorticotropic hormone (ACTH) and cerebrospinal fluid levels of corticotropin-releasing hormone (CRH), the two key upstream mediators of cortisol release, were observed, and individual differences in the extent of the lesion significantly predicted stress-related cortisol levels (Kalin et al., 2004). In conjunction with the FDG imaging results, these findings indicate a mechanistic role for the Ce in mediating the behavioral and pituitary–adrenal components of anxious temperament, as well as other fear-related behaviors, early in life.

Cortical and Subcortical Systems Interacting with Ce in Relation to Anxious Temperament

Psychiatric disorders likely reflect alterations in the coordinated activity of distributed functional circuits. While the results of our FDG and lesion studies suggest that the Ce is a key substrate for stable individual differences in anxious temperament, they do not directly address the larger functional network in which the Ce is embedded. To understand the long-range neural networks that may interact with the Ce in relation to anxious temperament, we used fMRI to assess functional connectivity of the Ce region. Based on work demonstrating the ability to reliably assess functional connectivity in anesthetized rhesus monkeys (Vincent et al., 2007), we used the Ce as a seed region to examine temporal correlations of the blood oxygen level-dependent (BOLD) signal in a subset of the monkeys from the large sample described earlier (Oler et al., 2010). By combining data from multiple modalities (FDG–PET and fMRI) we found that greater Ce glucose metabolism was associated with decreased functional coupling between the Ce and dlPFC, and that decreased functional coupling between the Ce and dlPFC was also associated with higher levels of anxious temperament (Birn et al., 2014). Decreased Ce–dlPFC connectivity was also observed in a sample of preadolescent children (ages 8–12) with anxiety disorders, further validating the monkey anxious temperament model, suggesting a role for altered dlPFC–amygdala functional coupling in the pathogenesis of childhood anxiety disorders and demonstrating that the modulatory influence of dlPFC on amygdalar function is evolutionarily conserved (Birn et al., 2014). Importantly, the monkey FDG–PET data provided evidence that elevated Ce metabolism statistically mediates the association between Ce and dlPFC connectivity and elevated anxious temperament (Birn et al., 2014). Thus, these functional connectivity data suggest that coordinated activity between the dlPFC and Ce is an important modulator of individual differences in the expression of anxious temperament. This highlights an important benefit of assessing functional connectivity, as findings are not constrained by direct neuroanatomical connections. Future studies aimed at directly modulating dlPFC–Ce functional connectivity would help in further understanding the role of dlPFC in regulating amygdala function and anxious temperament, as well as in children with anxiety disorders. In this regard, transcranial magnetic stimulation is a noninvasive strategy that could be used in both human and nonhuman primates to stimulate the dlPFC and examine downstream effects on amygdala function, as well as affect dlPFC–amygdala connectivity.

In addition to the amygdala, FDG–PET imaging studies suggest that anxious temperament reflects individual differences in a number of regions that include the anterior hippocampus, BST, anterior temporal cortex, and PAG. The caudal orbitofrontal cortex (OFC) also appears to play a role (FDR q < .05, corrected; unpublished analyses of the sample [n = 238] described by Oler et al., 2010). Furthermore, aspiration lesions of the OFC reduce freezing in response to the NEC challenge (Kalin, Shelton, & Davidson, 2007). Importantly, whole-brain FDG–PET imaging provided evidence suggesting that the reduction in freezing observed in OFC-lesioned animals reflects an indirect consequence of lesion-induced alterations in the extended amygdala. Specifically, OFC lesions reduced NEC-related metabolism in the BST (Fox et al., 2010). It is important to emphasize that while OFC lesions attenuate freezing and decrease BST metabolism, the correlation between BST activity and freezing behavior, evident prior to the lesions, remained significant after the lesions (Fox et al., 2010). This suggests that decreased freezing behavior in OFC-lesioned animals was directly related to decreased activity in the BST, and supports previously reported findings that individual differences in BST metabolic activity are predictive of individual differences in freezing and/or anxious temperament in young monkeys (Kalin et al., 2005; Fox et al., 2008). Thus, future studies examining the mechanistic role of BST in primate anxiety should employ selective BST lesion techniques similar to those described earlier and in other chapters in this volume, to dissociate the selective role that this component of the extended amygdala may play in normal and pathological anxiety.

Concluding Remarks and Future Directions

The functional neuroimaging data in intact animals and behavioral data from Ce-lesioned animals reviewed here extend prior studies on the function of the Ce. First, we demonstrated a mechanistic role for the Ce in the behavioral and pituitary–adrenal components of anxious temperament using selective ibotenic acid lesions. Then, building on earlier studies, we demonstrated that Ce metabolism strongly predicts individual differences in anxious temperament. In this large sample, we demonstrated that polymorphisms in the CRH receptor system are associated with heightened anxiety and elevated metabolic activity in the Ce in response to potential threat. In a subsample, we found that mRNA expression of neurodevelopment-related genes is decreased in the Ce of anxious monkeys, which suggests that learning-related neuroplasticity phenomena in the amygdala may be compromised in individuals with extreme anxious phenotypes. Additionally, we uncovered evidence suggesting that dorsolateral and orbital regions of the PFC influence anxious temperament-related activity within the extended amygdala. Taken together, these data indicate a role for a circuit centered on the extended amygdala, encompassing the Ce and BST, in establishing and maintaining normative and extreme anxiety early in life.

Future studies employing lesion or reversible inactivation techniques that target specific neuronal subpopulations will likely deepen our understanding of the amygdalar microcircuits that underlie primate anxious temperament. Furthermore, rapid immunohistochemical staining to identify specific cell populations for microdissection and subsequent deep RNA sequencing is a promising method for understanding the cell-specific molecular mechanisms related to anxious temperament. Gene delivery with viral vectors to induce or suppress expression of specific molecules is another technique with the potential to enrich our understanding of primate amygdalar microcircuit function and the role of the extended amygdala in temperamental anxiety. With the ultimate aim of developing more effective early-life interventions to treat and prevent anxiety-related psychopathology, it is our hope that such studies will shed light on the risk for anxiety-related psychopathology, as well as deepen our understanding of amygdala function and normal variation in temperament.

ACKNOWLEDGMENTS

We thank the personnel of the Harlow Center for Biological Psychology, HealthEmotions Research Institute, Waisman Laboratory for Brain Imaging and Behavior, and Wisconsin National Primate Center. This work was supported by the National Institutes of Health (Grant Nos. R01-MH046729, R01-MH081884, P50-MH084051, and R21-MH09258), the HealthEmotions Research Institute, and the University of Maryland, College Park.

REFERENCES

Adolphs, R. (2003). Is the human amygdala specialized for processing social information? *Annals of the New York Academy of Sciences, 985*, 326–340.

Adolphs, R., Gosselin, F, Buchanan, T. W., Tranel, D., Schyns, P., & Damasio, A. R. (2005). A mechanism for impaired fear recognition after amygdala damage. *Nature, 433*(7021), 68–72.

Adolphs, R., Tranel, D., & Damasio, A. R. (1998). The human amygdala in social judgment. *Nature, 393*(6684), 470–474.

Adolphs, R., Tranel, D., Damasio, A. R., & Damasio, H. (1994). Impaired recognition of emotion in facial expressions following bilateral damage to the human amygdala. *Letters to Nature, 372*, 669–672.

Aggleton, J. P., & Passingham, R. E. (1981). Syndrome produced by lesions of the amygdala in monkeys (*Macaca mulatta*). *Journal of Comparative and Physiological Psychology, 95*(6), 961–977.

Alheid, G. F., & Heimer, L. (1988). New perspectives in basal forebrain organization of special relevance for neuropsychiatric disorders: The striatopallidal, amygdaloid, and corticopetal components of substantia innominata. *Neuroscience, 27*(1), 1–39.

Almasy, L., & Blangero, J. (1998). Multipoint quantitative-trait linkage analysis in general pedigrees. *American Journal of Human Genetics, 62*(5), 1198–1211.

Alvarez, R. P., Chen, G., Bodurka, J., Kaplan, R., & Grillon, C. (2011). Phasic and sustained fear in humans elicits distinct patterns of brain activity. *NeuroImage, 55*(1), 389–400.

Amaral, D. G. (2002). The primate amygdala and the neurobiology of social behavior: Implications for understanding social anxiety. *Biological Psychiatry, 51*(1), 11–17.

Amaral, D. G. (2003). The amygdala, social behavior, and danger detection. *Annals of the New York Academy of Sciences, 1000*, 337–347.

American Psychiatric Association. (2013). *Diagnostic and statistical manual of mental disorders* (5th ed.). Arlington, VA: Author.

Avery, S. N., Clauss, J. A., Winder, D. G., Woodward, N., Heckers, S., & Blackford, J. U. (2014). BNST neurocircuitry in humans. *NeuroImage, 91*, 311–323.

Bechara, A., Tranel, D., Damasio, H., Adolphs, R., Rockland, C., & Damasio, A. R. (1995). Double dissociation of conditioning and declarative knowledge relative to the amygdala and hippocampus in humans. *Science, 269*, 1115–1116.

Beesdo, K., Bittner, A., Pine, D. S., Stein, M. B., Hofler, M., Lieb, R., et al. (2007). Incidence of social anxiety disorder and the consistent risk for secondary depression in the first three decades of life. *Archives of General Psychiatry, 64*(8), 903–912.

Benca, R. M., Obermeyer, W. H., Shelton, S. E., Droster, J., & Kalin, N. H. (2000). Effects of amygdala lesions on sleep in rhesus monkeys. *Brain Research, 879*(1–2), 130–138.

Benca, R. M., Obermeyer, W. H., Thisted, R. A., & Gillin, J. C. (1992). Sleep and psychiatric disorders: A meta-analysis. *Archives of General Psychiatry, 49*(8), 651–668; discussion 669–670.

Bernd, P. (2008). The role of neurotrophins during early development. *Gene Expression, 14*(4), 241–250.

Biederman, J., Hirshfeld-Becker, D. R., Rosenbaum, J. F., Herot, C., Friedman, D., Snidman, N., et al. (2001). Further evidence of association between behavioral inhibition and social anxiety in children. *American Journal of Psychiatry, 158*(10), 1673–1679.

Birn, R. M., Shackman, A. J., Oler, J. A., Williams, L. E., McFarlin, D. R., Rogers, G. M., et al. (2014). Evolutionarily conserved prefrontal–amygdalar dysfunction in early-life anxiety. *Molecular Psychiatry, 19*(8), 915–922.

Blackford, J. U., Avery, S. N., Cowan, R. L., Shelton, R. C., & Zald, D. H. (2011). Sustained amygdala response to both novel and newly familiar faces characterizes inhibited temperament. *Social Cognitive and Affective Neuroscience, 6*, 621–629.

Blackford, J. U., & Pine, D. S. (2012). Neural substrates of childhood anxiety disorders: A review of neuroimaging findings. *Child and Adolescent Psychiatric Clinics of North America, 21*(3), 501–525.

Bogdan, R., Hyde, L. W., & Hariri, A. R. (2013). A neurogenetics approach to understanding individual differences in brain, behavior, and risk for psychopathology. *Molecular Psychiatry, 18*(3), 288–299.

Bradley, R. G., Binder, E. B., Epstein, M. P., Tang, Y., Nair, H. P., Liu, W., et al. (2008). Influence of child abuse on adult depression: Moderation by the corticotropin-releasing hormone receptor gene. *Archives of General Psychiatry, 65*(2), 190–200.

Brooker, R. J., Buss, K. A., Lemery-Chalfant, K., Aksan, N., Davidson, R. J., & Goldsmith, H. H. (2013). The development of stranger fear in infancy and toddlerhood: Normative development, individual differences, antecedents, and outcomes. *Developmental Science, 16*(6), 864–878.

Brown, S., & Schafer, E. A. (1888). An investigation into the functions of the occipital and temporal lobes of the monkey's brain. *Philosophical Transactions of the Royal Society of London B: Biological Sciences, 179*, 303–327.

Buhle, J. T., Silvers, J. A., Wager, T. D., Lopez, R., Onyemekwu, C., Kober, H., et al. (2014). Cognitive reappraisal of emotion: A meta-analysis of human neuroimaging studies. *Cerebral Cortex, 24*(11), 2981–2990.

Buss, K. A., Davidson, R, J., Kalin, N. H., & Goldsmith, H. H. (2004). Context-specific freezing and associated physiological reactivity as a dysregulated fear response. *Developmental Psychology, 40*(4), 583–594.

Buss, K. A., Schumacher, J. R. M., Dolski, I., Kalin, N. H., Goldsmith, H. H., & Davidson, R. J. (2003). Right frontal brain activity, cortisol, and withdrawal behavior in 6-month-old infants. *Behavioral Neuroscience, 117*, 11–20.

Bystritsky, A. (2006). Treatment-resistant anxiety disorders. *Molecular Psychiatry, 11*, 805–814.

Caspi, A., Hariri, A. R., Holmes, A., Uher, R., & Moffitt, T. E. (2010). Genetic sensitivity to the environment: The case of the serotonin transporter gene and its implications for studying complex diseases and traits. *American Journal of Psychiatry, 167*(5), 509–527.

Caspi, A., Moffitt, T. E., Newman, D. L., & Silva, P. A. (1996). Behavioral observations at age 3 years predict adult psychiatric disorders: Longitudinal evidence from a birth cohort. *Archives of General Psychiatry, 53*(11), 1033–1039.

Choi, J. M., Padmala, S., Spechler, P., & Pessoa, L. (2014). Pervasive competition between threat and reward in the brain. *Social Cognitive and Affective Neuroscience, 9*(6), 737–750.

Choi, J. S., & Kim, J. J. (2010). Amygdala regulates risk of predation in rats foraging in a dynamic fear environment. *Proceedings of the National Academy of Sciences USA, 107*(50), 21773–21777.

Christian, B. T., Fox, A. S., Oler, J. A., Vandehey, N. T., Murali, D., & Rogers, J., et al. (2009). Serotonin transporter binding and genotype in the nonhuman primate brain using [C-11]DASB PET. *NeuroImage, 47*(4), 1230–1236.

Chronis-Tuscano, A., Degnan, K. A., Pine, D. S., Perez-Edgar, K., Henderson, H. A., & Diaz, Y., et al. (2009). Stable early maternal report of behavioral inhibition predicts lifetime social anxiety disorder in adolescence. *Journal of the American Academy of Child and Adolescent Psychiatry, 48*, 928–935.

Chudasama, Y., Izquierdo, A., & Murray, E. A. (2009). Distinct contributions of the amygdala and hippocampus to fear expression. *European Journal of Neuroscience, 30*(12), 2327–2337.

Ciocchi, S., Herry, C., Grenier, F., Wolff, S. B., Letzkus, J. J., Vlachos, I., et al. (2010). Encoding of conditioned fear in central amygdala inhibitory circuits. *Nature, 468*(7321), 277–282.

Clauss, J. A., & Blackford, J. U. (2012). Behavioral inhibition and risk for developing social anxiety disorder: A meta-analytic study. *Journal of the American Academy of Child and Adolescent Psychiatry, 51*(10), 1066–1075.

Cloos, J. M., & Ferreira, V. (2009). Current use of benzodiazepines in anxiety disorders. *Current Opinion in Psychiatry, 22*(1), 90–95.

Davidson, R. J. (2002). Anxiety and affective style: Role of prefrontal cortex and amygdala. *Biological Psychiatry, 51*(1), 68–80.

Davidson, R. J., Kalin, N. S., & Shelton, S. (1993). Lateralized response to diazepam predicts temperamental style in rhesus monkeys. *Behavioral Neuroscience, 107*, 1106–1110.

Davidson, R. J., Kalin, N. H., & Shelton, S. E. (1992). Lateralized effects of diazepam on frontal brain electrical asymmetries in rhesus monkeys. *Biological Psychiatry, 32*, 438–451.

Davidson, R. J., & Rickman, M. (1999). Behavioral inhibition and the emotional circuitry of the brain: Stability and plasticity during the early childhood years. In L. A. Schmidt & J. Schulkin (Eds.), *Extreme fear, shyness, and social phobia: Origins, biological mechanisms, and clinical outcomes* (pp. 67–87). New York: Oxford University Press.

Davis, M. (2000). The role of the amygdala in conditioned and unconditioned fear and anxiety. In J. P. Aggleton (Ed.), *The amygdala: A functional analysis* (pp. 213–287). New York: Oxford University Press.

Davis, M., Walker, D. L., Miles, L., & Grillon, C. (2010). Phasic vs sustained fear in rats and humans: Role of the extended amygdala in fear vs anxiety. *Neuropsychopharmacology, 35*(1), 105–135.

de Haan, M., Gunnar, M. R., Tout, K., Hart, J., & Stansbury, K. (1998). Familiar and novel contexts yield different associations between cortisol and behavior among 2-year-old children. *Developmental Psychobiology, 33*(1), 93–101.

de Olmos, J. S., & Heimer, L. (1999). The concepts of the ventral striatopallidal system and extended amygdala: Advancing from the ventral striatum to the extended amygdala: Implications for neuropsychiatry and drug abuse. *Annals of the New York Academy of Sciences, 877,* 1–32.

Degnan, K. A., Almas, A. N., & Fox, N. A. (2010). Temperament and the environment in the etiology of childhood anxiety. *Journal of Child Psychology and Psychiatry, 51*(4), 497–517.

Dong, H. W., Petrovich, G. D., & Swanson, L. W. (2001). Topography of projections from amygdala to bed nuclei of the stria terminalis. *Brain Research Reviews, 38*(1–2), 192–246.

Duvarci, S., & Pare, D. (2014). Amygdala microcircuits controlling learned fear. *Neuron, 82*(5), 966–980.

Emery, N. J., Capitanio, J. P., Mason, W. A., Machado, C. J., Mendoza, S. P., & Amaral, D. G. (2001). The effects of bilateral lesions of the amygdala on dyadic social interactions in rhesus monkeys (*Macaca mulatta*). *Behavioral Neuroscience, 115*(3), 515–544.

Essex, M. J., Klein, M. H., Cho, E., & Kalin, N. H. (2002). Maternal stress beginning in infancy may sensitize children to later stress exposure: Effects on cortisol and behavior. *Biological Psychiatry, 52*(8), 776–784.

Essex, M. J., Klein, M. H., Slattery, M. J., Goldsmith, H. H., & Kalin, N. H. (2010). Early risk factors and developmental pathways to chronic high inhibition and social anxiety disorder in adolescence. *American Journal of Psychiatry, 167*(1), 40–46.

Etkin, A., Egner, T., Peraza, D. M., Kandel, E. R., & Hirsch, J. (2006). Resolving emotional conflict: A role for the rostral anterior cingulate cortex in modulating activity in the amygdala. *Neuron, 51*(6), 871–882.

Etkin, A., & Wager, T. D. (2007). Functional neuroimaging of anxiety: A meta-analysis of emotional processing in PTSD, social anxiety disorder, and specific phobia. *American Journal of Psychiatry, 164*(10), 1476–1488.

Everitt, B. J., Cardinal, R. N., Parkinson, J. A., & Robbins, T. W. (2003). Appetitive behavior: Impact of amygdala-dependent mechanisms of emotional learning. *Annals of the New York Academy of Sciences, 985*(1), 233–250.

Feinstein, J. S., Adolphs, R., Damasio, A., & Tranel, D. (2011). The human amygdala and the induction and experience of fear. *Current Biology, 21,* 1–5.

Fox, A. S., Oakes, T. R., Shelton, S. E., Converse, A. K., Davidson, R. J., & Kalin, N. H. (2005a). Calling for help is independently modulated by brain systems underlying goal-directed behavior and threat perception. *Proceedings of the National Academy of Sciences USA, 102,* 4176–4179.

Fox, A. S., Oler, J. A., Shelton, S. E., Nanda, S. A., Davidson, R. J., Roseboom, P. H., et al. (2012). Central amygdala nucleus (Ce) gene expression linked to increased trait-like Ce metabolism and anxious temperament in young primates. *Proceedings of the National Academy of Sciences USA, 109*(44), 18108–18113.

Fox, A. S., Shelton, S. E., Oakes, T. R., Converse, A. K., Davidson, R. J., & Kalin, N. H. (2010). Orbitofrontal cortex lesions alter anxiety-related activity in the primate bed nucleus of stria terminalis. *Journal of Neuroscience, 30*(20), 7023–7027.

Fox, A. S., Shelton, S. E., Oakes, T. R., Davidson, R. J., & Kalin, N. H. (2008). Trait-like brain activity during adolescence predicts anxious temperament in primates. *PLoS ONE, 3*(7), e2570.

Fox, N. A., Henderson, H. A., Marshall, P. J., Nichols, K. E., & Ghera, M. M. (2005b). Behavioral inhibition: Linking biology and behavior within a developmental framework. *Annual Review of Psychology, 56*, 235–262.

Gabriel, M., Burhans, L., & Kashef, A. (2003). Consideration of a unified model of amygdalar associative functions. *Annals of the New York Academy of Sciences, 985*(1), 206–217.

Galatzer-Levy, I. R., Bonanno, G. A., Bush, D. E., & LeDoux, J. E. (2013). Heterogeneity in threat extinction learning: substantive and methodological considerations for identifying individual difference in response to stress. *Frontiers in Behavioral Neuroscience, 7*, 55.

Gallagher, M. (2000). The amygdala and associative learning. In J. P. Aggleton (Ed.), *The amygdala: A functional analysis* (pp. 311–329). New York: Oxford University Press.

Gallagher, M., & Holland, P. C. (1994). The amygdala complex: Multiple roles in associative learning and attention. *Proceedings of the National Academy of Sciences USA, 91*, 11771–11776.

Gladstone, G. L., & Parker, G. B. (2006). Is behavioral inhibition a risk factor for depression? *Journal of Affective Disorders, 95*(1–3), 85–94.

Goswami, S., Rodriguez-Sierra, O., Cascardi, M., & Pare, D. (2013). Animal models of post-traumatic stress disorder: Face validity. *Frontiers in Neuroscience, 7*, 89.

Grupe, D. W., & Nitschke, J. B. (2013). Uncertainty and anticipation in anxiety: An integrated neurobiological and psychological perspective. *Nature Reviews Neuroscience, 14*(7), 488–501.

Grupe, D. W., Oathes, D. J., & Nitschke, J. B. (2013). Dissecting the anticipation of aversion reveals dissociable neural networks. *Cerebral Cortex, 23*(8), 1874–1883.

Gungor, N. Z., Yamamoto, R., & Paré, D. (2015) Optogenetic study of the projections from the bed nucleus of the stria terminalis to the central amygdala. *Journal of Neurophysiology, 114*, 2903–2911.

Hardee, J. E., Benson, B. E., Bar-Haim, Y., Mogg, K., Bradley, B. P., & Chen, G., et al. (2013). Patterns of neural connectivity during an attention bias task moderate associations between early childhood temperament and internalizing symptoms in young adulthood. *Biological Psychiatry, 74*(4), 273–279.

Hariri, A. R., & Holmes, A. (2006). Genetics of emotional regulation: The role of the serotonin transporter in neural function. *Trends in Cognitive Sciences, 10*(4), 182–191.

Haubensak, W., Kunwar, P. S., Cai, H., Ciocchi, S., Wall, N. R., Ponnusamy, R., et al. (2010). Genetic dissection of an amygdala microcircuit that gates conditioned fear. *Nature, 468*(7321), 270–276.

Heimer, L. (2003). A new anatomical framework for neuropsychiatric disorders and drug abuse. *American Journal of Psychiatry, 160*(10), 1726–1739.

Heimer, L., & Van Hoesen, G. W. (2006). The limbic lobe and its output channels: Implications for emotional functions and adaptive behavior. *Neuroscience and Biobehavioral Reviews, 30*(2), 126–147.

Hettema, J. M., Neale, M. D., & Kendler, K. S. (2001). A review and meta-analysis of the genetic epidemiology of anxiety disorders. *American Journal of Psychiatry, 158*(10), 1568–1578.

Hirshfeld-Becker, D. R., Biederman, J., Henin, A., Faraone, S. V., Davis, S., Harrington, K., et al. (2007). Behavioral inhibition in preschool children at risk is a specific predictor of middle childhood social anxiety: A five-year follow-up. *Journal of Developmental and Behavioral Pediatrics, 28*(3), 225–233.

Hirshfeld-Becker, D. R., Micco, J., Henin, A., Bloomfield, A., Biederman, J., & Rosenbaum, J. (2008). Behavioral inhibition. *Depression and Anxiety, 25*(4), 357–367.

Holmes, A., & Singewald, N. (2013). Individual differences in recovery from traumatic fear. *Trends in Neurosciences, 36*(1), 23–31.

Hyde, L. W., Bogdan, R., & Hariri, A. R. (2011). Understanding risk for psychopathology through imaging gene–environment interactions. *Trends in Cognitive Sciences, 15*(9), 417–427.

Jaenisch, R., & Bird, A. (2003). Epigenetic regulation of gene expression: How the genome integrates intrinsic and environmental signals. *Nature Genetics, 33*, 245–254.

Jahn, A. L., Fox, A. S., Abercrombie, H. C., Shelton, S. E., Oakes, T. R., Davidson, R. J., et al. (2010). Subgenual prefrontal cortex activity predicts individual differences in hypothalamic–pituitary–adrenal activity across different contexts. *Biological Psychiatry, 67*, 175–181.

Kagan, J., Reznick, J. S., & Snidman, N. (1988). Biological bases of childhood shyness. *Science, 240*(4849), 167–171.

Kalin, N. H. (2002). The neurobiology of fear. *Scientific American, 12*, 72–81.

Kalin, N. H. (2003). Nonhuman primate studies of fear, anxiety, and temperament and the role of benzodiazepine receptors and GABA systems. *Journal of Clinical Psychiatry, 64*(Suppl. 3), 41–44.

Kalin, N. H., Larson, C., Shelton, S. E., & Davidson, R. J. (1998a). Asymmetric frontal brain activity, cortisol, and behavior associated with fearful temperament in rhesus monkeys. *Behavioral Neuroscience, 112*, 286–292.

Kalin, N. H., & Shelton, S. (2000). The regulation of defensive behaviors in rhesus monkeys. In, R. J. Davidson (Ed.), *Anxiety, depression, and emotion* (pp. 50–68). New York: Oxford University Press.

Kalin, N. H., & Shelton, S. E. (1989). Defensive behaviors in infant rhesus monkeys: Environmental cues and neurochemical regulation. *Science, 243*, 1718–1721.

Kalin, N. H., &. Shelton, S. E. (2003). Nonhuman primate models to study anxiety, emotion regulation, and psychopathology. *Annals of the New York Academy of Sciences, 1008*, 189–200.

Kalin, N. H., Shelton, S. E., & Davidson, R. J. (2004). The role of the central nucleus of the amygdala in mediating fear and anxiety in the primate. *Journal of Neuroscience, 24*(24), 5506–5515.

Kalin, N. H., Shelton, S. E., & Davidson, R. J. (2007). Role of the primate orbitofrontal cortex in mediating anxious temperament. *Biological Psychiatry, 62*(10), 1134–1139.

Kalin, N. H., Shelton, S. E., Davidson, R. J., & Kelley, A. E. (2001). The primate amygdala mediates acute fear but not the behavioral and physiological components of anxious temperament. *Journal of Neuroscience, 21*(6), 2067–2074.

Kalin, N. H., Shelton, S. E., Fox, A. S., Oakes, T. R., & Davidson, R. J. (2005).

Brain regions associated with the expression and contextual regulation of anxiety in primates. *Biological Psychiatry, 58,* 796–804.

Kalin, N. H., Shelton, S. E., Fox, A. S., Rogers, J., Oakes, T. R., & Davidson, R. J. (2008). The serotonin transporter genotype is associated with intermediate brain phenotypes that depend on the context of eliciting stressor. *Molecular Psychiatry, 13*(11), 1021–1027.

Kalin, N. H., Shelton, S. E., Rickman, M., & Davidson, R. J. (1998b). Individual differences in freezing and cortisol in infant and mother rhesus monkeys. *Behavioral Neuroscience, 112*(1), 251–254.

Kalin, N. H., Shelton, S. E., & Turner, J. G. (1992). Effects of beta-carboline on fear-related behavioral and neurohormonal responses in infant rhesus monkeys. *Biological Psychiatry, 31*(10), 1008–1019.

Kapp, B. S., Frysinger, R. C., Gallagher, M., & Haselton, J. R. (1979). Amygdala central nucleus lesions: Effect on heart rate conditioning in the rabbit. *Physiology and Behavior, 23,* 1109–1117.

Kapp, B. S., Whalen, P. J., Supple, W. F., & Pascoe, J. P. (1992). Amygdaloid contributions to conditioned arousal and sensory information processing. In J. P. Aggleton (Ed.), *The amygdala: Neurobiological aspects of emotion, memory, and mental dysfunction* (pp. 229–254). New York: Wiley-Liss.

Kennedy, D. P., Glascher, J., Tyszka, J. M., & Adolphs, R. (2009). Personal space regulation by the human amygdala. *Nature Neuroscience, 12*(10), 1226–1227.

Kessler, R. C., Petukhova, M., Sampson, N. A., Zaslavsky, A. M., & Wittchen, H. U. (2012). Twelve-month and lifetime prevalence and lifetime morbid risk of anxiety and mood disorders in the United States. *International Journal of Methods in Psychiatric Research, 21,* 169–184.

Kling, A. (1968). Effects of amygdalectomy and testosterone on sexual behavior of male juvenile macaques. *Journal of Comparative and Physiological Psychology, 65*(3), 466–471.

Klüver, H., & Bucy, P. C. (1937). "Psychic blindness" and other symptoms following bilateral temporal lobectomy in rhesus monkeys. *American Journal of Physiology, 119,* 352–353.

Klüver, H., & Bucy, P. C. (1939). Preliminary analysis of functions of the temporal lobes in monkeys. *Archives of Neurology and Psychiatry, 42*(6), 979–1000.

LeDoux, J. E. (2000). Emotion circuits in the brain. *Annual Review of Neuroscience, 23,* 155–184.

Machado, C. J., & Bachevalier, J. (2008). Behavioral and hormonal reactivity to threat: Effects of selective amygdala, hippocampal or orbital frontal lesions in monkeys. *Psychoneuroendocrinology, 33*(7), 926–941.

Machado, C. J., Emery, N. J., Capitanio, J. P., Mason, W. A., Mendoza, S. P., & Amaral, D. G. (2008). Bilateral neurotoxic amygdala lesions in rhesus monkeys (*Macaca mulatta*): Consistent pattern of behavior across different social contexts. *Behavioral Neuroscience, 122*(2), 251–266.

McEwen, B. S., Eiland, L., Hunter, R. G., & Miller, M. M. (2012). Stress and anxiety: structural plasticity and epigenetic regulation as a consequence of stress. *Neuropharmacology, 62*(1), 3–12.

Mobbs, D., Yu, R., Rowe, J. B., Eich, H., FeldmanHall, O., & Dalgleish, T. (2010). Neural activity associated with monitoring the oscillating threat value of a tarantula. *Proceedings of the National Academy of Sciences USA, 107*(47), 20582–20586.

Murray, E. A., & Izquierdo, A. (2007). Orbitofrontal cortex and amygdala contributions to affect and action in primates. *Annals of the New York Academy of Sciences, 1121,* 273–296.

Oler, J. A., Birn, R. M., Patriat, R., Fox, A. S., Shelton, S. E., Burghy, C. A., et al. (2012). Evidence for coordinated functional activity within the extended amygdala of non-human and human primates. *NeuroImage, 61,* 1059–1066.

Oler, J. A., Fox, A. S., Shelton, S. E., Christian, B. T., Murali, D., Oakes, T. R., et al. (2009). Serotonin transporter availability in the amygdala and bed nucleus of the stria terminalis predicts anxious temperament and brain glucose metabolic activity. *Journal of Neuroscience, 29,* 9961–9966.

Oler, J. A., Fox, A. S., Shelton, S. E., Rogers, J., Dyer, T. D., Davidson, R. J., et al. (2010). Amygdalar and hippocampal substrates of anxious temperament differ in their heritability. *Nature, 466*(7308), 864–868.

O'Rourke, H., & Fudge, J. L. (2006). Distribution of serotonin transporter labeled fibers in amygdaloid subregions: Implications for mood disorders. *Biological Psychiatry, 60,* 479–490.

Otnaess, M. K., Djurovic, S., Rimol, L. M., Kulle, B., Kahler, A. K., Jonsson, E. G., et al. (2009). Evidence for a possible association of neurotrophin receptor (*NTRK-3*) gene polymorphisms with hippocampal function and schizophrenia. *Neurobiology of Disease, 34*(3), 518–524.

Paré, D., Quirk, G. J., & LeDoux, J. E. (2004). New vistas on amygdala networks in conditioned fear. *Journal of Neurophysiology, 92*(1), 1–9.

Paulus, M. P., Feinstein, J. S., Castillo, G., Simmons, A. N., & Stein, M. B. (2005). Dose-dependent decrease of activation in bilateral amygdala and insula by lorazepam during emotion processing. *Archives of General Psychiatry, 62*(3), 282–288.

Pfeifer, M., Goldsmith, H. H., Davidson, R. J., & Rickman, M. (2002). Continuity and change in inhibited and uninhibited children. *Child Development, 73,* 1474–1485.

Pribram, K. H., Reitz, S., McNeil, M., & Spevack, A. A. (1979). The effect of amygdalectomy on orienting and classical conditioning in monkeys. *Pavlovian Journal of Biological Science, 14*(4), 203–217.

Prior, M., Smart, D., Sanson, A., & Oberklaid, F. (2000). Does shy-inhibited temperament in childhood lead to anxiety problems in adolescence? *Journal of the American Academy of Child and Adolescent Psychiatry, 39*(4), 461–468.

Rickman, M. D., & Davidson, R. J. (1994). Personality and behavior in parents of tempermentally inhibited and uninhibited children. *Developmental Psychology, 30*(3), 346–354.

Rogers, J., Raveendran, M., Fawcett, G. L., Fox, A. S., Shelton, S. E., Oler, J. A., et al. (2013). CRHR1 genotypes, neural circuits and the diathesis for anxiety and depression. *Molecular Psychiatry, 18*(6), 700–707.

Rogers, J., Shelton, S. E., Shelledy, W., Garcia, R., & Kalin, N. H. (2008). Genetic influences on behavioral inhibition and anxiety in juvenile rhesus macaques. *Genes, Brain and Behavior, 7*(4), 463–469.

Rolls, E. T. (1984). Neurons in the cortex of the temporal lobe and in the amygdala of the monkey with responses selective for faces. *Human Neurobiology, 3*(4), 209–222.

Roseboom, P. H., Nanda, S. A., Fox, A. S., Oler, J. A., Shackman, A. J., Shelton, S. E., et al. (2014). Neuropeptide Y receptor gene expression in the primate amygdala predicts anxious temperament and brain metabolism. *Biological Psychiatry, 76*(11), 850–857.

Schmidt, L. A., Fox, N. A., Rubin, K. H., Sternberg, E. M., Gold, P. W., Smith, C. C., et al. (1997). Behavioral and neuroendocrine responses in shy children. *Developmental Psychobiology, 30*(2), 127–140.

Schwartz, C. E., Snidman, N., & Kagan, J. (1999). Adolescent social anxiety as an outcome of inhibited temperament in childhood. *Journal of the American Academy of Child and Adolescent Psychiatry, 38*(8), 1008–1015.

Schwartz, C. E., Wright, C. I., Shin, L. M., Kagan, J., & Rauch, S. L. (2003). Inhibited and uninhibited infants "grown up": Adult amygdalar response to novelty. *Science, 300*(5627), 1952–1953.

Shackman, A. J., Fox, A. S., Oler, J. A., Shelton, S. E., Davidson, R. J., & Kalin, N. H. (2013). Neural mechanisms underlying heterogeneity in the presentation of anxious temperament. *Proceedings of the National Academy of Sciences USA, 110*(15), 6145–6150.

Sokoloff, L., Reivich, M., Kennedy, C., Des Rosiers, M. H., Patlak, C. S., Pettigrew, K. D., et al. (1977). The [^{14}C]deoxyglucose method for the measurement of local cerebral glucose utilization: theory, procedure, and normal values in the conscious and anesthetized albino rat. *Journal of Neurochemistry, 28*(5), 897–916.

Somerville, L. H., Whalen, P. J., & Kelley, W. M. (2010). Human bed nucleus of the stria terminalis indexes hypervigilant threat monitoring. *Biological Psychiatry, 68*(5), 416–424.

Straube, T., Mentzel, H. J., & Miltner, W. H. (2007). Waiting for spiders: Brain activation during anticipatory anxiety in spider phobics. *NeuroImage, 37*(4), 1427–1436.

Swanson, L. W. (2003). The amygdala and its place in the cerebral hemisphere. *Annals of the New York Academy of Sciences, 985*, 174–184.

Terburg, D., Morgan, B. E., Montoya, E. R., Hooge, I. T., Thornton, H. B., Hariri, A. R., et al. (2012). Hypervigilance for fear after basolateral amygdala damage in humans. *Translational Psychiatry, 2*, e115.

Vincent, J. L., Patel, G. H., Fox, M. D., Snyder, A. Z., Baker, J. T., Van Essen, D. C., et al. (2007). Intrinsic functional architecture in the anaesthetized monkey brain. *Nature, 447*(7140), 83–86.

Viviani, R., Sim, E. J., Lo, H., Beschoner, P., Osterfeld, N., Maier, C., et al. (2010). Baseline brain perfusion and the serotonin transporter promoter polymorphism. *Biological Psychiatry, 67*(4), 317–322.

Walker, D. L., & Davis, M. (2008). Role of the extended amygdala in short-duration versus sustained fear: A tribute to Dr. Lennart Heimer. *Brain Structure and Function, 213*(1–2), 29–42.

Weiskrantz, L. (1956). Behavioral changes associated with ablation of the amgdaloid complex in monkeys. *Journal of Comparative Physiological Psychology, 49*, 381–391.

Whalen, P. J. (1998). Fear, vigilance, and ambiguity: Initial neuroimaging studies of the human amygdala. *Current Directions in Psychological Science, 7,* 177–188.

Whalen, P. J., & Phelps, E. A. E. (2009). *The human amygdala.* New York: Guilford Press.

Williamson, D. E., Coleman, K., Bacanu, S. A., Devlin, B. J., Rogers, J., Ryan, N. D., et al. (2003). Heritability of fearful-anxious endophenotypes in infant rhesus macaques: A preliminary report. *Biological Psychiatry, 53*(4), 284–291.

Wolff, S. B., Grundemann, J., Tovote, P., Krabbe, S., Jacobson, G. A., Muller, C., et al. (2014). Amygdala interneuron subtypes control fear learning through disinhibition. *Nature, 509*(7501), 453–458.

Yehuda, R., & LeDoux, J. (2007). Response variation following trauma: A translational neuroscience approach to understanding PTSD. *Neuron, 56*(1), 19–32.

Zaborszky, L., Hoemke, L., Mohlberg, H., Schleicher, A., Amunts, K., & Zilles, K. (2008). Stereotaxic probabilistic maps of the magnocellular cell groups in human basal forebrain. *NeuroImage, 42*(3), 1127–1141.

Zola-Morgan, S., Squire, L. R., Alvarez-Royo, P., & Clower, R. P. (1991). Independence of memory functions and emotional behavior: Separate contributions of the hippocampal formation and the amygdala. *Hippocampus, 1*(2), 207–220.

CHAPTER 9

Monkeys without an Amygdala

ELISABETH A. MURRAY
SARAH E. V. RHODES

In monkeys, life without an amygdala involves an inflexible adherence to long-standing preferences, poor adaptation to changing wants and needs, and deficient attention to biologically significant events. Compared to normal monkeys, for example, individuals without an amygdala show a blunted reaction to threats, and their sensory cortex fails to respond normally to emotional facial gestures of other monkeys. These impairments arise because the amygdala modulates sensory-processing and decision-making systems for crucial biological functions such as foraging, harm avoidance, and social behavior, and it does so based on updated valuations that depend on current internal states.

Although the amygdala evolved in our ancient vertebrate ancestors and plays a fundamental role in the behavior of humans and other animals, its precise functions remain enigmatic in any species. Research on monkeys has contributed to ideas about the amygdala for as long as anyone has studied either monkeys or the amygdala. According to Klüver and Bucy (1939), for example, as influenced by the later findings of Weiskrantz (1956), life without an amygdala would consist of binge eating, promiscuous sexuality, and a tendency to put just about anything into one's mouth. Fortunately for people with serious amygdala dysfunction, this view has little validity. Klüver and Bucy could not make selective lesions, as neuropsychologists do today. If they had, they might have realized that many components of the so-called Klüver–Bucy syndrome result from damage to structures outside the amygdala.

More recent research on the monkey amygdala has focused on learning and emotion. The amygdala has, for example, been considered a center for negative emotions, especially fear (LeDoux, 2003), as well as a mediator of reward-based learning (Balleine & Killcross, 2006). According to these ideas, life without an amygdala would be a fearless and ignorant one. Although the amygdala plays a role in both learning and emotion, on their own, these ideas do not capture amygdala function very well. Research on monkeys has revealed that the amygdala contributes to several kinds of motivated learning, but not all kinds (Baxter & Murray, 2002). Likewise, the amygdala plays an important role in both positive and negative emotions, not just negative ones (Braesicke et al., 2005; Izquierdo, Suda, & Murray, 2005; Parkinson et al., 2001).

In this chapter, we review some recent advances in understanding the life of monkeys without an amygdala, focusing on three behaviors that are fundamental to their biological success: foraging choices, defensive actions, and social responses. These studies involve the behavioral or physiological effects of selective excitotoxic lesions of the amygdala. Where possible, we compare and contrast these effects with those caused by lesions of the orbitofrontal cortex (OFC). The amygdala and the OFC have long been thought to function cooperatively in learning, emotion, and reward processing. As we shall see, this cooperation is less consistent than often is assumed.

Foraging Behavior

Our internal environment constantly changes, and the same thing happens in monkeys. These changes generate hunger, among other drives, that maintain homeostasis. The key to satisfying these wants and needs is the relative value that we attach to available resources, such as the nutrients that reduce hunger. Recent research implicates the amygdala in keeping track of the value of foods—often referred to as "rewards," "reinforcers," or "outcomes" in the psychology literature—as valuations change with alterations in internal states. As such, the amygdala plays a key role in foraging choices. Normally, we think of foraging as an activity involving movements of the whole body, as an animal moves among patches of resources. More generally, however, "foraging choices" involve any action to acquire resources, including picking and choosing among the objects and actions associated with foods.

The Devaluation Test

We focus in this chapter on monkey research, but we begin with an example from functional magnetic resonance imaging (fMRI) in humans. One such study shows that activation in the amygdala reflects the current value of foods and odors associated with different images (Gottfried,

O'Doherty, & Dolan, 2003). The participants had previously learned to associate images with two distinct food odors, such as peanut butter and vanilla. During testing, they ate either a peanut butter sandwich or vanilla ice cream, and then went into the MRI scanner. The idea was that if they had eaten vanilla ice cream, for example, then the value of vanilla odor would decrease temporarily, relative to the smell of peanut butter. In agreement with this idea, activations in both the amygdala and the OFC decreased when participants viewed images associated with vanilla odor, compared to those associated with peanut butter odor. These findings showed that some aspect of neural processing had changed in these two structures after the value of the vanilla odor had decreased due to the consumption of vanilla ice cream.

Functional neuroimaging findings tell us that a region is activated to a greater or lesser extent, not that it is vital to a particular behavior. The study of monkeys with anatomically selective brain lesions allows us to probe neural mechanisms at a causal level; if lesions of discrete brain areas result in disruption of a particular behavior, then it follows that that region plays a critical role in some aspect of that behavior. The studies described below demonstrate that the amygdala indeed makes a causal contribution to the updating of food valuations, but only under certain circumstances.

Like the neuroimaging study just described, monkey studies of value updating have used a procedure known as "reinforcer devaluation," sometimes called simply "the devaluation procedure." In these experiments, the current value of a food reward is reduced by selective satiation, which is achieved by allowing the monkey to eat as much of a single type of food as it wants in one sitting. Once one kind of food has been devalued in this way, we can assess subsequent changes in foraging choices.

This research typically involves choices among relatively simple objects to obtain food, which might seem trivial compared to the choices made by humans. People, for example, choose among investments, careers, political ideologies, religions, and potential spouses (sometimes several times each). We believe, however, that our findings from monkeys tell us something fundamental about value-based decision making in any species. And the precise way in which we conduct these experiments has advantages over alternative research approaches. In our experiments, we examine the way in which value guides choices in relative isolation from other factors that influence choices, such as the history of success or failure of those choices, the amount of effort required, and so forth.

In considering our results, it is important to recognize at the outset that monkeys with amygdala lesions exhibit normal or nearly normal appetite and food preferences (Aggleton & Passingham, 1981; Izquierdo & Murray, 2007; Machado & Bachevalier, 2007; Machado, Emery, Mason, & Amaral, 2010; Murray, Gaffan, & Flint, 1996; cf. Agustín-Pavón,

Parkinson, Man, & Roberts, 2011). That is, after an amygdala lesion, monkeys prefer the same foods in about the same order of preference as before the lesion, and they eat a normal amount. In addition, they have intact satiety mechanisms, becoming sated in a normal manner after consuming a particular food and later avoiding that food when choosing between it and some alternative (Izquierdo & Murray, 2007; Machado & Bachevalier, 2007).

Although food preferences and appetite are not altered by amygdala damage, these lesions do affect how changes in food value influence a choice among objects (Baxter, Parker, Lindner, Izquierdo, & Murray, 2000; Machado & Bachevalier, 2007; Málková, Gaffan, & Murray, 1997; Murray & Izquierdo, 2007). In a typical devaluation experiment, illustrated in Figure 9.1, monkeys learn about a large number of objects and their associated food rewards. The choice of one set of objects is rewarded with one type of food (e.g., a peanut), and the choice of another set of objects is rewarded with another type of food (e.g., an M&M). The choice of yet additional objects is not rewarded at all. So monkeys learn to choose the food-associated objects over the alternatives and thereby learn the object–food pairings. After experience with the object–food pairings, the monkeys are fed to satiety on one of the two foods to temporarily devalue it, and shortly thereafter, we test the monkeys for their object preferences. Normal monkeys show a "devaluation effect," which consists of shifting their choices to objects associated with the food of currently higher value, thus avoiding objects associated with the devalued food. Monkeys with amygdala lesions, however, fail to shift their choice preferences in this manner. Figure 9.2 (left) summarizes findings from one such study (Izquierdo & Murray, 2007). The height of the bars represents the "difference score," which measures the decrease in choosing objects associated with a devalued food relative to baseline choices. ("Baseline" refers to the choice preferences of the same monkeys when they were not sated on either of the two foods.) The higher the bar, the greater the sensitivity to changes in food value. Monkeys with selective excitotoxic lesions of the amygdala are relatively insensitive to changes in the current, up-to-date value of foods associated with objects.

Relatively recent work has explored the mechanisms of devaluation effects and the impairments that follow amygdala lesions. One possibility is that without an amygdala, monkeys can no longer use their current internal state, satiety in this case, to guide object choices. Results from our laboratory have ruled out this idea (Rhodes, Charles, Howland, & Murray, 2012). In this experiment, monkeys were either hungry or thirsty, and while in these states, they learned that certain objects were associated with food, others with water, and still others with neither food nor water. Obviously, hungry monkeys should choose food-related objects, and thirsty monkeys should choose water-related objects. Monkeys with amygdala lesions learned and performed this task normally. Although this is a "negative result," meaning that the lesions had no effect on behavior, our findings tell us something important all the same. Monkeys without an amygdala can still represent information about their internal states and use that information to guide choices among objects. So the amygdala-lesion effect on the devaluation test must result from an impairment in updating valuations rather than representing internal states per se.

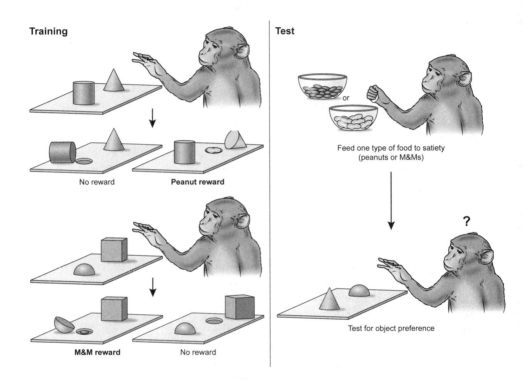

FIGURE 9.1. Object devaluation test procedure. During the training phase, monkeys learn a large set of visual discrimination problems. On each trial, two objects are presented—one object is always baited and the other is never baited. The left–right position of the baited object followed a pseudorandom order, and over several sessions, monkeys learn to displace only those objects that overlie food rewards. Half of the baited objects always cover one food, such as a peanut (top), and the other half always cover an alternate food, such as an M&M (bottom). During the test phase, monkeys are prefed one type of food to satiety in order to temporarily lower its value. Pairs of rewarded objects (made up of objects associated with each of the two food rewards) are then presented to the monkeys, and the monkeys are required to choose between them. Normal monkeys show a devaluation effect, whereby they will displace the object associated with the higher valued food over the one associated with the temporarily devalued food.

Additional studies have revealed more details about the mechanisms of devaluation effects and the amygdala's contribution. In one study, injection of a gamma-aminobutyric acid ($GABA_A$) agonist (muscimol) into the basolateral amygdala temporarily inactivated it either before or after the selective satiation procedure (Wellman, Gale, & Málková, 2005). When muscimol was injected *before* selective satiation, amygdala neurons were inactive during both the selective satiation procedure and the choice tests. In this case, the monkeys showed a greatly depressed devaluation effect. In contrast, when muscimol was injected *after* selective satiation, the amygdala neurons were active during the selective satiation procedure but not during the choice tests. In this case, the monkeys performed normally, as they did when isotonic saline was injected into the same brain location. Two conclusions follow from these results. First, the basolateral amygdala plays a necessary role in registering changes in reward value. Second, the basolateral amygdala is necessary for the process of updating these valuations as satiation develops, but not for its influence on object choices after the updating has occurred.

As illustrated in Figure 9.2 (left), monkeys with selective OFC lesions show the same behavior in the devaluation task as those with amygdala lesions (Rudebeck, Saunders, Prescott, Chau, & Murray, 2013b). Indeed,

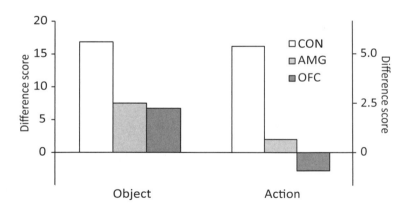

FIGURE 9.2. Results of devaluation testing on the Object task (left), and the Action task (right). The bars represent the difference score on the two tasks; the greater the difference score, the greater the devaluation effect. Note that the scores were calculated differently in the two tasks (see text), hence the different scales. Both amygdala and OFC lesions depress the devaluation effect, resulting in a difference score that is abnormally small. CON, unoperated control monkeys; AMG, monkeys with bilateral lesions of the amygdala; OFC, monkeys with bilateral lesions of the orbitofrontal cortex. Left: Data from Izquierdo and Murray (2007) and Rudebeck et al. (2013b); right: data from Rhodes and Murray (2013).

the amygdala and the OFC work together to enable the current, updated value of a reinforcer to influence behavior. Functional disconnection—achieved by removal of the amygdala in one hemisphere and the removal of the OFC in the other, together with section of the forebrain commissures—disrupts the devaluation effect just as much as bilateral lesions of either area (Baxter et al., 2000).

Although so far we have discussed linking *objects* with updated reward value, the amygdala makes a similar contribution to linking *actions* with updated reward value (Rhodes & Murray, 2013). In this task, illustrated in Figure 9.3, we first trained monkeys to learn two different actions, each linked to a different kind of food. One action, called a "tap," required the monkeys to repeatedly touch a colored square on the monitor screen to produce one kind of food reward, such as M&Ms. The other action, called a "hold," required persistent contact of an identical stimulus and produced a different kind of food reward, such as peanuts. After the monkeys had learned these action–food pairings, just as for the object–food pairings described earlier, they were allowed to consume one of the two foods to satiety. Shortly thereafter, they were given the opportunity to make either a "tap" or a "hold" movement. We performed this procedure under extinction, which means that we withheld rewards during testing. Although this undoubtedly disappointed the monkeys, it helped us interpret the results.

Normal monkeys showed a typical devaluation effect, indicating the ability to flexibly choose actions in line with the updated reward valuations, just as monkeys can choose objects on that basis. However, monkeys with bilateral lesions of the amygdala exhibited significantly depressed devaluation effects, indicating an impaired ability to link actions with current, updated food value and to choose actions on that basis. For example, despite being sated on M&Ms, monkeys with amygdala lesions continued to work toward obtaining more M&Ms, and they did so at the same rate as they worked toward obtaining peanuts, which had their normal value. Figure 9.2 (right) summarizes these findings.

As was the case for the object-based devaluation test, lesions of the OFC produced effects similar to those observed after amygdala lesions. Thus, whatever the amygdala and the OFC contribute to choice behavior, it involves choices among actions as well as among objects.

Interpretation

Our results indicate that the amygdala makes a causal contribution to updating the predicted value of rewards, and that it does so both for choices between objects and choices between actions. Although the results are qualitatively similar for the action- and object-based devaluation tasks, we note that the difference scores are calculated differently.

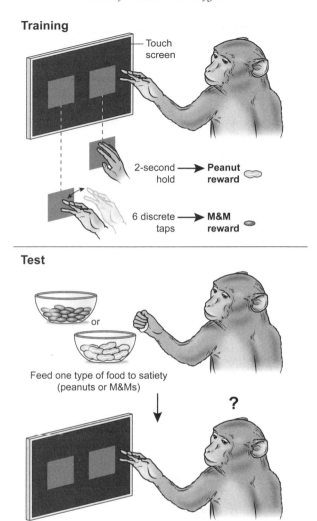

Training

Touch screen

2-second hold → **Peanut reward**

6 discrete taps → **M&M reward**

Test

or

Feed one type of food to satiety
(peanuts or M&Ms)

?

Test for response preference

FIGURE 9.3. Action devaluation test procedure. During the training phase, monkeys learn to make tap and hold responses to designated buttons on a touch screen in order to obtain different rewards, such as a peanut and an M&M—one for each of the two response types. During the test phase, monkeys are prefed one type of food to satiety in order to temporarily lower its value. They are then tested under extinction for their preference for the tap or hold response. Normal monkeys show a devaluation effect, whereby they make the response associated with the higher valued food over the one associated with the temporarily devalued food. For example, if a tap response was followed by the delivery of a peanut, and a hold response was followed by an M&M, then prefeeding on peanuts would result in a shift in response preference to hold.

The difference scores for the object task contrast preferences after satiation with those during baseline sessions, whereas scores for the action task contrast the number of actions associated with the higher-valued versus lower-valued food within sessions. This difference makes it difficult to compare results from these two kinds of experiments quantitatively, but the basic result is the same.

Taken together, results from the devaluation tests lead to several conclusions. The amygdala, in cooperation with the OFC, plays a causal role in making foraging choices based on the updated value of the rewards predicted to follow from those choices; the choices could be among objects or actions; these effects do not depend on an ability of monkeys to use their current internal state to guide choices; and the amygdala makes its contribution during the updating process, not afterward, when monkeys use these updated valuations to make choices.

We do not know how the amygdala makes these contributions to foraging choices, but we can engage in some informed speculation. One possibility is that the amygdala contributes a valuation feature to OFC's representation of specific, predicted outcomes, such as peanuts. The literature on the perception and memory of objects often appeals to neurons or networks that "bind" features from different sensory modalities or submodalities into a single, conjunctive representation. For example, the "object" in our object-based devaluation task might be a red cone. Somewhere, presumably in the temporal cortex, neurons represent the conjunction of "red" and "cone shaped" as a coherent whole. The objects used in our devaluation task had many more than two features, also called "dimensions," but the principle is the same regardless of the number. Through training on the task, the monkeys learned the object–food pairings, for example, that a red cone is associated with peanuts. Like the red cone, the brain represents peanuts as a conjunction of features: shape, texture, taste, and so forth. Perhaps the amygdala adds an additional feature dimension to the representation of peanuts, such as the neural equivalent of "highly desirable." When faced with a choice between a red cone and a blue hemisphere in the baseline condition, the red cone elicits a specific outcome representation that includes the feature "highly desirable," which beats the competition. So the monkey chooses the red cone. As the monkey consumes peanuts to satiety, the amygdala downgrades this feature of OFC's peanut representation to "desirable," then "neutral," "less than neutral," and finally "disgusting." Then, in the probe tests, the red cone elicits a representation that includes the feature "disgusting," which loses to the competition. So the monkey avoids the red cone and chooses the blue hemisphere. After this updating has occurred, the amygdala is no longer necessary, until—as it inevitably will—the value of peanuts changes again.

An alternative mechanism appeals to representations of yet higher dimensionality. Rather than separate, associated representations of the red cone and peanuts, perhaps the OFC represents the conjunction of all of the relevant features combined: "red–cone–oblong–crunchy texture–savory taste–highly desirable." The amygdala's contribution during satiation would be the same in this case: to update the palatability and motivation dimension of this representation from "highly desirable" to "disgusting." However, if this were the case, we would predict an impairment for object–food and object–water pairings, which does not occur. The representation "red–cone–water–highly desirable" versus "red–cone–water–unwanted now" should depend on valuation updating by the amygdala, and it does not.

A third possibility is that the palatability and motivation dimension is conjointly represented with the test object, but not the outcome, as "red–cone–desirable outcome" or "red–cone–undesirable outcome." These kinds of representations would be adequate for discrimination reversal tasks, but as we explain in the next section, we can rule out this possibility, at least for joint amygdala–OFC functions.

The Object Reversal Test

Updated valuations of foods and other rewards are one important factor in making foraging choices, but another involves which objects or other stimuli signal resource availability. In the psychology literature, the former concept is commonly referred to as "valuation" and "devaluation," with the terms "contingency" or "stimulus–reward contingency" used for the latter. In choosing among coffee shops, for example, it is vital to know both that the Starbucks logo indicates the availability of a Grande Mocha Frappuccino®, and to know the subjective value of a Grande Mocha Frappuccino® to oneself at the moment of decision. What if, someday, Starbucks and Dunkin' Donuts switched their menus, and thereafter only Dunkin' Donuts and not Starbucks sold Grande Mocha Frappuccinos? It would make sense then to change one's choice to Dunkin' Donuts. No matter how highly one valued a Starbucks Grande Mocha Frappuccino, it would make no sense to continue to visit Starbucks, because the drink you crave is no longer there. This is the principle underlying object reversal learning and the key way in which it differs from the devaluation task.

One might think that these two aspects of stimulus–reward association are so closely related that they depend on the same neural mechanisms. Indeed, in the literature, terms such as "reward," "reinforcement," "outcome," "valuation," and "utility" are sometimes used interchangeably. And all of them can be "updated" based on changing circumstances. But to presage the results discussed next, the evidence from monkeys shows that whereas updating valuations depends on the amygdala, updating stimulus–reward contingencies does not.

The role of different brain regions in maintaining up-to-date knowledge of the relationship between different objects and food availability has been teased apart by object reversal learning experiments, called "reversal learning" for short. Importantly, whereas devaluation tasks examine the ability of animals to respond flexibly to changes in food value, reversal learning tasks examine the ability of animals to respond flexibly to changes in stimulus–reward contingencies when the value of the food outcome is fixed. In simple terms, devaluation tasks probe what a resource is worth at the moment, whereas reversal learning relates to the likelihood of resource availability.

In a typical reversal learning task, monkeys first learn to discriminate a single pair of objects. One object hides a food reward, such as a peanut, but the other does not. In order to earn food on each trial, monkeys must learn which object signals food availability. Once the monkey has learned to select the correct (rewarded) object of the pair, and to avoid the unrewarded object, the object–food pairings are reversed. Now the object that signaled food no longer does so, and vice versa, as illustrated in Figure 9.4. This procedure can be repeated for a series of several reversals. The measure of interest is the number of errors made before reaching a predetermined (criterion) level of performance after each reversal, typically about 90% correct. Unsurprisingly, monkeys can not only learn the initial object–food pairing, but they can also adapt to multiple reversals, quickly altering their behavior in keeping with the current stimulus–reward contingency. In addition, with each subsequent reversal, monkeys become more adept at switching their choice, making fewer errors after stimulus–reward contingencies switch. Figure 9.5 summarizes these results in normal monkeys based on findings from our laboratory (Izquierdo & Murray, 2007; Rudebeck et al., 2013b).

Contrary to earlier findings based on aspiration lesions of the amygdala (Jones & Mishkin, 1972; Schwartzbaum & Poulos, 1965), we and others have found that fiber-sparing excitotoxic lesions of the amygdala fail to disrupt performance on reversal learning (Izquierdo & Murray, 2007; Kazama & Bachevalier, 2009). In fact, a reanalysis of the data showed that amygdala lesions lead to a significant facilitation in reversal learning, due to the operated monkeys benefiting more than controls from correctly performed trials that immediately follow an error (Rudebeck & Murray, 2008).

Notably, the history of research on OFC contributions to reversal learning parallels that of amygdala contributions in some respects. Contrary to earlier findings based on aspiration lesions of the OFC (Izquierdo, Suda, & Murray, 2004; Jones & Mishkin, 1972; Meunier, Bachevalier,

Acquisition

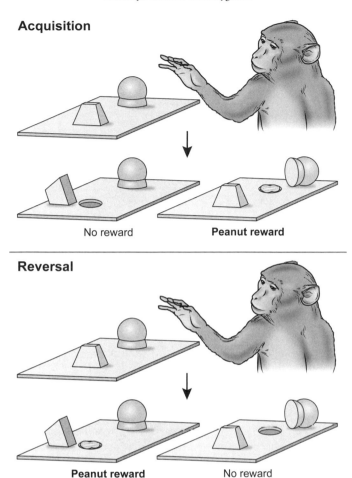

Reversal

FIGURE 9.4. Object reversal test procedure. During the acquisition phase, monkeys learn to discriminate a single pair of objects The two objects are always presented together; one object of the pair is always baited with a specific food, such as a peanut, whereas the other is always unbaited. The left–right position of the baited object followed a pseudorandom order, and over several sessions, monkeys learn to displace only the object that overlies the food reward. During the reversal phase, this object–reward pairing is switched. Accordingly, the object that was baited during acquisition no longer covers food, and the object that was unbaited is now rewarded.

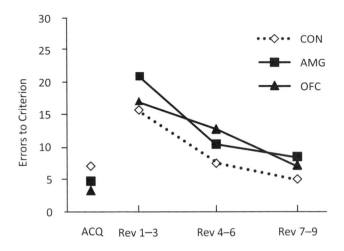

FIGURE 9.5. Results of the object reversal task. Errors to a predetermined level of performance (Criterion) for the initial phase of learning (Acquisition, or ACQ) and nine subsequent serial reversals, grouped into blocks of three (Rev 1–3, Rev 4–6, Rev 7–9). The slight differences seen in the curves were not statistically significant; neither amygdala nor OFC lesions cause impairments on the reversal test. CON, unoperated control monkeys; AMG, monkeys with bilateral lesions of the amygdala; OFC, monkeys with bilateral lesions of the orbitofrontal cortex. Data from Izquierdo and Murray (2007) and Rudebeck et al. (2013b).

& Mishkin, 1997), we found that fiber-sparing, excitotoxic lesions of the entire OFC fail to disrupt performance on reversal learning (Rudebeck et al., 2013b).

Interpretation

Earlier studies indicated that without an amygdala, monkeys were impaired at switching their foraging choices based on changes in stimulus–reward contingencies. These conclusions were based on findings from monkeys that sustained brain damage not only to the amygdala but also to nearby regions. More recent studies of reversal learning have demonstrated that selective, fiber-sparing amygdala lesions cause little or no impairment—and sometimes facilitate performance. Taken together with the negative findings from monkeys without an OFC, the findings overturn a long-held view about amygdala and OFC function: that these regions are essential for flexible learning of stimulus–reward contingencies. We return to this point in the section, "Defensive Behavior," below.

    We caution, however, against overly rigid conclusions along these lines, because we so far have investigated only deterministic (as opposed to probabilistic) learning, and only relatively early in learning. Indeed, some preliminary data from our laboratory suggest that lesions of the amygdala may disrupt reversal learning in animals with extensive training (Lucas et al., 2014). Thus, amygdala damage might sometimes impair reversal learning, depending on levels of choice uncertainty. In addition, the amygdala might be important for stimulus–reward learning in other settings, for example, in Pavlovian conditioning paradigms. Nevertheless, the fact that monkeys with complete lesions of the amygdala perform many versions of the reversal learning task normally demonstrates that, under some circumstances, the amygdala does not play a necessary role in learning about stimulus–reward contingencies.

Defensive Behavior

Defensive behavior is the subject of considerable research because it potentially bears on anxiety, posttraumatic stress, and other mental health disorders. The contribution of the amygdala to the generation and expression of defensive behaviors is well known (Paré, Quirk, & LeDoux, 2004).

Most advances in understanding the neural bases of defensive responses have come from research on rodents; by comparison, relevant work on monkeys is limited. Studies implicating the amygdala in the generation of appropriate defensive responses in adult monkeys have capitalized on innate responses to predators, threatening conspecifics, social stimuli of varying types, and the fear-potentiated startle paradigm, which is based on the enhancement of startle reflexes that occurs when subjects anticipate danger (Antoniadis, Winslow, Davis, & Amaral, 2007; Kalin, Shelton, Davidson, & Kelley, 2001; Mason, Capitanio, Machado, Mendoza, & Amaral, 2006; Meunier, Bachevalier, Murray, Málková, & Mishkin, 1999; Zola-Morgan, Squire, Alvarez-Royo, & Clower, 1991).

The Snake Test

One method to assess defensive behavior—and, presumably, the accompanying emotion of fear—draws on the reactions exhibited by macaque monkeys in the presence of snakes. In their natural habitat, snakes are one of the biggest threats to monkeys, especially young ones. No one knows how many monkeys succumb to snake predation, but some estimates have indicated that half or more of young monkeys fail to reach maturity in the wild (Fichtel, 2012). Consistent with the idea that predation by snakes was a selective pressure leading to special mechanisms for identification and detection of snakes, Nelson, Shelton, and Kalin (2003) demonstrated an innate fear of snakes in monkeys that had never seen them previously.

In our own studies, we compared unlearned responses of monkeys to spiders, as well as snakes, as a window on the neural bases of emotion—or, at least, defensive reactions. Although spiders do not prey on monkeys, they seem to produce innate avoidance responses in these animals, just as they do in some people. Using a task adapted from Mineka, Kier, and Price (1980), we pitted approach responses to obtain food against defensive responses engendered by a snake or spider, contrasted with responses to neutral objects, as illustrated in Figure 9.6. Our main measure of interest is food-retrieval latency, and we predicted that the presence of a snake or spider (relative to a neutral object) would slow a monkey's retrieval of the food. On each trial of these tests, monkeys are confronted with a rectangular transparent box containing either one of several neutral objects, a rubber snake, or a rubber spider. A small piece of food is placed on the top of the box, near the edge farthest from the monkey. The monkey is allowed to retrieve the food at its own pace, within a limit of 30 seconds. The test is run only every other day for five days, so exposure to the snake and spider is relatively limited.

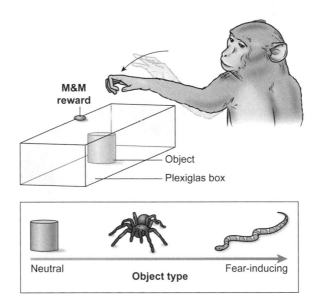

FIGURE 9.6. Snake test procedure. On each trial, monkeys are presented with a clear Plexiglas box. Inside the box is placed an object that ranges from neutral to fear inducing; the monkey is allowed to retrieve a food reward, such as an M&M, located on the far edge of the box. In order to obtain the food, the monkey must reach over the object. Control monkeys take longer to reach over a fear-inducing object to retrieve the food—sometimes failing to reach at all—compared to a neutral object.

Figure 9.7 summarizes findings from two such studies, one looking at the effect of amygdala lesions and the other of OFC lesions. The height of the bars shows the mean food-retrieval latency for the five exposures each to the snake, spider, and eight neutral objects. On trials with neutral objects, all monkeys retrieved the food quickly, in just 2–3 seconds. In contrast, on trials with rubber snakes, normal monkeys hesitated for long periods and in many cases failed to retrieve the food altogether. As they hesitated, the monkeys expressed a variety of defensive responses, including withdrawal, head aversion, eye aversion, and freezing (Izquierdo et al., 2005).

Monkeys with amygdala lesions showed no such reactions. They retrieved the food very quickly when faced with snakes, with roughly the same latency as on trials with neutral objects. This effect was all the more striking given that on many trials, monkeys with amygdala lesions stared at the snake or tried to grasp it before retrieving the food (Chudasama, Izquierdo, & Murray, 2009), behaviors that delayed food retrieval. Trials with the rubber spider yielded an intermediate effect on food-retrieval latency in normal monkeys, and a mild but significant reduction in food-retrieval latency in monkeys without an amygdala (Izquierdo et al., 2005).

For comparison, we studied monkeys with excitotoxic lesions of the OFC on the snake test. Unlike monkeys with amygdala lesions, and unlike monkeys with aspiration lesions of the OFC (Izquierdo et al., 2005;

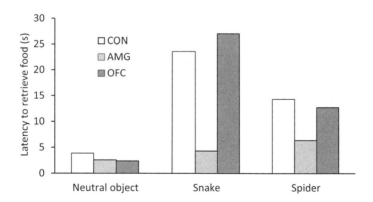

FIGURE 9.7. Results from the snake test. The plot shows monkey's latencies to retrieve food (in seconds) when exposed to either a neutral object, a rubber snake, or a rubber spider. Monkeys with amygdala lesions show faster retrieval of food compared to both monkeys with OFC lesions and controls, presumably because of reduced fear of both snakes and spiders. CON, unoperated control monkeys; AMG, monkeys with bilateral lesions of the amygdala; OFC, monkeys with bilateral lesions of the orbitofrontal cortex. Data from Izquierdo et al. (2005) and Rudebeck et al. (2013b).

Rudebeck, Buckley, Walton, & Rushworth, 2006), they behaved like normal monkeys (Rudebeck et al., 2013b).

Interpretation

Before the snake test, the monkeys in our experiment had had experience with cognitive tasks administered in a similar testing situation. As a result, they knew that displacing objects would often lead to food rewards. When exposure to the snake and spider is assessed on a background of monkeys' expectation of obtaining food in a given situation, as done in our experiments, it provides a sensitive measure of the monkey's emotional, defensive responses to snakes.

Our results show that the amygdala, but not the OFC, plays a causal role in generating normal defensive behavior. Because aspiration lesions of the OFC, but not selective, fiber-sparing lesions of OFC, yield effects similar to those of amygdala lesions (Izquierdo et al., 2005), the amygdala presumably interacts with frontal cortical regions outside the OFC in mediating the defensive responses to the rubber snake.

Importantly, the effects on food-retrieval latency can be dissociated from those involving other defensive responses, such as freezing, piloerection, and head or eye aversion. Following perirhinal cortex lesions, monkeys showed normal levels of freezing, piloerection, and head/eye aversion to the snake but not the usual reluctance to reach over the snake for food (Chudasama, Wright, & Murray, 2008). A detailed discussion of this finding is beyond the scope of this chapter, but the abnormally short food-retrieval latencies after perirhinal cortex lesions may result from the loss of visual inputs to frontal areas outside the OFC or to disruption of a network involving the perirhinal cortex, the basolateral amygdala, and some part of the frontal cortex.

These new results from the reversal learning and snake tests, taken together, overturn some commonly held ideas about cooperation between the amygdala and the OFC. The older studies were based on the effects of relatively unselective aspiration lesions of the OFC and the amygdala, and they seemed to indicate that amygdala and OFC damage almost always produced similar results. According to these studies, both kinds of lesions yield severe impairments on reversal learning, as well as altered emotional responding (Jones & Mishkin, 1972; Izquierdo et al., 2004, 2005). In addition, the older literature sometimes emphasizes a relationship between performance on reversal learning and the emotional disturbances that follow amygdala damage in monkeys (Aggleton & Passingham, 1981) and OFC damage in humans (Rolls, Hornak, Wade, & McGrath, 1994).

Findings based on selective lesions lead to very different conclusions. In these studies, lesions of the amygdala and the OFC avoid damage to nearby pathways and cortical areas. Instead of depending on a cooperative interaction between the amygdala and the OFC, selective lesions show that reversal learning depends on neither the amygdala nor the OFC. For instance, the temporal lobe substrate for reversal learning appears to be the entorhinal and perirhinal areas, not the amygdala (Murray, Gaffan, & Baxter, 1998); and the frontal lobe substrate lies somewhere outside the OFC (Rudebeck et al., 2013b). Furthermore, although normal defensive responding does depend on the amygdala, it does not require the OFC (Rudebeck et al., 2013b).

Social Behavior

Other chapters in this book deal with the amygdala's role in social behavior in detail (Bliss-Moreau, Moadab, & Amaral, Chapter 6, and Bachevalier, Sanchez, Raper, Stephens, & Wallen, Chapter 7). Accordingly, here we focus on responses to emotions signaled from monkey to monkey through facial gestures.

Viewing Facial Expressions of Emotion

Another window on life without an amygdala is provided by studies of cortical responses to socially important visual signals. These studies involve fMRI, and they require monkeys to view images of monkey faces, presented one at a time. Under these conditions, both the amygdala and the inferior temporal cortex show greater activation during the viewing of facial expressions of emotion relative to neutral facial expressions (Hadj-Bouziane, Bell, Knusten, Ungerleider, & Tootell, 2008). These results indicate that activity in the amygdala and the inferior temporal cortex is modulated by socially relevant facial expressions of emotion in macaques, as it is in humans (Vuillemieuer, Richardson, Armony, Driver, & Dolan, 2004).

Because the amygdala and the inferior temporal cortex are reciprocally connected with each other (Ghashghaei & Barbas, 2002; Price & Amaral, 1981), we conducted a study to determine whether the amygdala might be essential for modulation of activations in the inferior temporal cortex. Specifically, we examined the effects of amygdala removals on fMRI activation in the inferior temporal cortex during the passive viewing of faces. The most striking difference between intact hemispheres and hemispheres with amygdala lesions involves responses to lip smack expressions, an affiliative gesture among macaques. Normally, the inferior temporal cortex shows an enhanced activation to lip-smacking faces as contrasted with neutral ones. After amygdala lesions, however, this enhanced activation does not occur.

Not all of these monkeys had the exact same degree of amygdala damage in these experiments; each had some remaining (spared) amygdala, ranging from an estimated 5 to 35% of its total volume. We found that damage to the anterior part of the amygdala disrupted the socioemotional modulation of activation in anterior parts of the inferior temporal cortex, whereas damage to posterior amygdala did so in posterior parts. This was especially true for cortical responses to fear grimaces and open-mouth threats.

Other studies have provided evidence of causal contributions of the amygdala to the processing of social signals. In macaque monkeys, for example, preliminary data indicate that the amygdala is essential for attending to facial expressions. The task required monkeys to shift their gaze from a central spot of light on a monitor screen to a peripheral spot. On some trials, a fragment of a face image (the eyes, nose or mouth) appeared at the central location at the same time as the target appeared in the periphery. On other trials, a nonsocial image (a scrambled face) appeared instead. Normal monkeys shifted gaze more slowly when presented with a social stimulus than with a nonsocial one, but monkeys with amygdala lesions showed much less slowing relative to controls (Dal Monte, Costa, Noble, Murray, & Averbeck, 2015). These data provide further evidence that the amygdala plays a crucial role in attending to social signals and modulating the behavioral responses related to them.

Interpretation

Importantly, in the fMRI study, the amygdala lesions did not alter activation in inferior temporal cortex in response to neutral faces. When contrasted with the effects of socially relevant stimuli on fMRI activation of the inferior temporal cortex, the findings summarized here support the idea that the amygdala modulates responses to socially important signals, including those related to faces, social threats, fear, and conflict.

Conclusions

The findings reviewed in this chapter reveal the influence of the amygdala on several kinds of behavior, including foraging choices based on updated valuations, defensive behaviors (e.g., snake avoidance), and social behaviors (e.g., attending to facial expressions of emotion).

Nevertheless, life goes on without an amygdala, and monkeys with amygdala lesions are normal in many ways. They have no gross impairment in visual perception, as evidenced by their normal rates of acquisition of visual discrimination problems (Málková et al., 1997; Izquierdo

& Murray, 2007). And they can learn normally in many tasks (Baxter & Murray, 2002), as exemplified by their intact performance in reversal learning, at least under many conditions. The amygdala has more specific functions.

A key clue to this specific function comes from four neurophysiological experiments, each involving changes in neuronal activity after lesions or inactivations of the amygdala. First, neurons in the gustatory cortex of rats lose the ability to signal palatability, although they continue encoding the basic sensory features of taste, such as salty, sweet, bitter, and sour sensations (Piette, Baez-Santiago, Reid, Katz, & Moran, 2012). Second, neurons in the nucleus accumbens of rats respond less than they normally do to an acoustic stimulus that indicates reward availability following a bar press (Ambroggi, Ishikawa, Fields, & Nicola, 2008). Third, neurons in the OFC of rats show less encoding of predicted rewards when they discharge in response to odor cues associated with those rewards (Schoenbaum, Setlow, Saddoris, & Gallagher, 2003). And fourth, neurons in the OFC of monkeys decrease their encoding of reward quantity, as signaled by a visual cue (Rudebeck, Mitz, Chacko, & Murray, 2013a). In each case, the amygdala appears to enhance activity in other brain regions in response to biologically important stimuli. The results on cortical activations for facial expressions of emotion lead to the same conclusion.

Taken together, the findings summarized in this chapter suggest that the amygdala contributes a valuation element to representations of special biological importance—elsewhere in the brain—updated in accord with current biological wants and needs. The effects of this influence would depend on what kind of information each target brain area represents: specific outcomes and the object or actions associated with them; the threat posed by predators (e.g., snakes) or irritants (e.g., spiders); or social signals sent by conspecifics. Life without an amygdala removes these influences, so behavior tends to lack its special relationship with the most biologically significant stimuli and their value at any given moment. In monkeys, this means making foraging choices based on outdated valuations of the outcomes associated with objects or actions; deficiencies in the normal defensive responses to both existential threats and minor irritants; and failing to pay special attention to communicative gestures in one's social circle, among other behaviors important to the life of primates.

ACKNOWLEDGMENT

This work was supported by the Intramural Research Program of the National Institute of Mental Health.

REFERENCES

Antoniadis, E. A., Winslow, J. T., Davis, M., & Amaral, D. G. (2007). Role of the primate amygdala in fear-potentiated startle: Effects of chronic lesions in the rhesus monkey. *Journal of Neuroscience, 27*(28), 7386–7396.

Agustín-Pavón, C., Parkinson, J., Man, M. S., & Roberts, A. C. (2011). Contribution of the amygdala, but not orbitofrontal or medial prefrontal cortices, to the expression of flavour preferences in marmoset monkeys. *European Journal of Neuroscience, 34*(6), 1006–1017.

Aggleton, J. P., & Passingham, R. E. (1981). Syndrome produced by lesions of the amygdala in monkeys (*Macaca mulatta*). *Journal of Comparative and Physiological Psychology, 95*(6), 961–977.

Ambroggi, F., Ishikawa, A., Fields, H. L., & Nicola, S. M. (2008). Basolateral amygdala neurons facilitate reward-seeking behavior by exciting nucleus accumbens neurons. *Neuron, 59*(4), 648–661.

Balleine, B. W., & Killcross, S. (2006). Parallel incentive processing: An integrated view of amygdala function. *Trends in Neuroscience, 29*(5), 272–279.

Baxter, M. G., & Murray, E. A. (2002). The amygdala and reward. *Nature Reviews Neuroscience, 3*(7), 563–573.

Baxter, M. G., Parker, A., Lindner, C. C., Izquierdo, A. D., & Murray, E. A. (2000). Control of response selection by reinforcer value requires interaction of amygdala and orbital prefrontal cortex. *Journal of Neuroscience, 20*(11), 4311–4319.

Braesicke, K., Parkinson, J. A., Reekie, Y., Man, M. S., Hopewell, L., Pears, A., et al. (2005). Autonomic arousal in an appetitive context in primates: A behavioural and neural analysis. *European Journal of Neuroscience, 21*(6), 1733–1740.

Chudasama, Y., Izquierdo, A., & Murray, E. A. (2009). Distinct contributions of the amygdala and hippocampus to fear expression. *European Journal of Neuroscience, 30*(12), 2327–2337.

Chudasama, Y., Wright, K. S., & Murray, E. A. (2008). Hippocampal lesions in rhesus monkeys disrupt emotional responses but not reinforcer devaluation effects. *Biological Psychiatry, 63*(11), 1084–1091.

Dal Monte, O., Costa, V. D., Noble, P., Murray, E. A., & Averbeck, B. B. (2015). Amygdala lesions in rhesus macaques decrease attention to threat. *Nature Communications, 6.*

Fichtel, C. (2012). Predation. In J. C. Mitani, J. Call, P. M. Kappeler, R. A. Palombit, & J. Silk (Eds.), *The evolution of primate societies* (pp. 169–194). Chicago: University of Chicago Press.

Ghashghaei, H. T., & Barbas, H. (2002). Pathways for emotion: interactions of prefrontal and anterior temporal pathways in the amygdala of the rhesus monkey. *Neuroscience, 115*(4), 1261–1279.

Gottfried, J. A., O'Doherty, J., & Dolan, R. J. (2003). Encoding predictive reward value in human amygdala and orbitofrontal cortex. *Science, 301*(5636), 1104–1107.

Hadj-Bouziane, F., Bell, A. H., Knusten, T. A., Ungerleider, L. G., & Tootell, R. B. (2008). Perception of emotional expressions is independent of face selectivity in monkey inferior temporal cortex. *Proceedings of the National Academy of Sciences, 105*(14), 5591–5596.

Izquierdo, A., & Murray, E. A. (2007). Selective bilateral amygdala lesions in rhesus monkeys fail to disrupt object reversal learning. *Journal of Neuroscience, 27*(5), 1054–1062.

Izquierdo, A., Suda, R. K., & Murray, E. A. (2004). Bilateral orbital prefrontal cortex lesions in rhesus monkeys disrupt choices guided by both reward value and reward contingency. *Journal of Neuroscience, 24*(34), 7540–7548.

Izquierdo, A., Suda, R. K., & Murray, E. A. (2005). Comparison of the effects of bilateral orbital prefrontal cortex lesions and amygdala lesions on emotional responses in rhesus monkeys. *Journal of Neuroscience, 25*(37), 8534–8542.

Jones, B., & Mishkin, M. (1972). Limbic lesions and the problem of stimulus–Reinforcement associations. *Experimental Neurology, 36*(2), 362–377.

Kalin, N. H., Shelton, S. E., Davidson, R. J., & Kelley, A. E. (2001). The primate amygdala mediates acute fear but not the behavioral and physiological components of anxious temperament. *Journal of Neuroscience, 21*(6), 2067–2074.

Kazama, A., & Bachevalier, J. (2009). Selective aspiration or neurotoxic lesions of orbital frontal areas 11 and 13 spared monkeys' performance on the object discrimination reversal task. *Journal of Neuroscience, 29*(9), 2794–2804.

Klüver, H., & Bucy, P. C. (1939). Preliminary analysis of functions of the temporal lobes in monkeys. *Archives of Neurology and Psychiatry, 42*(6), 979–1000.

LeDoux, J. (2003). The emotional brain, fear, and the amygdala. *Cellular and Molecular Neurobiology, 23*(4–5), 727–738.

Lucas, D. R., III, Costa, V. D., Dal Monte, O., Rudebeck, P. H., Murray, E. A., & Averbeck, B. B. (2014, November). *Amygdala lesions compromise reinforcement learning to impact behavioral flexibility.* Poster presented at the Society for Neuroscience Annual Meeting, Washington, DC.

Machado, C. J., & Bachevalier, J. (2007). The effects of selective amygdala, orbital frontal cortex or hippocampal formation lesions on reward assessment in nonhuman primates. *European Journal of Neuroscience, 25*(9), 2885–2904.

Machado, C. J., Emery, N. J., Mason, W. A., & Amaral, D. G. (2010). Selective changes in foraging behavior following bilateral neurotoxic amygdala lesions in rhesus monkeys. *Behavioral Neuroscience, 124*(6), 761–772.

Málková, L., Gaffan, D., & Murray, E. A. (1997). Excitotoxic lesions of the amygdala fail to produce impairment in visual learning for auditory secondary reinforcement but interfere with reinforcer devaluation effects in rhesus monkeys. *Journal of Neuroscience, 17*(15), 6011–6020.

Mason, W. A., Capitanio, J. P., Machado, C. J., Mendoza, S. P., & Amaral, D. G. (2006). Amygdalectomy and responsiveness to novelty in rhesus monkeys (*Macaca mulatta*): Generality and individual consistency of effects. *Emotion, 6*(1), 73–81.

Meunier, M., Bachevalier, J., & Mishkin, M. (1997). Effects of orbital frontal and anterior cingulate lesions on object and spatial memory in rhesus monkeys. *Neuropsychologia, 35*(7), 999–1015.

Meunier, M., Bachevalier, J., Murray, E. A., Málková, L., & Mishkin, M. (1999). Effects of aspiration versus neurotoxic lesions of the amygdala on emotional responses in monkeys. *European Journal of Neuroscience, 11*(12), 4403–4418.

Mineka, S., Keir, R., & Price, V. (1980). Fear of snakes in wild- and laboratory-reared rhesus monkeys (*Macaca mulatta*). *Animal Learning and Behavior, 8*(4), 653–663.

Murray, E. A., Gaffan, D., & Baxter, M. G. (1998). Monkeys with rhinal cortex damage or neurotoxic hippocampal lesions are impaired on spatial scene learning and object reversals. *Behavioral Neuroscience, 112*(6), 1291–1303.

Murray, E. A., Gaffan, E. A., & Flint, R. W. (1996). Anterior rhinal cortex and amygdala: Dissociation of their contributions to memory and food preference in rhesus monkeys. *Behavioral Neuroscience, 110*(1), 30–42.

Murray, E. A., & Izquierdo, A. (2007). Orbitofrontal cortex and amygdala contributions to affect and action in primates. *Annals of the New York Academy of Sciences, 1121*, 273–296.

Nelson, E. E., Shelton, S. E., & Kalin, N. H. (2003). Individual differences in the responses of naive rhesus monkeys to snakes. *Emotion, 3*(1), 3–11.

Paré, D., Quirk, G. J., & LeDoux, J. E. (2004). New vistas on amygdala networks in conditioned fear. *Journal of Neurophysiology, 92*(1), 1–9.

Parkinson, J. A., Crofts, H. S., McGuigan, M., Tomic, D. L., Everitt, B. J., & Roberts, A. C. (2001). The role of the primate amygdala in conditioned reinforcement. *Journal of Neuroscience, 21*(19), 7770–7780.

Piette, C. E., Baez-Santiago, M. A., Reid, E. E., Katz, D. B., & Moran, A. (2012). Inactivation of basolateral amygdala specifically eliminates palatability-related information in cortical sensory responses. *Journal of Neuroscience, 32*(29), 9981–9991.

Price, J. L., & Amaral, D. G. (1981). An autoradiographic study of the projections of the central nucleus of the monkey amygdala. *Journal of Neuroscience, 1*(11), 1242–1259.

Rhodes, S. E. V., Charles, D. P., Howland, E. J., & Murray, E. A. (2012). Amygdala lesions in rhesus monkeys fail to disrupt object choices based on internal context. *Behavioral Neuroscience, 126*(2), 270–278.

Rhodes, S. E. V., & Murray, E. A. (2013). Differential effects of amygdala, orbital prefrontal cortex, and prelimbic cortex lesions on goal-directed behavior in rhesus macaques. *Journal of Neuroscience, 33*(8), 3380–3389.

Rolls, E. T., Hornak, J., Wade, D., & McGrath, J. (1994). Emotion-related learning in patients with social and emotional changes associated with frontal lobe damage. *Journal of Neurology, Neurosurgery, and Psychiatry, 57*(12), 1518–1524.

Rudebeck, P. H., Buckley, M. J., Walton, M. E., & Rushworth, M. F. (2006). A role for the macaque anterior cingulate gyrus in social valuation. *Science, 313*(5791), 1310–1312.

Rudebeck, P. H., Mitz, A. R., Chacko, R. V., & Murray, E. A. (2013a). Effects of amygdala lesions on reward-value coding in orbital and medial prefrontal cortex. *Neuron, 80*(6), 1519–1531.

Rudebeck, P. H., & Murray, E. A. (2008). Amygdala and orbitofrontal cortex lesions differentially influence choices during object reversal learning. *Journal of Neuroscience, 28*(33), 8338–8343.

Rudebeck, P. H., Saunders, R. C., Prescott, A. T., Chau, L. S., & Murray, E. A. (2013b). Prefrontal mechanisms of behavioral flexibility, emotion regulation and value updating. *Nature Neuroscience, 16*(8), 1140–1145.

Schoenbaum, G., Setlow, B., Saddoris, M. P., & Gallagher, M. (2003). Encoding predicted outcome and acquired value in orbitofrontal cortex during cue sampling depends upon input from basolateral amygdala. *Neuron, 39*(5), 855–867.

Schwartzbaum, J. S., & Poulos, D. A. (1965). Discrimination behavior after amygdalectomy in monkeys: Learning set and discrimination reversals. *Journal of Comparative and Physiological Psychology, 60*(3), 320–328.

Vuilleumier, P., Richardson, M. P., Armony, J. L., Driver, J., & Dolan, R. J. (2004). Distant influences of amygdala lesion on visual cortical activation during emotional face processing. *Nature Neuroscience, 7*(11), 1271–1278.

Weiskrantz, L. (1956). Behavioral changes associated with ablation of the amygdaloid complex in monkeys. *Journal of Comparative and Physiological Psychology, 49*(4), 381–391.

Wellman, L. L., Gale, K., & Málková, L. (2005). GABA$_A$-mediated inhibition of basolateral amygdala blocks reward devaluation in macaques. *Journal of Neuroscience, 25*(18), 4577–4586.

Zola-Morgan, S., Squire, L. R., Alvarez-Royo, P., & Clower, R. P. (1991). Independence of memory functions and emotional behavior: Separate contributions of the hippocampal formation and the amygdala. *Hippocampus, 1*(2), 207–220.

CHAPTER 10

Consequences of Developmental Bilateral Amygdala Lesions in Humans

RALPH ADOLPHS

The amygdala is involved in a host of cognitive functions, tied together by some common themes. Those functions include perception, attention, memory, and decision making. The themes revolve around biological relevance, saliency, emotion, and social communication. While the vast majority of studies on the functions of the human amygdala come from functional neuroimaging studies, a handful of rare patients with lesions to the amygdala have provided particularly provocative insights into the essential functions of the amygdala, and have stimulated specific hypotheses to pursue further. One key distinction, however, is whether these lesions were sustained early in development or in adulthood. This distinction is reflected in differences in the types and severity of behavioral changes that are seen, and is likely attributable, at least in part, to secondary changes that are distal to the amygdala lesions themselves. Here I review these findings and suggest key challenges for the future: better delineation of the lesions, concurrent neuroimaging to quantify systems-level changes following amygdala lesions, and comparisons across different ages.

Developmental versus Adult-Onset Lesions

The consequences of developmental-onset lesions are likely to offer some profound differences in comparison to otherwise anatomically similar lesions that have an adult onset. This is an issue to which I return throughout this chapter. For instance, there is a discrepancy between conclusions regarding the human amygdala's role in conscious experience of emotions derived from developmental-onset versus adult-onset lesions (see last section of this chapter and Todd, Anderson, & Phelps, Chapter 13, this volume). Similarly, there are differences between adult-onset and developmental onset lesions of the amygdala in monkeys and rats (cf. Sarro & Sullivan, Chapter 4, and Bliss-Moreau, Moadab, & Amaral, Chapter 6, this volume). On the one hand, what distinguishes developmental-onset lesions can be seen as a matter of lesion duration (Dijkhuizen et al., 2001). On the other hand, there is so much more possibility for plasticity and reorganization during development that one would expect considerably greater distal changes following a lesion early in life rather than later in life, even once mere duration has been controlled for—the so-called "Kennard principle" that earlier onset is associated with increased opportunity for plasticity (Dennis, 2010; Kennard, 1942).

There are numerous clear examples of this issue (Kolb, Mychasiuk, Williams, & Gibb, 2011). For instance, it is well known that the possibility for language recovery following left-hemispheric lesions is often greater if the lesions are sustained early in development (Marsh & Hillis, 2006). Indeed, in the extreme example, complete hemispherectomy, if sustained early in life, can yield a remarkable sparing of the functions normally associated with the lesioned hemisphere (Umeda & Funakoshi, 2014), and age of the surgery is correlated with extensive white-matter reorganization related to the spared functions (Choi, Vining, Mori, & Bastian, 2010).

Yet the consequences of some developmental-onset lesions are, intriguingly, more severe rather than less severe than their adult-onset counterparts. This appears to be the case for lesions of the ventromedial prefrontal cortex (Anderson, Damasio, Tranel, & Damasio, 2000; Eslinger, Grattan, Damaso, & Damasio, 1992), and may well be the case also for lesions of the amygdala. In both cases, these types of brain damage share two factors in common. Both are lesions that impact social and emotional functioning. Both are also generally studied as bilateral lesions rather than as unilateral lesions, a factor that is known to exacerbate dysfunction in the case of the prefrontal cortex (Eslinger, Flaherty-Craig, & Benton, 2004) as well as the amygdala (Adolphs, Tranel, & Damasio, 2001). Likely for both of these reasons, the consequences of developmental-onset damage in these structures in many respects appear more severe, particularly in the domain of social and emotional processing, than those for the adult-onset equivalents. This issue is also of critical importance to understanding the role of the amygdala in psychiatric developmental disorders; for instance, amygdala dysfunction has been implicated not only in autism spectrum disorders (Amaral, Schumann, & Nordahl, 2008) but also seems to be reported fairly ubiquitously across neurodevelopmental disorders (Schumann, Bauman, & Amaral, 2011).

In understanding systems-level changes following developmental amygdala lesions, it is critical not to conflate "plasticity" with "improvement." Not only has the Kennard principle, as such, been questioned (i.e., it is not universally the case that there is increased plasticity with younger age of onset of the lesion), but it has also been stressed that the reorganization due to "plasticity" (itself a complex and multilevel construct) could give rise to pathology in its own right rather than invariable improvement in function (Dennis et al., 2013). This "dark side" of plasticity (Elbert & Heim, 2001) has been acknowledged to play as big a role as in compensation and recovery (Pascual-Leone, Amedi, Fregni, & Merabet, 2005). Indeed, one of the earliest dissociations of structural reorganization from functional recovery clearly showed that greater plasticity could be associated with poorer function (interestingly, also, for a subcortical structure, the hamster midbrain) (Schneider, 1974).

The factors that determine whether early plastic changes improve or are detrimental to functional recovery are not understood, although the vague concept of "imbalance" is often invoked (Menon, 2013). The idea is that plastic and possibly locally compensatory changes following damage result in a systems-level imbalance in function (the case of autism is a good example of these ideas, in which imbalance between excitatory and inhibitory neuronal processing, or between bottom-up and top-down processing, or between underconnectivity and overconnectivity at different spatial scales, is often hypothesized). There is even some direct evidence supporting the idea of "pathological plasticity" at distal locations following damage elsewhere: A second lesion can improve function following a primary lesion! (Kapur, 1996). While much more experimental work in animal models is needed to understand the principles of distal plasticity, and how they relate to systems-level function, the broad conclusions from this work for our purposes are clear. The consequences of amygdala lesions (like any brain lesions) cannot be understood simply by investigating the functioning of the lesioned structure in isolation. We need to focus on the distal structures that used to be structurally and functionally connected to the lesion site, the age at which the lesion occurred, the time elapsed since the lesion occurred, and the present age of the patient. This systems-level and lifespan-plasticity view of the functional consequences of brain lesions is also likely to account for much of the variability in outcome following focal brain lesions (once sheer neuroanatomical lesion variability has been accounted for). Adding to the complexity in the case of emotional and social functions, of course, is the fact that focal lesions impact not only other parts of the brain but can also be thought of as catalyzing a developmental trajectory that incorporates interactions with the environment and with other people with whom the young patient interacts (Eslinger et al., 2004).

Distal Changes Following Developmental Amygdala Lesions

Turning to the topic of this chapter then: What are the consequences of developmental-onset amygdala lesions? A first description of this complex topic might begin with a description of the anatomy of damage within the amygdala, a topic I address in the following section. No less important is a description of the whole-brain anatomical changes that might arise from developmental amygdala lesions, picking up from the themes discussed in the preceding section.

We undertook such an investigation a few years ago with collaborators at the University of Iowa (Boes et al., 2012). In that study, we investigated two rare patients with developmental-onset bilateral amygdala lesions due to Urbach–Wiethe disease (UWD; see next section). Although the analysis we used in that study was a whole-brain one, the findings fit very well with regional predictions that one would have hypothesized. Specifically, there were changes in cortical thickness in those regions that have the densest connectivity with the amygdala (Amaral, Price, Pitkanen, & Carmichael, 1992; Öngür & Price, 2000): ventral temporal cortices and ventromedial prefrontal cortex (Figure 10.1). It is fascinating that while some of these changes corresponded to a reduction in cortical thickness, others, particularly in regions of medial prefrontal cortex and anterior cingulate cortex, actually corresponded to an increase in cortical thickness (an observation also in line with what is seen in monkeys with amygdala lesions; D. G. Amaral, personal communication, 2013). It is also interesting to note that cortical thickness changes dramatically in many of these particular regions over childhood (Khundrakpam et al., 2013), and one would therefore expect that there could be large differences in the kinds of effects we observed, depending on the precise age at which the amygdala lesions are sustained.

The functions of the regions highlighted in Figure 10.1 are known to intersect in many respects with the putative functions of the amygdala. Of particular note is the circuit encompassing the ventromedial prefrontal cortex, dorsomedial thalamus, and amygdala: all these structures are interconnected, and experimental disconnections of them in animal studies can reproduce many of the behavioral impairments that are seen following focal lesions to either of the structures in isolation (Gaffan & Murray, 1990; Gaffan, Murray, & Fabre-Thorpe, 1993). It is thus perhaps not surprising also to find abnormal modulations of one structure in functional magnetic resonance imaging (fMRI) when another of these structures is selectively lesioned. For instance, patients with developmental bilateral amygdala lesions show abnormal blood oxygenation level-dependent (BOLD)-fMRI signal in sectors of medial prefrontal cortex

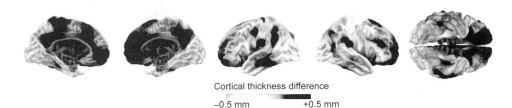

Cortical thickness difference

−0.5 mm   +0.5 mm

FIGURE 10.1. Changes in cortical thickness in subject S. M., who has long-standing bilateral lesions of the amygdala. Changes are relative to the distribution measured in an age- and gender-matched group of 20 healthy participants. When considered together with another patient with bilateral amygdala lesions (who was compared to her own independent set of controls), two regions stood out as significantly different (increased) in terms of their cortical thickness: the medial prefrontal cortex, and the ventral temporal cortex. From Boes et al. (2012). Copyright 2012 by Ralph Adolphs. Reprinted by permission.

during a reward learning task (Hampton, Adolphs, Tyszka, & O'Doherty, 2007); conversely, patients with selective bilateral damage to the ventromedial prefrontal cortex show an abnormal BOLD signal in the amygdala (Motzkin, Philippi, Wolf, Baskaya, & Koenigs, 2015). Clearly, lesioning the amygdala has network-level effects, both structurally and functionally, and these are the most apparent for those distal structures that normally are most intimately connected with the amygdala.

There are other ways in which amygdala lesions influence the response of distal regions, not so much due to the direct loss of inputs from the amygdala, but rather through the recruitment of compensatory cognitive strategies of solving tasks that might normally rely on the amygdala. For instance, responses to fearful faces often elicit a mirroring of the motor representations required to produce such an expression on one's own face—one route that is hypothesized to provide us with knowledge about how other people feel from looking at their faces (by "simulation"). In one study of a patient with bilateral amygdala lesions, this mechanism appeared to be recruited, as deduced from BOLD signal in cortical regions thought to implement such a "simulation" routine. And, indeed, the patient's compensatory cortical activation went hand in hand with compensatory performance on a task requiring the recognition of fear from faces (Mihov et al., 2013; see also Patin & Hurlemann, Chapter 11, this volume).

The distal consequences of amygdala lesions are of particular interest in a developmental context, because numerous studies point to a broad modulatory role for the amygdala; that is, a wealth of data suggests that the amygdala itself prominently modulates processing elsewhere in the brain, with examples ranging from fear conditioning in animals (Maren, Yap, & Goosens, 2001) to attention (Holland & Gallagher, 1999), to emotional modulation of declarative memory in humans (McGaugh, 2004). Given the previously mentioned findings of long-term structural changes in sectors of prefrontal and temporal cortex, then, it would be important to take these into consideration when interpreting perceptual, attentional, emotional, and decision-making processes that might be affected by bilateral amygdala lesions, especially in a developmental context (Skuse, Morris, & Lawrence, 2003). In the following survey of all of these cognitive domains, it will be important to keep in mind, and it is a major challenge to all future interpretations, to what extent dysfunction can be attributed to amygdala damage per se, and to what extent it can be attributed to dysfunction in distal structures normally interconnected with the amygdala.

Anatomy of Amygdala Damage

Bilateral damage to the human amygdala can arise from a number of etiologies. Perhaps the most common are a variety of inflammatory diseases, including *Herpes simplex* encephalitis and limbic encephalitis. These etiologies almost always result in adult-onset lesions, and they are invariably nonspecific to the amygdala. Typical consequences of these diseases include profound emotional changes; dense anterograde amnesia; and, if the lesion encroaches substantially into surrounding cortex, also a significant, often category-specific agnosia (Damasio, Eslinger, Damasio, Van Hoese, & Cornell, 1985; Stefanacci, Buffalo, Schmolck, & Squire, 2000). While the amygdala is often completely and bilaterally lesioned in these patients, isolating the contributions made by the amygdala damage from damage to surrounding structures is essentially impossible, making the value of such lesions to our knowledge of amygdala function per se problematic.

Very rarely nowadays, bilateral amygdala lesions are made neurosurgically. The most famous case here is, of course, the late patient H. M.—famous for his contributions to our knowledge of the functions of the hippocampus, but not so much the amygdala (Corkin, 1984). Lesions restricted to the amygdala have been made neurosurgically in some cases for psychosurgical treatment of aggression (Lee et al., 1998; Mpakopoulou, Gatos, Brotis, Paternakis, & Fountas, 2008), performed exceedingly rarely nowadays but popular historically (Fountas & Smith, 2007). Regardless of the details, all these cases have one large shortcoming: The very reason such an invasive treatment was selected in the first place—the reason for the neurosurgical lesion—is that the patients were severely ill to begin with (with long-standing epilepsy or severe psychiatric illness).

Perhaps the "cleanest" case involving neurosurgical lesions is that described by Anderson and Phelps (1998, 2000, 2001, 2002; see Todd, Anderson, & Phelps, Chapter 13, this volume), which involved a complex etiology including epilepsy, sclerosis, as well as surgery. This rare case had a mixture of damage, some of which was sustained earlier in life, and some later. Some neurosurgical cases, however, clearly had childhood-onset lesions: There are large series of children from Japan and India with neurosurgical bilateral amygdala lesions for psychiatric treatment, usually for very aggressive behavior but also for severe intellectual disabilities (Narabayashi, Nagao, Saito, Yoshida, & Nagahata, 1963). It is doubtful that all of the neurosurgical cases are entirely selective for the amygdala (for one thing, mere surgical access to the amygdala would require some damage to surrounding structures).

Of course, by far the most common surgical amygdala lesions in humans are unilateral: surgical resections for the treatment of medically refractory epilepsy. Due to their unilateral nature, deficits attributable specifically to the amygdala are typically considerably weaker (or nonexistent) compared to bilateral amygdala lesions (e.g., Adolphs et al., 2001). Due to the premorbid epilepsy, as well as typically partial resection of the hippocampus, it is also difficult to attribute dysfunction specifically to the amygdala (although, to some extent, this can be disentangled by quantifying the relative proportion of damage to the hippocampus and amygdala; rare resections that damage only the amygdala and spare the hippocampus are also occasionally encountered; cf. Cordeiro, Wagner, Trippel, Zentner, & Schulze-Bonhage, 2011).

One particular kind of etiology produces the most consistent developmental-onset amygdala lesions: genetic mutations in the gene encoding the structural protein extracellular matrix protein 1 (*ECM1*; Chan, Liu, Hamada, Sethuraman, & McGrath, 2007; Hamada et al., 2002). The gene is located on chromosome 1 and has at least three splice variants that are expressed ubiquitously in the body; it appears to play a primary role in the development and maintenance of epidermal tissue. While a variety of different mutations in this gene result in amygdala lesions (offering important genotypic variability whose phenotypic consequences remain to be mapped in detail), they generally produce a fairly consistent constellation of cognitive, behavioral, and physiological changes known as Urbach–Wiethe Disease (UWD) (Hofer, 1973; Thornton et al., 2008), or "lipoid proteinosis" in America. Patients with UWD often present to dermatology clinics, since the phenotype prominently affects epithelial tissue, resulting in abnormal healing of skin lesions and abnormal thickening of the vocal cords (producing a hoarse voice). In many patients there is evidence of occasional and mild seizure-like symptoms that bear some resemblance to the auras associated with medial temporal lobe epilepsy, although typically without generalization, and without loss of consciousness. The disease is exceedingly rare; since its first description in 1929, only about 300 cases have been published world-wide, with at least a dozen different specific mutations.

It remains unknown at what age amygdala lesions develop in UWD, although some evidence suggests that the lesions form progressively in childhood (Appenzeller et al., 2006). Based on a variety of evidence, including autobiographical reports of childhood, we have suggested that lesions in one well-studied patient (S. M.) manifested around age 10 (Feinstein, Adolphs, Damasio, & Tranel, 2011), although this may well vary across different patients (and could vary with specific genotype). In any case, given the genetic nature of the disease and its clear establishment early in life, the amygdala lesions produced should be considered "developmental." To our knowledge, no patient with UWD has ever been studied "before" and "after" the establishment of amygdala lesions, indeed leaving open the possibility that some or all of the damage is congenital.

While the first cognitive neuroscience studies of patients with UWD reported a very small handful of case studies (Babinsky et al., 1993; Tranel & Hyman, 1990), a series of 10 or more patients has now been reported (Siebert, Markowitsch, & Bartel, 2003; Thornton et al., 2008). The amygdalae in these patients exhibits abnormal T1- and T2-weighted signals on structural MRI scans, changes in T2* susceptibility, a near-absence in blood flow measured with resting-state 14-fluorodeoxyglucose (FDG) positron emission tomography (PET), and profound reduction in T2*-weighted BOLD in fMRI studies (cf. Bach, Talmi, Hurlemann, Patin, & Dolan, 2011b; Becker et al., 2012; Buchanan, Tranel, & Adolphs, 2009). On computed tomographic (CT) scans, the amygdalae show up as highly radio-opaque regions, consistent with postmortem examinations of the medial temporal lobe in patients with UWD that find extensive calcification, especially of the blood vessels, and severe necrosis in adjacent tissue (Holtz, 1962; Meenan et al., 1978). Taken together, the neurofunctional data unequivocally demonstrate dysfunction of the amygdala consistent with a lesion. Yet this general consensus leaves open a critical and currently unresolved question: Is the lesion complete? Does it affect all nuclei of the amygdala?

Amygdala Subnuclei

The amygdala consists of a collection of interacting nuclei (Amaral et al., 1992; Pitkanen et al., 1997; Schumann, Vargas, & Lee, Chapter 2, this volume), and studies in nonhuman animals generally distinguish lesions to specific nuclei. With the widespread availability of high-resolution MRI tools, this poses the question of whether the functions of distinct subdivisions of the amygdala might also be distinguishable in humans with UWD.

This issue has been addressed recently in perhaps the most detail by Jack van Honk and colleagues (see van Honk, Terburg, Thornton, Stein, & Morgan, Chapter 12, this volume; Morgan, Terburg, Thornton, Stein, & van Honk, 2012; Terburg et al., 2012; van Honk, Eisenegger, Terburg, Stein, & Morgan, 2013), who documented several patients with UWD who have amygdala lesions that are incomplete. Not only are the lesions incomplete but they are also systematically incomplete, appearing to spare the most centromedial sectors of the amygdala, while clearly lesioning most of the basolateral complex. Variability in the precise distribution of damage across amygdala nuclei could well account for some of the reported variability of cognitive dysfunctions across studies. No less important is the delineation of the damage beyond the immediate boundaries of the amygdala: Not only is white matter affected but portions of adjacent entorhinal cortex in many patients appear lesioned as well. While these issues are perhaps unsurprising given the nature of the disease, and given the resolution afforded by standard MRI, they are particularly important given the different functions of spatially very proximal regions in the medial temporal lobe and their tight interaction. The issue is well recognized, for instance, in optogenetic studies of the amygdala in rodents: Manipulations of the basolateral amygdala produce behavioral changes that are different from manipulations to the very terminals that neurons from the basolateral amygdala make onto sectors of the centromedial amygdala (Tye et al., 2011). In humans, differences in how UWD lesions impact different sectors of the amygdala may translate into abnormalities that can go in opposite directions: insensitivity to fear (Feinstein et al., 2011), or hypervigilance to it (Terburg et al., 2012), all depending on exactly which nuclei of the amygdala are damaged (see van Honk et al., Chapter 12, this volume). Given the complex interconnectivity among amygdala subnuclei (Pitkanen, Savander, & LeDoux, 1997), understanding the precise extent of lesions in patients with UWD is a future topic of the highest priority.

What are the options for addressing the resolution required to obtain such data? With the advent of human MRI at 7 tesla (T) and higher, it is not an insurmountable difficulty with structural MRI alone. Higher-resolution structural imaging will reveal new details that can be mapped onto MR atlases of amygdala nuclei (Amunts et al., 2005), and ultrahigh-field MRI permits some delineation between amygdala nuclei in single subjects (Solano-Castiella et al., 2011). fMRI will no doubt contribute to this as well, although given the well-known difficulty of obtaining good BOLD signal from the amygdala, together with the fundamental physiological limitations of BOLD imaging, this may be insufficient to resolve functional differences if constrained to signals within the amygdala itself. Perhaps the most promising is a network approach, according to which different amygdala nuclei can be identified by their differential patterns of large-scale connectivity with other brain regions—a macroscopic network-level differentiation that can work even with fMRI (e.g., Bickart, Hollenbeck, Barrett, & Dickerson, 2012; Roy et al., 2009). In such an approach, different subregions of the amygdala are used as functional "seed" regions, and one can then examine the BOLD signal in voxels over the rest of the brain for the strength of the correlations in BOLD signal time course between those distal voxels and the seed regions. The approach has been used to segment nuclei of the thalamus by their pattern of connectivity with neocortex (Johansen-Berg et al., 2005), and once requisite signal-to-noise is obtained, the same approach could be applied to the amygdala (e.g., Mishra, Rogers, Chen, & Gore, 2013). Analogous segmentation of amygdala nuclei can, of course, be done on the basis of structural connectivity patterns as well, using diffusion-weighted MRI *in vivo* (Bach, Behrens, Garrido, Weiskopf, & Dolan, 2011a; Saygin, Osher, Augustinack, Fischl, & Gabrieli, 2011; Solano-Castiella et al., 2010).

The most common functional parcellation scheme ends up with three regions within the human amygdala (Bzdok, Laird, Zilles, Fox, & Eickhoff, 2012): a basolateral one with connections to higher-order sensory cortices that includes visual inputs to the amygdala; a centromedial one concerned with autonomic and attentional functions; and a superficial one devoted to olfactory input. Some variations on this scheme (Bickart et al., 2012) include prominent connections with the orbitofrontal cortex in relation to the ventral and lateral regions of the amygdala, consistent with higher-level perceptual processing, including processing of socially relevant signals; connections with ventromedial prefrontal cortex (vmPFC) and anterior cingulate cortex in relation to more basomedial parts of the amygdala, hypothesized to subserve affiliative behaviors; and connections with hypothalamus and brainstem for the dorsal amygdala (corresponding to the centromedial nucleus), with a hypothesized role prioritizing threat-related behaviors. Clearly, the eventual parcellation will need to become more fine-grained, but even at this coarse level, it is apparent that important distinctions in terms of both connectivity profile and behavioral function can be delineated. These make specific predictions regarding the deficits that would be seen following lesions of the amygdala that disproportionately affect certain nuclei.

Functional Roles for the Amygdala

Most of the functional roles assigned to the human amygdala as a consequence of developmental lesions are generally aligned with studies in animals, as well as human fMRI data. That said, this "alignment" is certainly not a simple match with conclusions derived from the different types of studies. There is also a tension regarding how best to report the results from lesion studies: On the one hand, one would like to derive generalizations that should hold across groups of lesion patients (e.g., Adolphs et al., 1999b); on the other, there is something to be said for a detailed characterization of single-case studies that offer particularly striking dissociations (e.g., Adolphs, Tranel, Damasio, & Damasio, 1994), although, of course, these may be idiosyncratic.

A summary of functional roles for the amygdala as gleaned from the single-case studies of subject S. M., the most thoroughly studied subject with developmental bilateral amygdala lesions arising from UWD, is given in Table 10.1 (cf. Adolphs, 2010). All of these findings need to be qualified by their dependence on a case study, and also relative to the specific stimuli and tasks that were used. What conclusions can be drawn from these studies, and how well do they fit with other human lesion studies, fMRI studies, and studies of the amygdala in animals? This large question is summarized in Table 10.2, and I comment on it briefly here.

TABLE 10.1. Summary of Deficits in Subject S. M.

- Impaired in judging fear from static facial expressions
- Insensitivity to the degree of fear shown in faces
- Reduced conditioned skin conductance responses in Pavlovian fear conditioning
- Reduced augmentation of declarative memory by emotional arousal
- Increased judgment of the trustworthiness of faces
- Increased judgment of the approachability of faces
- Increased approach behavior to a real person
- Lack of a feeling of personal space
- Reduced judgment of arousal for negatively valenced stimuli
- Increased preferences for abstract visual stimuli
- Lack of loss aversion to money
- Intact ability to discriminate between facial expressions of emotion
- Intact ability to judge emotions from voices
- Impaired ability to judge emotions from music
- Impaired on the Baron-Cohen "mind in the eyes" task
- Less impaired in recognizing emotions from scenes when faces are erased
- Mildly impaired in recognizing other negative emotions, but not happiness
- Impaired in fixating, and utilizing information from, the eye region of faces
- Tends to look at the mouth rather than the eyes when looking at a real person
- Impaired emotional declarative memory for the gist, but not the details, of a story
- Lack of an experience of fear in real life
- Lack of an experience of fear in response to movies, snakes, spiders, or haunted houses
- Impaired reward learning and complex decision making
- Intact ability to recognize fear from body posture and pointlight walkers
- Intact ability to detect rapidly or subliminally presented fear stimuli
- Intact ability to experience fear through interoceptive stimuli (CO_2 inhalation)

S. M. remains, by far, the single person with bilateral developmental amygdala lesions who has been investigated in the most detail. She has developmental-onset lesions that appear to encompass most of the amygdala and parts of entorhinal cortex, resulting from UWD. From Adolphs (2010). Copyright 2010 by John Wiley and Sons. Reprinted by permission.

TABLE 10.2. How Well Do Findings from S. M. Fit with Other Studies of the Amygdala?

S. M.	Other lesions	fMRI	Animals
Social perception	Y	Y	Y
Facial emotion recognition	Y	Y	?
Fear recognition	Y	Y/N	?
Pavlovian fear conditioning	Y	Y	Y
Emotional declarative memory	Y	Y	Y
Positivity/approach bias	Y	Y/N	Y
Social attention	?	Y	Y
Fixating on eyes in faces	?	Y	?
Using eye information from faces	?	?	?
Decision making/reward learning	?	Y	Y
Personal space	?	?	?
Conscious experience of emotion	?	Y/N	?

Note. Deficits reported in S. M. appear in the leftmost column. The right three columns indicate whether similar deficits are observed in other lesion patients, consistent with fMRI activation of the amygdala in healthy individuals, or consistent with the literature from animal studies. Y/N/?, yes, no, insufficient data.

There is a strong consensus for the amygdala's role in social perception (first three rows in Table 10.2). In subject S. M. (Adolphs, Tranel, & Damasio, 1998; Adolphs et al., 1994) as well as other patients with bilateral amygdala lesions (Adolphs et al., 1999b; Anderson & Phelps, 2000), there are deficits in social judgments made from faces, with more variable patterns of impairments with respect to other kinds of stimuli, such as scenes (Adolphs & Tranel, 2003) and auditory stimuli (Adolphs & Tranel, 1999a; Anderson & Phelps, 1998). However, so far, only in subject S. M. has this impairment been linked to a failure to make use of, and to fixate on, the eye region of faces (Adolphs et al., 2005), even though there is other evidence that the amygdala plays a role in fixations onto faces from human fMRI studies (Gamer & Büchel, 2009; Kliemann, Dziobek, Hatri, Baudewig, & Heekeren, 2012). Most striking, and most specific, is S. M.'s profound insensitivity to fear shown in facial expressions (Adolphs et al., 1994): When spontaneously describing fear faces, she very rarely uses the word "fear," instead misrecognizing the faces as angry (and other emotions). When asked explicitly to rate the intensity of fear shown in faces,

S. M. ascribes to them unusually low ratings of fear intensity. Perhaps simplest and most telling, on many occasions, she states that she simply does not know what kind of emotion is shown on a fearful face. All of these striking impairments in the case of fear occur against the backdrop of an otherwise relatively intact ability to recognize and rate other emotions from facial expressions. While this pattern of a disproportionate impairment in recognizing fear has been found across a number of subjects with bilateral amygdala lesions (Adolphs et al., 1999b), it has never been seen with the severity and the specificity shown in S. M. It is also important to note here some patients with UWD who have partial amygdala lesions instead show an exaggerated sensitivity to fear in faces when those are dynamic—just the opposite of what is seen in S. M. (see Terburg et al., 2012; van Honk et al., Chapter 12, this volume).

One would like to situate the findings on social perception in the context of the amygdala's connectivity, especially with temporal visual cortices. One of the first studies to examine this issue found an influence of amygdala lesions (from medial temporal sclerosis, not from UWD) on evoked BOLD-fMRI signal in the temporal visual cortex (Vuilleumier, Richardson, Armony, Driver, & Dolan, 2004). Specifically, BOLD signal evoked by attention to faces as compared to houses is modulated in visual cortices by the emotional expression shown on the face: Fear faces elicit greater signal. This specific modulation by fear faces in temporal cortices was reported to be absent in those patients who had lesions of the amygdala (this same study was also an example of how differential lesions to the amygdala or hippocampus could be quantified in a group). However, this finding has not been replicated in more recent work that investigated the same question in patients with unilateral amygdala lesions from temporal lobectomy (Edmiston et al., 2013), discrepancies that could well arise from the very different etiologies of the patients studied (notably including different ages of onset of the amygdala lesions, which were likely early in the Vuilleumier et al. [2004] study, but may have been mostly adult-onset in the study by Edmiston et al. [2013]). The anatomical demonstration of feedback connections from the primate amygdala to all visual cortices, including striate cortex (Amaral & Price, 1984; Freese & Amaral, 2005, 2006), suggests that these projections may mediate the functional role of modulating perceptual processing, contributing to aspects of social attention.

These findings suggest a modulatory role for the amygdala in cortical processing, but it remains unclear at what point in time such an effect might be mediated. A classical view of the amygdala's role here envisions a rapid subcortical route of visual input to the amygdala, via the superior colliculus and pulvinar thalamus, which could then modulate cortical processing already at its earliest stages. However, our view is that the human amygdala contributes to social perception and face processing primarily not via a rapid, subcortically mediated route, but rather through slower cycles of both feedforward and reentrant processing involving connections with neocortex (Pessoa & Adolphs, 2010; see Figure 10.2). Such an elaborative role, in which amygdala and neocortex jointly process the social meaning of stimuli, is consistent with not only the long response latencies of single neurons recorded in the human amygdala but also more detailed electrophysiological studies indicating that amygdala neurons fire in phase synchrony with an induced theta rhythm (Rey, Fried, & Quiroga, 2014). While the theta rhythm is generated relatively early following stimulus onset, it takes a few cycles to become fully established, reflecting coherent processing between a likely large ensemble of cortices. Only once established does it elicit phase-triggered spikes from neurons within the amygdala, likely accounting for the long latencies seen in single-unit studies of amygdala neurons recorded in surgical patients (Mormann et al., 2008; see Figure 10.3). Event-related potential (ERP) studies in patients with amygdala pathology also support the idea that the amygdala influences cortical processing at multiple temporal scales, including epochs more than 500 ms from the onset of emotional stimuli (Rotshtein et al., 2010). All these findings,

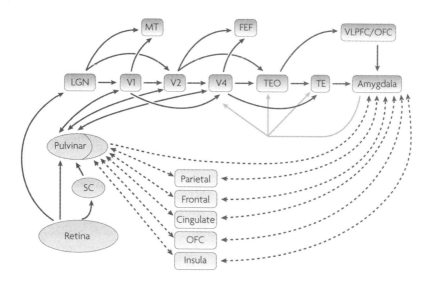

FIGURE 10.2. Connectivity of the amygdala with cortical and subcortical visual structures. From Pessoa and Adolphs (2010). Reprinted with permission of Nature Publishing Group.

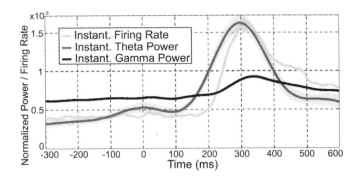

FIGURE 10.3. Time course of electrophysiological response to stimuli recorded in the human amygdala with depth electrode. While theta-band power responds with a relatively short latency, actual spikes from amygdala neurons require considerably more time to show changes in their firing rate, due to phase-locking to the induced theta rhythm. This finding is consistent with the idea that amygdala neurons only respond once a stable sensory representation has been established through the ensemble of neocortex that provides input to the amygdala. From Rey, Fried, and Quiroga (2014). Copyrght 2014 by Elsevier. Reprinted by permission.

then, suggest that the mechanism by which amygdala lesions may impact the judgments of emotional and social stimuli depends on the amygdala's extended connectivity with neocortex: cycles of visual input and modulation with temporal cortices, and context-dependent information from the prefrontal cortex. At the same time, processing within these cortical targets of the amygdala, as we saw in Figure 10.1, is also likely altered itself, possibly accounting for some of the abnormal behaviors and judgments listed in Table 10.1.

One important domain that needs to be investigated in more detail in humans is the amygdala's role in attention. While attentional effects have been dissociated from emotional effects, with only the latter showing a clear dependency on the amygdala, in human fMRI studies (Vuilleumier & Driver, 2007), the amygdala clearly plays a role in attention as well. A number of animal studies indicate that amygdala lesions impair attentional processes (Holland & Gallagher, 1999; Holland, Han, & Gallagher, 2000), and studies in rats have linked the amygdala to mediating a kind of "surprise" signal that can motivate learning (Roesch, Calu, Esber, & Schoenbaum, 2010). This particular attention signal appears to derive from the dopaminergic midbrain (Esber et al., 2012), which projects to the basolateral amygdala, and possibly then modulates cortical function via outputs from the central nucleus. The central nucleus of the amygdala projects to the cholinergic basal forebrain, and disconnection of these two structures impairs the ability to maintain task performance under increasing attentional loads (Holland, 2007). In some human patients with amygdala lesions, there is a failure to boost attention to emotional stimuli in the attentional blink paradigm (Anderson & Phelps, 2001; Todd et al., Chapter 13, this volume; but also see Bach et al., 2011b), and some of the abnormal eye fixations that such patients make onto faces can be interpreted as a deficit in aspects of stimulus-triggered visual attention (Kennedy & Adolphs, 2010). One approach that would seem highly valuable to incorporate into future studies with these patients is to vary attentional load across tasks parametrically, permitting a characterization of how attention may interact with impaired task performances (for an example, see Wang, Xu, Jiang, Zhao, Hurlemann, et al., 2014). Equally important, different types of attention need to be more fully explored. The issue is of particular interest, since integrated accounts of amygdala function, and of the consequences of amygdala lesions, often revolve around constructs that would appear prominently to include attentional effects (unpredictability, social function, saliency, relevance, to name just a few; see Adolphs, 2010, for review).

Finally, amygdala lesions in humans also impair a host of roles that are quite well established from animal and fMRI studies: Pavlovian fear conditioning (Bechara et al., 1995), emotional modulation of declarative memory (Adolphs, Cahill, Schul, & Babinsky, 1997; Cahill, Babinsky, Markowitsch, & McGaugh, 1995), and other aspects of reward learning and decision making (Bechara, Damasio, & Damasio, 2003; De Martino, Camerer, & Adolphs, 2010; Hsu, Bhatt, Adolphs, Tranel, & Camerer, 2005) all are compromised by amygdala lesions (cf. Table 10.2). The extent to which any of these might show differences depending on whether the amygdala is lesioned developmentally or in adulthood remains to be investigated.

The Human Amygdala's Role in the Conscious Experience of Fear

While the amygdala clearly participates in processing stimuli that are both appetitive and aversive (as borne out by fMRI [Hamann, Ely, Hoffman, & Kilts, 2002] and in electrophysiological studies [Paton, Belova, Morrison, & Salzman, 2006]), lesion studies in both animals (Choi & Kim, 2010; also see Kim, Choi, & Lee, Chapter 5, this volume) and humans strongly argue for a disproportionately important role with respect to aversive stimuli. Patient S. M. shows a positive bias in interpreting other people's faces (Adolphs, Russell, & Tranel, 1999a; Adolphs et al., 1998), as she does in judging a variety of nonsocial visual stimuli (Adolphs & Tranel, 1999b);

she also shows a lack of loss aversion to money (De Martino et al., 2010), and a behavioral tendency to approach other people (Kennedy, Gläscher, Tyszka, & Adolphs, 2009; see Figure 10.4). Very broadly, then, there is a bias exaggerating appetitive processing and reducing aversive processing. Does this bias extend to S. M.'s experience of emotions?

Perhaps no other aspect of emotion is as difficult to investigate as conscious experience. Most psychological accounts of emotion focus on conscious experience (Barrett, Mesquita, Ochsner, & Gross, 2007; Scherer, 2000), as does the layperson's concept of emotion. Joe LeDoux (2012) has famously argued from this fact that we should not apply our ordinary emotion concepts to the study of nonhuman animals, since it will invariably attribute findings from animal studies with unwarranted conscious experiences of emotion. Yet this state of affairs has always seemed deeply puzzling to me. After all, much the same could be said for the study of memory, or vision, for that matter. If you ask people on the street what "memory" is, their concept will highlight the conscious experience of recollection; if you ask them what "vision" is, their concept will highlight the conscious experience of seeing. Yet in neither case does this prevent scientists from using the word "memory" when they study aspects of it in *Aplysia*, or "vision," when they study it in flies. The prescription in all of these cases, including emotion, seems straightforward: Just be clear that the conscious experience is a distinct aspect; some species, under some circumstances, may have conscious experiences of the process you are studying, but that is a separate and empirical question.

This distinction between conscious experiences of emotions ("feelings") and all the other aspects of emotion was already made forcefully by Antonio Damasio (1999, 2003), and I have argued for it as well (Anderson & Adolphs, 2014; Tsuchiya & Adolphs, 2007). If one accepts

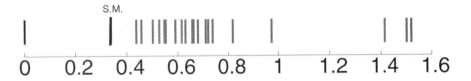

FIGURE 10.4. Impaired personal space in patient S. M. Participants were asked to walk toward the experimenter and stop when they felt it natural to do so. Mean interpersonal distance from this protocol is plotted, in meters, on the *x*-axis, representing the experimenter standing at the origin, the patient S. M. (with a mean interpersonal distance <0.4 m), then all the control subjects. S. M.'s interpersonal distance was less than that of any control, and she did not report any feeling of uncomfortableness when her personal space was invaded. Reprinted with permission of Nature Publishing Group from Kennedy, Gläscher, Tyszka, and Adolphs (2009).

this distinction, then it is certainly a large and entirely open question to what extent the amygdala contributes to the conscious experience of emotion. Although it contributes to myriad aspects of emotion (autonomic responses, perception, memory, etc.), it remains a distinct possibility that all of these contributions are not essential to the conscious experience of feeling an emotion. S. M. is unable to recognize facial expressions of fear, unable to show Pavlovian fear conditioning, unable to modulate declarative emotional memories related to fear. Can she experience fear?

The answer to this question has turned out to be fascinating and highly revealing about the role of the amygdala in conscious experience of emotions (see Feinstein, Adolphs, & Tranel, Chapter 1, this volume, for the full details). S. M.'s basic personality can be gleaned already from the constellation of impairments that have been reported: She is generally cheerful and trusting, a profile that in psychological assessment comes across as resilient to life stressors (Tranel, Gullickson, Koch, & Adolphs, 2006). Although S. M. exhibits profound alterations in eyetracking to faces (Adolphs et al., 2005) and in interpersonal approach behaviors (Kennedy et al., 2009; see Figure 10.4), which are reminiscent of aspects of autism spectrum disorder, subjects with amygdala lesions from UWD do not in any way meet criteria for autism (Paul, Corsello, Tranel, & Adolphs, 2010). If you met S. M., then, you might notice slightly unusual aspects of her social behavior, but without further information, you would not be inclined to conclude that she cannot experience fear.

Feinstein et al. (2011; Chapter 1, this volume) detail the effects of bilateral amygdala lesions in S. M. on the conscious experience of fear. In short, across a broad array of dependent measures (questionnaires, ratings of films, behavior in a haunted house or in response to live spiders and snakes), S. M. shows a remarkable absence of any of the verbal reports or behaviors that we would normally take as sufficient to attribute an experience of fear to a person. When asked about her experiences in questionnaires, she consistently endorses abnormally low ratings of any experiences related to fear (Figure 10.5).

A role for the amygdala in the experience of fear is, of course, not at all a new idea. Older studies of electrical stimulation in animals and humans already suggested as much. Behavioral changes following amygdala lesions in species ranging from rodents (Choi & Kim, 2010) to monkeys (Mason, Capitanio, Machado, Mendoza, & Amaral, 2006) to humans (Kennedy et al., 2009) are all consistent with a reduction in the experience of fear and anxiety, but, of course, in the animal cases, we cannot ascertain this with certainty, since the animals cannot report on their experiences. As detailed by Feinstein et al. (Chapter 1, this volume), S. M. provides compelling evidence for a lack of fear induced by exteroceptive stimuli that would normally evoke feelings of fear, across a wide range of stimuli and situations.

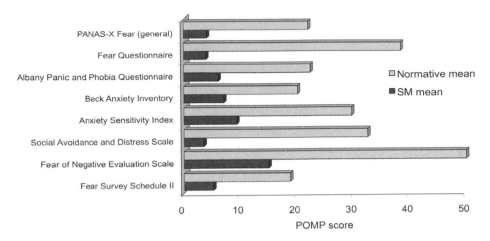

FIGURE 10.5. Lack of fear experience in S. M. Plotted are the mean scores on a variety of fear-related questionnaires, as the percent of maximum possible (POMP). S. M.'s scores were considerably lower that those of the controls for every questionnaire. In this same study, S. M. showed lack of fear also from horror movies, snakes, spiders, and haunted houses, which supports the argument that the amygdala is required for exteroceptive induction of fear. Importantly, S. M. is able to experience fear when it is induced through interoceptive stimuli (carbon dioxide inhalation, which induces a feeling of suffocation) From Feinstein, Adolphs, Damasio, and Tranel (2011). Copyright 2011 by Elsevier. Reprinted by permission.

Yet one very surprising, and very important, contrast came from a recent investigative study of S. M., as well as two other patients with bilateral amygdala lesions resulting from UWD. That study found that fear, indeed panic, could be induced through an interoceptive stimulus: carbon dioxide inhalation (Feinstein et al., 2013). In healthy individuals, inhaling carbon dioxide causes a sense of suffocation, and many people in fact experience panic attacks through this experience (which is otherwise, with a single breath, entirely harmless). This set of studies in the same UWD subject (S. M.) thus shows a striking dissociation: complete failure to induce fear through a large variety of stimuli in the environment (films, snakes, spiders), but intact and likely even exaggerated fear induced through interoception (carbon dioxide inhalation). The dissociation offers a fairly specific role for the amygdala in the experience of fear: It is required to induce fear through exteroceptive stimuli, but not through interoceptive stimuli. Consequently, the amygdala cannot itself be essential to experiencing fear as such, but rather provides a specific bottleneck for how fear can be induced (and is then presumably mediated by other structures, including neocortex).

There is a further wrinkle in comparison with other patients with bilateral amygdala lesions, at least some of whom appear to have a relatively normal experience of fear (Anderson & Phelps, 2002). The differences between the studies could be attributable to many factors, including the age of onset of the lesion, the precise extent of the lesion (and in particular involvement of specific amygdala nuclei, as noted earlier), as well as interaction with individual differences in personality. However, one big factor that certainly would be important to try to address in future studies is simply the differences in the experimental assessment of fear experience. Anderson and Phelps used a single, self-rated questionnaire, the Positive and Negative Affect Schedule (PANAS), which assesses long-term experience of emotions without a particular focus on fear, without a focus on phasic fear, and without any experimental manipulation actually to induce fear whatsoever. By contrast, Feinstein et al. (2011) used a large range of questionnaires focused specifically on the assessment of fear and anxiety, and experimentally attempted to induce fear with stimuli such as movies, snakes, spiders, and haunted houses, as well as through autobiographical recall of traumatic real-life events. These methodological differences are so extreme that it would be premature to make any direct comparison between the two studies until a more convergent set of dependent measures can be obtained.

Open Questions

Several open questions, in addition to the ones raised earlier, would serve to broaden our understanding of developmental amygdala damage. For instance, it will be important to connect the amygdala's role during development both to neurodevelopmental disorders such as autism (Schumann et al., 2011) and to variance in social behavior across individual differences in healthy individuals (Bickart, Wright, Dautoff, Dickerson, & Barrett, 2010). Further detailed studies of patients with developmental-onset lesions of the amygdala will be critical points of comparison in this regard, and the ideal studies would make direct comparisons between such patients and individual-difference dimensions in healthy individuals, as well as with people with autism spectrum disorder (for an example of the latter, see Birmingham, Cerf, & Adolphs, 2011).

Equally important is the need to provide not only a more detailed characterization of the functional lesion within the amygdala (see van Honk et al., Chapter 12, this volume), but also of its functional consequences elsewhere in the brain, an issue I detailed at the outset of this chapter. Combining lesion studies with high-resolution fMRI will be an important direction for future work, complementing the largely behavior-based lesion studies to date (e.g., Mihov et al., 2013).

Putting together all these pieces to glean a single "function" for the amygdala (Adolphs, 2010) may be misguided. Instead, the answer may be that, depending on the precise extent of the lesion, the age of onset of the lesion, and other individual differences, this may result in variable changes in brain function elsewhere that in turn explain the cognitive and behavioral deficits reported in papers. Perhaps the single most important recommendation for future studies is to encourage groups toward more collaboration. If patients with developmental-onset lesions, those with adult-onset lesions, and patients with variable extents of lesions can be studied using the same stimuli, tasks, and dependent measures, we will be in the best position to assemble a fuller picture of the functional role of this complex structure in human cognition and behavior. This issue is especially pertinent in the case of patients with bilateral amygdala lesions, given their rarity.

We can conclude with some hypotheses that seem reasonable in light of the extant data, together with prescriptions for experiments to test them.

1. *The human amygdala is important for social judgments from faces.* It furthermore appears particularly critical for judgments related to threat assessment. It is also likely that this role is highly context-dependent. Developmental bilateral amygdala lesions cause deficits in this domain, although there are large individual differences.

Experiments should aim for richer, more ecologically valid, yet quantitative studies that could parametrically vary social dimensions that can be judged from faces. Essentially all studies—fMRI, electrophysiological, or lesion—have used (usually static) faces presented on a computer monitor. Extending this work to real people's faces under a particular socially relevant context would be not only challenging but also very necessary if we are to understand the amygdala's role in this domain.

Some further important experiments need to add eyetracking, in order to better understand whether the amygdala serves a primarily attentional or motivational role in directing fixations to faces, or relevant features of faces, or whether it serves a role in more elaborated social judgments once faces and features have been fixated. Of course, both may be the case, but they may well map onto different amygdala nuclei.

2. *The human amygdala is important for reward learning.* This role appears diverse, encompassing both simple Pavlovian fear conditioning and more complex aspects of decision making observed in real life and

on tasks such as the Iowa Gambling Task. There is perhaps the best agreement across studies that developmental bilateral amygdala lesions impair this domain, but considerable further work remains to be done.

Experiments should aim to test patients with bilateral amygdala lesions on a broader array of more formal reward learning tasks. Are they differentially impaired on habit-based versus goal-directed learning? Learning with respect to reward versus punishment? Many of the behavioral tasks that have been done with monkeys turn out to be extremely difficult to get to work in a valid fashion in humans, and will require some ingenuity and perseverance.

3. *The human amygdala plays a role in the conscious experience of fear.* The amygdala may be particularly important for generating anxiety or fear-related feelings, although these could be diminished or exaggerated following lesions, depending on the precise amygdala nuclei that are damaged. This topic is, of course, of the highest relevance also to understanding the amygdala's role in mood and anxiety disorders.

This very interesting hypothesis has broad support from a variety of sources but definitely needs more exploration. There is now a wealth of rodent studies that indicate changes in fear behaviors following optogenetic manipulation; of course, they do not and cannot address conscious experience but should serve to further refine predictions for the human amygdala. Human lesion studies will need to map out conscious experience of emotions in richer detail (an issue as tricky practically as ethically). And once again, combining such studies with fMRI (as has been done in some studies of healthy individuals; e.g., Mobbs, Yu, Rowe, Eich, FeldmanHall, & Dalgleish, 2010) will be valuable in order to obtain a full picture of how amygdala damage may influence the induction of fear experience via modulations of distal cortical targets.

I conclude by emphasizing perhaps three issues of the highest priority that would cut across all studies. The first is the role of development: The ideal experiments would be longitudinal and follow young patients with UWD across the lifespan. This is a tall order, but families with UWD who have young children do exist, particularly in South Africa, as studied by Jack van Honk and colleagues. The second issue is to delineate better the extent of the lesions, both structurally and functionally. Right now, our neuroanatomical precision in human studies is woefully inadequate, and far behind what is commonly accepted in animal studies involving amygdala lesions. Third is to conduct all behavioral studies, insofar as possible, with concurrent whole-brain fMRI. We will only be able to understand the consequences of developmental bilateral amygdala lesions once we understand how they influence function in the rest of the brain.

ACKNOWLEDGMENT

This work was supported by a Conte Center from the National Institute of Mental Health.

REFERENCES

Adolphs, R. (2010). What does the amygdala contribute to social cognition? *Annals of the New York Academy of Sciences, 1191*, 42–61.

Adolphs, R., Cahill, L., Schul, R., & Babinsky, R. (1997). Impaired declarative memory for emotional material following bilateral amygdala damage in humans. *Learning and Memory, 4*, 291–300.

Adolphs, R., Gosselin, F., Buchanan, T. W., Tranel, D., Schyns, P., & Damasio, A. R. (2005). A mechanism for impaired fear recognition after amygdala damage. *Nature, 433*, 68–72.

Adolphs, R., Russell, J. A., & Tranel, D. (1999a). A role for the human amygdala in recognizing emotional arousal from unpleasant stimuli. *Psychological Science, 10*, 167–171.

Adolphs, R., & Tranel, D. (1999a). Intact recognition of emotional prosody following amygdala damage. *Neuropsychologia, 37*, 1285–1292.

Adolphs, R., & Tranel, D. (1999b). Preferences for visual stimuli following amygdala damage. *Journal of Cognitive Neuroscience, 11*, 610–616.

Adolphs, R., & Tranel, D. (2003). Amygdala damage impairs emotion recognition from scenes only when they contain facial expressions. *Neuropsychologia, 41*, 1281–1289.

Adolphs, R., Tranel, D., & Damasio, A. R. (1998). The human amygdala in social judgment. *Nature, 393*, 470–474.

Adolphs, R., Tranel, D., & Damasio, H. (2001). Emotion recognition from faces and prosody following temporal lobectomy. *Neuropsychology, 15*, 396–404.

Adolphs, R., Tranel, D., Damasio, H., & Damasio, A. (1994). Impaired recognition of emotion in facial expressions following bilateral damage to the human amygdala. *Nature, 372*, 669–672.

Adolphs, R., Tranel, D., Hamann, S., Young, A., Calder, A., Anderson, A., et al. (1999b). Recognition of facial emotion in nine subjects with bilateral amygdala damage. *Neuropsychologia, 37*, 1111–1117.

Amaral, D. G., & Price, J. L. (1984). Amygdalo-cortical projections in the monkey (*Macaca fascicularis*). *Journal of Comparative Neurology, 230*, 465–496.

Amaral, D. G., Price, J. L., Pitkanen, A., & Carmichael, S. T. (1992). Anatomical organization of the primate amygdaloid complex. In J. P. Aggleton (Ed.), *The amygdala: Neurobiological aspects of emotion, memory, and mental dysfunction* (pp. 1–66). New York: Wiley-Liss.

Amaral, D. G., Schumann, C. M., & Nordahl, C. W. (2008). Neuroanatomy of autism. *Trends in Neurosciences, 31*, 137–145.

Amunts, K., Kedo, O., Kindler, M., Pieperhoff, P., Mohlberg, H., Shah, N. J., et al. (2005). Cytoarchitectonic mapping of the human amygdala, hippocampal region and entorhinal cortex: Intersubject variability and probability maps. *Anatomy and Embryology, 210*, 343–352.

Anderson, A. K., & Phelps, E. A. (1998). Intact recognition of vocal expressions of fear following bilateral lesions of the human amygdala. *NeuroReport, 9,* 3607–3613.

Anderson, A. K., & Phelps, E. A. (2000). Expression without recognition: Contributions of the human amygdala to emotional communication. *Psychological Science, 11,* 106–111.

Anderson, A. K., & Phelps, E. A. (2001). Lesions of the human amygdala impair enhanced perception of emotionally salient events. *Nature, 411,* 305–309.

Anderson, A. K., & Phelps, E. A. (2002). Is the human amygdala critical for the subjective experience of emotion?: Evidence of intact dispositional affect in patients with amygdala lesions. *Journal of Cognitive Neuroscience, 14,* 709–720.

Anderson, D. J., & Adolphs, R. (2014). A framework for investigating emotion across species. *Cell, 157*(1), 187–200.

Anderson, S. W., Damasio, H., Tranel, D., & Damasio, A. R. (2000). Long-term sequelae of prefrontal cortex damage acquired in early childhood. *Developmental Neuropsychology, 18,* 281–296.

Appenzeller, S., Chaloult, E., Velho, P., de Souza, E. M., Araujo, V. Z., Cendes, F., et al. (2006). Amygdalae calcifications associated with disease duration in lipoid proteinosis. *Journal of Neuroimaging, 16,* 154–156.

Babinsky, R., Calabrese, P., Durwen, H. F., Markowitsch, H. J., Brechtelsbauer, D., Heuser, L., et al. (1993). The possible contribution of the amygdala to memory. *Behavioral Neurology, 6,* 167–170.

Bach, D. R., Behrens, T. E., Garrido, L., Weiskopf, N., & Dolan, R. (2011a). Deep and superficial amygdala nuclei projections revealed *in vivo* by probabilistic tractography. *Journal of Neuroscience, 31,* 618–623.

Bach, D. R., Talmi, D., Hurlemann, R., Patin, A., & Dolan, R. J. (2011b). Automatic relevance detection in the absence of a functional amygdala. *Neuropsychologia, 49,* 1302–1305.

Barrett, L. F., Mesquita, B., Ochsner, K., & Gross, J. J. (2007). The experience of emotion. *Annual Review of Psychology, 58,* 373–403.

Bechara, A., Damasio, H., & Damasio, A. R. (2003). Role of the amygdala in decision-making. *Annals of the New York Academy of Sciences, 985,* 356–369.

Bechara, A., Tranel, D., Damasio, H., Adolphs, R., Rockland, C., & Damasio, A. R. (1995). Double dissociation of conditioning and declarative knowledge relative to the amygdala and hippocampus in humans. *Science, 269,* 1115–1118.

Becker, B., Mihov, Y., Scheele, D., Kendrick, K. M., Feinstein, J. S., Matusch, A., et al. (2012). Fear processing and social networking in the absence of a functional amygdala. *Biological Psychiatry, 72,* 70–77.

Bickart, K. C., Hollenbeck, M. C., Barrett, L. F., & Dickerson, B. C. (2012). Intrinsic amygdala-cortical functional connectivity predicts social network size in humans. *Journal of Neuroscience, 32,* 14729–14741.

Bickart, K. C., Wright, C. I., Dautoff, R. J., Dickerson, B. C., & Barrett, L. F. (2010). Amygdala volume and social network size in humans. *Nature Neuroscience, 14,* 163–164.

Birmingham, E., Cerf, M., & Adolphs, R. (2011). Comparing social attention in autism and amygdala lesions: Effects of stimulus and task conditions. *Social Neuroscience, 6,* 420–435.

Boes, A. D., Mehta, S., Rudrauf, D., van der Plas, E., Grabowski, T., Adolphs,

R., et al. (2012). Changes in cortical morphology resulting from long-term amygdala damage. *Social Cognitive and Affective Neuroscience, 7*(5), 588–595.

Buchanan, T. W., Tranel, D., & Adolphs, R. (2009). The human amygdala in social function. In P. W. Whalen & L. Phelps (Eds.), *The human amygdala* (pp. 289–320). New York: Oxford University Press.

Bzdok, D., Laird, A. R., Zilles, K., Fox, P. T., & Eickhoff, S. B. (2012). An investigation of the structural, connectional, and functional subspecialization in the human amygdala. *Human Brain Mapping, 34,* 3247–3266.

Cahill, L., Babinsky, R., Markowitsch, H. J., & McGaugh, J. L. (1995). The amygdala and emotional memory. *Nature, 377,* 295–296.

Chan, I., Liu, L., Hamada, T., Sethuraman, G., & McGrath, J. A. (2007). The molecular basis of lipoid proteinosis: Mutations in extracellular matrix protein 1. *Experimental Dermatology, 16,* 881–890.

Choi, J.-S., & Kim, J. J. (2010). Amygdala regulates risk of predation in rats foraging in a dynamic fear environment. *Proceedings of the National Academy of Sciences, 107,* 21773–21777.

Choi, J. T., Vining, E. P. G., Mori, S., & Bastian, A. J. (2010). Sensorimotor function and sensorimotor tracts after hemispherectomy. *Neuropsychologia, 48,* 1192–1199.

Cordeiro, J. G., Wagner, K., Trippel, M., Zentner, J., & Schulze-Bonhage, A. (2011). Superselective anterior temporal resection in mesial temporal lobe epilepsy. *Epileptic Disorders, 13,* 284–290.

Corkin, S. (1984). Lasting consequences of bilateral medial temporal lobectomy: Clinical course and experimental findings in H. M. *Seminars in Neurology, 4,* 249–259.

Damasio, A. (2003). *Looking for Spinoza: Joy, sorrow, and the feeling brain.* Orlando, FL: Harcourt.

Damasio, A. R. (1999). *The feeling of what happens: Body and emotion in the making of consciousness.* New York: Harcourt Brace.

Damasio, A. R., Eslinger, P. J., Damasio, H., Van Hoesen, G. W., & Cornell, S. (1985). Multimodal amnesic syndrome following bilateral temporal and basal forebrain damage. *Archives of Neurology, 42,* 252–259.

De Martino, B., Camerer, C. F., & Adolphs, R. (2010). Amygdala damage eliminates monetary loss aversion. *Proceedings of the National Academy of Sciences, 107,* 3788–3792.

Dennis, M. (2010). Margaret Kennard (1899–1975): Not a "principle" of brain plasticity but a founding mother of developmental neuropsychology. *Cortex, 46,* 1043–1059.

Dennis, M., Spiegler, B. J., Juranek, J. J., Bigler, E. D., Snead, O. C., & Fletcher, J. M. (2013). Age, plasticity, and homeostasis in childhood brain disorders. *Neuroscience and Biobehavioral Reviews, 37,* 2760–2773.

Dijkhuizen, R. M., Ren, J., Mandeville, J. B., Wu, O., Ozdag, F. M., Moskowitz, M. A., et al. (2001). Functional magnetic resonance imaging of reorganization in rat brain after stroke. *Proceedings of the National Academy of Sciences, 98,* 12766–12771.

Edmiston, E. K., McHugo, M., Dukic, M. S., Smith, S. D., Abou-Khalil, B., Eggers, E., et al. (2013). Enhanced visual cortical activation for emotional stimuli is preserved in patients with unilateral amygdala resection. *Journal of Neuroscience, 33,* 11023–11031.

Elbert, T., & Heim, S. (2001). A light and a dark side. *Nature, 411,* 139.

Esber, G. R., Roesch, M. R., Bali, S., Trageser, J., Bissonette, G. B., Puche, A. C., et al. (2012). Attention-related Pearce–Kay–Hall signals in basolateral amygdala require the midbrain dopaminergic system. *Biological Psychiatry, 72,* 1012–1019.

Eslinger, P., Flaherty-Craig, C. V., & Benton, A. L. (2004). Developmental outcomes after early prefrontal cortex damage. *Brain and Cognition, 55,* 84–103.

Eslinger, P. J., Grattan, L. M., Damasio, H., & Damasio, A. R. (1992). Developmental consequences of childhood frontal lobe damage. *Archives of Neurology, 49,* 764–769.

Feinstein, J. S., Adolphs, R., Damasio, A., & Tranel, D. (2011). The human amygdala and the induction and experience of fear. *Current Biology, 21,* 34–38.

Feinstein, J. S., Buzza, C., Hurlemann, R., Follmer, R. L., Dahdaleh, N. S., Coryell, W. H., et al. (2013). Fear and panic in humans with bilateral amygdala damage. *Nature Neuroscience, 16,* 270–272.

Fountas, K. N., & Smith, J. R. (2007). Historical evolution of stereotactic amygdalotomy for the management of severe aggression. *Journal of Neurosurgery, 106,* 710–713.

Freese, J. L., & Amaral, D. G. (2005). The organization of projections from the amygdala to visual cortical areas TE and V1 in the macaque monkey. *Journal of Comparative Neurology, 486,* 295–317.

Freese, J. L., & Amaral, D. G. (2006). Synaptic organization of projections from the amygdala to visual cortical areas TE in the macaque monkey. *Journal of Comparative Neurology, 496,* 655–667.

Gaffan, D., & Murray, E. A. (1990). Amygdalar interaction with the mediodorsal nucleus of the thalamus and the ventromedial prefrontal cortex in stimulus–reward associative learning in the monkey. *Journal of Neuroscience, 10,* 3479–3493.

Gaffan, D., Murray, E. A., & Fabre-Thorpe, M. (1993). Interaction of the amygdala with the frontal lobe in reward memory. *European Journal of Neuroscience, 5,* 968–975.

Gamer, M., & Büchel, C. (2009). Amygdala activation predicts gaze toward fearful eyes. *Journal of Neuroscience, 29,* 9123–9126.

Hamada, T., McLean, W. H., Ramsay, M., Ashton, G. H., Nanda, A., Jenkins, T., et al. (2002). Lipoid proteinosis maps to 1q21 and is caused by mutations in the extracellular matrix protein 1 gene (*ECM1*). *Human Molecular Genetics, 11,* 833–840.

Hamann, S. B., Ely, T. D., Hoffman, J. M., & Kilts, C. D. (2002). Ecstasy and agony: Activation of the human amygdala in positive and negative emotion. *Psychological Science, 13,* 135–141.

Hampton, A., Adolphs, R., Tyszka, J. M., & O'Doherty, J. (2007). Contributions of the amygdala to reward expectancy and choice signals in human prefrontal cortex. *Neuron, 55,* 545–555.

Hofer, P.-A. (1973). Urbach–Wiethe disease: A review. *Acta Dermato-Venereologica, 53,* 5–52.

Holland, P. C. (2007). Disconnection of the amygdala central nucleus and the substantia innominata/nucleus basalis magnocellularis disrupts performance in a sustained attention task. *Behavioral Neuroscience, 121,* 80–89.

Holland, P. C., & Gallagher, M. (1999). Amygdala circuitry in attentional and representational processes. *Trends in Cognitive Sciences, 3,* 65–73.

Holland, P. C., Han, J.-S., & Gallagher, M. (2000). Lesions of the amygdala central nucleus alter performance on a selective attention task. *Journal of Neuroscience, 20,* 6701–6706.

Holtz, K. H. (1962). Über Gehirn und Augenveränderungen bei Hyalinosis cutis et mucosae (Lipoidproteinose) mit Autopsiebefund [On brain and eye abnormalities in hyalinosis cutis et mucosae (lipoid proteinosis) including autopsy findings]. *Archiv für Klinische und Experimentelle Dermatologie, 214,* 289–306.

Hsu, M., Bhatt, M., Adolphs, R., Tranel, D., & Camerer, C. F. (2005). Neural systems responding to degrees of uncertainty in human decision-making. *Science, 310,* 1680–1683.

Johansen-Berg, H., Behrens, T. E., Sillery, E., Ciccarelli, O., Thompson, A. J., Smith, S. M., & Matthews, P. M. (2005). Functional–anatomical validation and individual variation of diffusion tractography-based segementation of the human thalamus. *Cerebral Cortex, 15,* 31–39.

Kapur, N. (1996). Paradoxical functional facilitation in brain–behavior research. *Brain, 119,* 1775–1790.

Kennard, M. (1942). Cortical reorganization of motor function. *Archives of Neurology, 48,* 227–240.

Kennedy, D. P., & Adolphs, R. (2010). Impaired fixation to eyes following amygdala damage arises from abnormal bottom-up attention. *Neuropsychologia, 48,* 3392–3398.

Kennedy, D. P., Gläscher, J., Tyszka, J. M., & Adolphs, R. (2009). Personal space regulation by the human amygdala. *Nature Neuroscience, 12,* 1226–1227.

Khundrakpam, B. S., Reid, A., Brauer, J., Carbonell, F., Lewis, J., Ameis, S., et al. (2013). Developmental changes in organization of structural brain networks. *Cerebral Cortex, 23,* 2072–2085.

Kliemann, D., Dziobek, I., Hatri, A., Baudewig, J., & Heekeren, H. R. (2012). The role of the amygdala in atypical gaze on emotional faces in autism spectrum disorders. *Journal of Neuroscience, 32,* 9469–9476.

Kolb, B., Mychasiuk, R., Williams, P., & Gibb, R. (2011). Brain plasticity and recovery from early cortical injury. *Developmental Medicine and Child Neurology, 53,* 4–8.

LeDoux, J. (2012). Rethinking the emotional brain. *Neuron, 73,* 653–676.

Lee, G. P., Bechara, A., Adolphs, R., Arena, J., Meador, K. J., Loring, D. W., et al. (1998). Clinical and physiological effects of stereotaxic bilateral amygdalotomy for intractable aggression. *Journal of Neuropsychiatry and Clinical Neurosciences, 10,* 413–420.

Maren, S., Yap, S. A., & Goosens, K. A. (2001). The amygdala is essential for the development of neuronal plasticity in the medial geniculate nucleus during auditory fear conditioning in rats. *Journal of Neuroscience, 21,* RC135.

Marsh, E. B., & Hillis, A. E. (2006). Recovery from aphasia following brain injury: The role of reorganization. *Progress in Brain Research, 157,* 143–156.

Mason, W. A., Capitanio, J. P., Machado, C . J., Mendoza, S. P., & Amaral, D. G.

(2006). Amygdalectomy and responsiveness to novelty in rhesus monkeys: Generality and individual consistency of effects. *Emotion, 6,* 73–81.

McGaugh, J. L. (2004). The amygdala modulates the consolidation of memories of emotionally arousing experiences. *Annual Review of Neuroscience, 27,* 1–28.

Meenan, F. O. C., Bowe, S. D, Dinn, J. J., McCabe, M., McCullen, O., Masterson, J. G., et al. (1978). Lipoid proteinosis: A clinical, pathological and genetic study. *Quarterly Journal of Medicine, 188,* 549–561.

Menon, V. (2013). Developmental pathways to functional brain networks: Emerging principles. *Trends in Cognitive Sciences, 17,* 627–640.

Mihov, Y., Kendrick, K. M., Becker, B., Zschernack, J., Reich, H., Maier, W., et al. (2013). Mirroring fear in the absence of a functional amygdala. *Biological Psychiatry, 73,* e9–e11.

Mishra, A., Rogers, B. P., Chen, L. M., & Gore, J. C. (2013). Functional connectivity-based parcellation of amygdala using self-organized mapping: A data driven approach. *Human Brain Mapping, 35,* 1247–1260.

Mobbs, D., Yu, R., Rowe, J. B., Eich, H., FeldmanHall, O., & Dalgleish, T. (2010). Neural activity associated with monitoring the oscillating threat value of a tarantula. *Proceedings of the National Academy of Sciences, 47,* 20582–20586.

Morgan, B., Terburg, D., Thornton, H. B., Stein, D. J., & van Honk, J. (2012). Paradoxical facilitation of working memory after basolateral amgydala damage. *PLoS ONE, 7,* e38116.

Mormann, F., Kornblith, S., Quiroga, R. Q., Kraskov, A., Cerf, M., Fried, I., et al. (2008). Latency and selectivity of single neurons indicate hierarchical processing in the human medial temporal lobe. *Journal of Neuroscience, 28,* 8865–8872.

Motzkin, J. C., Philippi, C. L., Wolf, R. C., Baskaya, M. K., & Koenigs, M. (2014). Ventromedial prefrontal cortex is critical for the regulation of amygdala activity in humans. *Biological Psychiatry, 77*(3), 276–284.

Mpakopoulou, M., Gatos, J., Brotis, A., Paternakis, K. N., & Fountas, K. N. (2008). Stereotactic amygdalotomy in the management of severe aggressive behavioral disorders. *Neurosurgery Focus, 25,* E6.

Narabayashi, H., Nagao, T., Saito, Y., Yoshida, M., & Nagahata, M. (1963). Stereotaxic amygdalotomy for behavioral disorders. *Archives of Neurology, 9,* 11–26.

Öngür, D., & Price, J. L. (2000). The organization of networks within the orbital and medial prefrontal cortex of rats, monkeys, and humans. *Cerebral Cortex, 10,* 206–219.

Pascual-Leone, A., Amedi, A., Fregni, F., & Merabet, L. B. (2005). The plastic human brain cortex. *Annual Review of Neuroscience, 28,* 377–401.

Paton, J. J., Belova, M. A., Morrison, S. E., & Salzman, C. D. (2006). The primate amygdala represents the positive and negative value of visual stimuli during learning. *Nature, 439,* 865–870.

Paul, L. K., Corsello, C., Tranel, D., & Adolphs, R. (2010). Does bilateral damage to the human amygdala produce autistic symptoms? *Journal of Neurodevelopmental Disorders, 2,* 165–173.

Pessoa, L., & Adolphs, R. (2010). Emotion processing and the amygdala: from a "low road" to "many roads" of evaluating biological significance. *Nature Reviews Neuroscience, 11,* 773–782.

Pitkanen, A., Savander, V., & LeDoux, J. E. (1997). Organization of intra-amygdaloid circuitries in the rat: An emerging framework for understanding functions of the amygdala. *Trends in Neurosciences, 20,* 517–523.

Rey, H. G., Fried, I., & Quiroga, R. Q. (2014). Timing of single-neuron and local field potential responses in the human medial temporal lobe. *Current Biology, 24,* 299–304.

Roesch, M. R., Calu, D. J., Esber, G. R., & Schoenbaum, G. (2010). Neural correlates of variations in event processing during learning in basolateral amygdala. *Journal of Neuroscience, 30,* 2490–2495.

Rotshtein, P., Richardson, M. P., Winston, J. S., Kiebel, S. J., Vuilleumier, P., Eimer, M., Driver, J., et al. (2010). Amygdala damage affects event-related potentials for fearful faces at specific time windows. *Human Brain Mapping, 31,* 1089–1105.

Roy, A. K., Shehzad, Z., Margulies, D. S., Kelly, A. M. C., Uddin, L. Q., Gotimer, K., et al. (2009). Functional connectivity of the human amygdala using resting state fMRI. *NeuroImage, 45,* 614–626.

Saygin, Z. M., Osher, D. E., Augustinack, J., Fischl, B., & Gabrieli, J. D. E. (2011). Connectivity-based segmentation of human amygdala nuclei using probabilistic tractography. *NeuroImage, 56,* 1353–1361.

Scherer, K. R. (2000). Psychological models of emotion. In J. C. Borod (Ed.), *The neuropsychology of emotion* (pp. 137–162). New York: Oxford University Press.

Schneider, G. E. (1974). Anomalous axonal connections implicated in sparing and alteration of function after early lesions. *Neurosciences Research Program Bulletin, 12,* 222–228.

Schumann, C. M., Bauman, M. D., & Amaral, D. G. (2011). Abnormal structure or function of the amygdala is a common component of neurodevelopmental disorders. *Neuropsychologia, 49,* 745–759.

Siebert, M., Markowitsch, H. J., & Bartel, P. (2003). Amygdala, affect and cognition: Evidence from 10 patients with Urbach–Wiethe disease. *Brain, 126,* 2627–2637.

Skuse, D., Morris, J. S., & Lawrence, K. (2003). The amygdala and development of the social brain. *Annals of the New York Academy of Sciences, 1008,* 91–101.

Solano-Castiella, E., Anwander, A., Lohmann, G., Weiss, M., Docherty, C., Geyer, S., et al. (2010). Diffusion tensory imaging segments the human amygdala *in vivo. NeuroImage, 49,* 2958–2965.

Solano-Castiella, E., Schäfer, A., Reimer, E., Türke, E., Pröger, T., Lohmann, G., et al. (2011). Parcellation of human amygdala *in vivo* using ultra high field structural MRI. *NeuroImage, 58,* 741–748.

Stefanacci, L., Buffalo, E. A., Schmolck, H., & Squire, L. R. (2000). Profound amnesia after damage to the medial temporal lobe: a neuroanatomical and neuropsychological profile of patient E. P. *Journal of Neuroscience, 20,* 7024–7036.

Terburg, D., Morgan, B. E., Montoya, E. R., Hooge, I. T., Thornton, H. B., Hariri, A. R., et al. (2012). Hypervigilance for fear after basolateral amygdala damage. *Translational Psychiatry, 2,* e115.

Thornton, H. B., Nel, D., Thornton, D., van Honk, J., Baker, G. A., & Stein, D. J. (2008). The neuropsychiatry and neuropsychology of lipoid proteinosis. *Journal of Neuropsychiatry and Clinical Neuroscience, 20,* 86–92.

Tranel, D., Gullickson, G., Koch, M., & Adolphs, R. (2006). Altered experience of emotion following bilateral amygdala damage. *Cognitive Neuropsychiatry, 11*, 219–232.

Tranel, D., & Hyman, B. T. (1990). Neuropsychological correlates of bilateral amygdala damage. *Archives of Neurology, 47*, 349–355.

Tsuchiya, N., & Adolphs, R. (2007). Emotion and consciousness. *Trends in Cognitive Sciences, 11*, 158–167.

Tye, K. M., Prakash, R., Kim, S.-Y., Fenno, L. E., Grosenick, L., Zarabi, H., et al. (2011). Amygdala circuitry mediating reversible and bidirectional control of anxiety. *Nature, 471*, 358–362.

Umeda, T., & Funakoshi, K. (2014). Reorganization of motor circuits after neonatal hemidecortication. *Neuroscience Research, 78*, 30–37.

van Honk, J., Eisenegger, C., Terburg, D., Stein, D. J., & Morgan, B. (2013). Generous economic investments after basolateral amygdala damage. *Proceedings of the National Academy of Sciences, 110*, 2506–2510.

Vuilleumier, P., & Driver, J. (2007). Modulation of visual processing by attention and emotion: Windows on causal interactions between human brain regions. *Philosophical Transactions of the Royal Society B: Biological Sciences, 362*, 837–855.

Vuilleumier, P., Richardson, M. P., Armony, J. L., Driver, J., & Dolan, R. J. (2004). Distant influences of amygdala lesion on visual cortical activation during emotional face processing. *Nature Neuroscience, 7*, 1271–1278.

Wang, S., Xu, J., Jiang, M., Zhao, Q., Hurlemann, R., & Adolphs, R. (2014). Autism spectrum disorder but not amygdala lesions impairs social attention in visual search. *Neuropsychologia, 63*, 259–274.

CHAPTER 11

Behavioral Consequences and Compensatory Adaptations after Early Bilateral Amygdala Damage in Monozygotic Twins

ALEXANDRA PATIN
RENÉ HURLEMANN

A. M. and B. G., monozygotic twins diagnosed with Urbach–Wiethe disease (UWD), both present with selective bilateral amygdala lesions. The twins share a common genotype, as well as upbringing, and therefore provide a superb opportunity to examine possible compensatory mechanisms to work around their lesions. In this chapter, we open with a description of possible mechanisms of compensation and a detailed introduction of A. M. and B. G. We then examine findings from studies exploring learning and memory, reward and risk taking, autonomic response, emotional processing, and altruistic punishment, and discuss both the areas affected by the amygdala damage and the areas in which the twins are similar to healthy controls, despite the task's probable reliance on an intact amygdala under healthy conditions. In a final discussion, we discuss how these latter findings can be interpreted against the background of amygdala lesions, and suggest that they are indicative of compensatory processes taking place. We furthermore examine how individual differences between the twins could illustrate varying levels of compensation, and what consequences these differences could have in the everyday lives of the twins, as well as other patients with amygdala lesions.

In contrast to earlier ideas of the amygdala as a single, homogeneous structure, integrated in the limbic system and merely taking part in the activity surrounding it, the amygdala has emerged as one of the most complex and widely interconnected structures in the brain. Its cytoarchitectonics, chemoarchitectonics, and fiber connections (Brockhaus,

1938, 1940) set it apart as a key center of emotional processing (Barbas, 1995; Pessoa, 2008; Swanson, 2003). On the one hand, the amygdala is crucial for the formation of implicit and—via its modulatory impact on the hippocampus—explicit emotional memories, as well as early, preattentive detection of emotional stimuli. Fear conditioning and fear extinction are two clinically relevant manifestations of this pivotal role in emotional learning and memory. On the other hand, cognitive abilities (e.g., perception, attention, and decision making) have all been found to be modulated in one vital way or another by the amygdala (Aggleton, 2000; LeDoux, 2007; Phelps, 2004; Seymour & Dolan, 2008; Swanson & Petrovich, 1998). Furthermore, the amygdala has been implicated in aggressive, maternal, sexual, and consummatory behaviors (LeDoux, 2007). Such a diverse repertoire of behavioral and cognitive effects is likely a by-product of the diverse collection of nuclei that comprise the amygdala, which can be roughly organized into three general divisions: the superficial (corticoid) subregion, the centromedial subregion, and the basolateral amygdala (Amunts et al., 2005; Heimer et al., 1999).

Pharmacological imaging studies are useful in exploring the short-term influence of changed amygdala behavior on otherwise healthy brains (Patin & Hurlemann, 2011). Propranolol, a relatively nonselective, beta-noradrenergic receptor antagonist, is traditionally used by musicians or actors to combat stage fright and performance anxiety (Brantigan, Brantigan, & Joseph, 1982; Tyrer, 1988). It also decreased the amygdala's response to negative, emotionally charged pictures from the International Affective Picture System (IAPS; van Stegeren et al., 2005), as well as to emotional faces, which evoked the strongest response in the basolateral amygdala in the placebo group (Hurlemann et al., 2010b). In an opposite effect, the selective noradrenaline reuptake inhibitor reboxetine was shown actually to induce an exaggerated response to fearful faces in the right basolateral amygdala (Onur et al., 2009), providing further support for the basolateral amygdala's central role in processing emotions. Interestingly, surrounding amygdala subregions and other more distal brain regions do not appear to compensate for the sudden changes in basolateral amygdala activity seen in pharmacological studies.

So what are the defining criteria that allow compensation for the functional loss of a vital neural region? In healthy organisms, "synaptogenesis" (the formation of new synapses) and "neurogenesis" (the formation of new neurons) continue throughout life. Studying for an examination, learning a language, or mastering the violin all require the growth of new neurons and connectivity changes often localized to task-specific regions (e.g., the hippocampus to commit the new task to memory, the motor cortices to coordinate new movements involved in the task).

The plasticity of the brain is perhaps in part due to a fundamental mechanism of compensation, for example following a lesion. This is, however, a relatively new idea. Long a dogma of neuroscience was the notion that we age shortly following our birth, characterized by the famous diagnosis by Ramón y Cajál in 1913: "Once the development was ended, the founts of growth and regeneration of axons and dendrites dried up irrevocably. In the adult centers, the nerve paths are something fixed, ended, and immutable. Everything may die, nothing may be regenerated" (Colucci-D'Amato, Bonavita, & di Porzio, 2006; Ramón y Cajál, 1913–1914). It is therefore perhaps no surprise that the initial suggestion of adult neurogenesis would be met with disapproval within the neuroscience field (Colucci-D'Amato et al., 2006). Nevertheless, neurogenesis has become a highly promising direction and has been found in the hippocampus and olfactory bulb (Altman, 1963; Altman & Das, 1965; Doetsch, Garcia-Verdugo, & Alvarez-Buylla, 1999; Seri, Garcia-Verdugo, McEwen, & Alvarez-Buylla, 2001), and more recently, the striatum (Ernst et al., 2014; Kempermann, 2014). Early findings suggested enormous potential for therapeutic regeneration following a major stroke (Arvidsson, Collin, Kirik, Kokaia, & Lindvall, 2002). These findings, while not conclusive proof of morphological compensation following a lesion, point to the possibility of the brain's plasticity being a powerful mechanism for functional recovery, perhaps alongside or in concert with other highly visible plasticity mechanisms, such as synaptic plasticity and long-term potentiation (LTP) and depression (LTD).

Lesions of the brain result in greater or lesser impairments, based not only on their location and size but also on the time of their occurrence and recuperation. When it comes to the amygdala, there are several types of clinically documented amygdala lesions springing from a variety of sources, such as herpes encephalitis, neurosurgery for intractable temporal lobe epilepsy, stroke, craniocerebral injury, and so forth. The vast majority of these acquired amygdala lesions are unilateral and/or the damage extends into other structures outside the amygdala, thus not allowing for a clear experimental isolation of amygdala function. There is, however, a genetic illness capable of causing selective bilateral amygdala dysfunction. This illness, known as Urbach–Wiethe disease (UWD), was discovered in 1929 and is extremely rare (Urbach & Wiethe, 1929; see Box 11.1 for details on UWD).

A. M. and B. G. are monozygotic twins who were diagnosed with UWD late in childhood, following a grand mal seizure in B. G. at age 12. Both A. M. and B. G. experience epileptic auras as often as twice a month, although A. M. has never suffered a real seizure (Becker, Mihov, Scheele, Kendrick, Feinstein, et al., 2012). Recent genetic findings in A. M. and B. G. show a novel homozygous missense mutation in exon 7 and a resulting switch from tryptophan 237 to arginine (c.709T >C; p.W237R). The p.Trp237Arg extracellular matrix protein 1 gene (*ECM1*) mutation is

BOX 11.1. Urbach–Wiethe Disease

Urbach–Wiethe disease (UWD; also called lipoid proteinosis or hyalinosis cutis et mucosae) is a rare, autosomal recessive genodermatosis often involving bilateral calcification of the amygdala. Since the discovery of amygdala calcifications in patients with UWD, it has served as a stable model of lesions that allows unique insight into the functional workings of the amygdala. The disease has been noted in fewer than 300 cases since it was initially reported (Di Giandomenico et al., 2006). Symptoms include periodic acid–Schiff (PAS) stain-positive hyaline residue in the skin, mucous, and visceral areas, resulting in hoarse cries and later a hoarse voice, skin lesions, and papules around the eyes (see Figure 11.1) (Appenzeller et al., 2006; Caro, 1978; Hamada, 2002). Although symptoms typically appear from a very young age (Di Giandomenico et al., 2006), patients live an average lifespan (Appenzeller et al., 2006).

The cause of the disease lies in six distinct loss-of-function mutations in the extracellular matrix protein 1 gene (*ECM1*) on chromosome 1q21 (Hamada et al., 2002), most commonly at exons 6 and 7 (Hamada et al., 2003). Newer findings, however, suggest that UWD appears to be the result of any of the 41 separate mutations that can cause loss of function (Chan, Liu, Hamada, Sethuraman, & McGrath, 2007). The gene's exact functions are not entirely understood in healthy individuals. The disease has been found to follow both a quasi-dominant pedigree inheritance (Rosenthal & Duke, 1967) and a recessive pattern (Gordon, Gordon, & Botha, 1969). These differences can be reconciled with the explanation that the gene is pleiotropic and recessive in clinical terms but dominant in the context of selection (Stine & Smith, 1990).

Despite the progress in genomic mapping, the exact underlying mechanism of the disease is unclear. Two leading theories have suggested that UWD is either a mucopolysaccharide metabolism dysfunction (Moynahan, 1966) or a lysosomal storage disease, mainly due to vacuolization in the cytoplasm of dermal fibroblasts (Bauer, Santa-Cruz, & Eisen, 1981). Epilepsy is a typical complication of UWD, and the intracranial calcifications that occur in the area of the amygdala are found in 50–75% of patients (Appenzeller et al., 2006). The calcifications may show a slow progression throughout life, but the time course has not yet been found for certain.

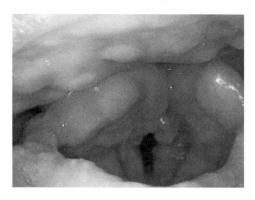

FIGURE 11.1. A view of the laryngopharynx in a patient with UWD. Recognizable are the vocal folds surrounding the opening to the trachea. In contrast to the normally smooth and straight surfaces of the laryngopharynx, the uneven, bumpy surfaces and discolorations caused by periodic acid–Schiff (PAS) stain positive hyaline plaques typical of UWD are apparent here in the patient B. G. UWD is partly characterized by such hyaline residue in the skin, mucous, and visceral areas, which results in hoarse cries and a hoarse voice later in life, as well as skin lesions and papules around the eyes (Appenzeller et al., 2006; Caro, 1978; Hamada, 2002). Patients A. M. and B. G. both display these symptoms, in addition to neurological symptoms. Photograph courtesy of Prof. Dr. Goetz Schade, Director of the Department of Phoniatrics and Pediatric Audiology, University Hospital of Bonn, Germany.

likely an underlying source of pathological changes in the twins' phenotype (Becker et al., 2012). In a novel approach, we used stereotaxic cytoarchitectonics probabilistic maps placed over the twins' structural magnetic resonance imaging (MRI) scans to show that the calcifications in the twins with UWD enveloped the basolateral amygdala (BLA; Amunts et al., 2005; Hurlemann et al., 2007b), and we have followed up on the twins' amygdala calcifications since. Recent scans of the twins' brains revealed not only a striking similarity of their lesion size but also that the BLA is completely calcified, along with parts of the rostral anterior and ventral cortical amygdala regions, and caudally in the lateral and medial regions of the central nucleus and amygdala–hippocampal transition region (Becker et al., 2012) (see Plates 11.1 and 11.2 on color insert).

Early experiments in monkeys involving experimental lesions of the temporal lobe (including the amygdala) resulted in Klüver–Bucy syndrome, characterized by hypersexuality, hyperorality, and visual agnosia, among other symptoms (Afifi & Bergman, 2005; Ozawa et al., 1997; Salloway, Malloy, & Cummings, 1997). Interestingly, the behavioral phenotype of the twins is remarkably different from Klüver–Bucy syndrome, and both are functioning remarkably well given their complex disease and brain damage. Both successfully completed 13 years of schooling and apprenticeship training, currently have jobs, are married with children, and are free of any mental disorders.

Currently, A. M. and B. G. are the only known monozygotic twins in the world with UWD. They have allowed themselves to be studied under numerous paradigms and countless tasks since they first started volunteering for psychological studies in 2001. The twins are so important and unique precisely because they offer the only true opportunity to explore compensation in the amygdala. Both their nature and their nurture are presumably highly similar in every way, because they share an identical genotype and were raised together throughout their entire lives. Their amygdala lesions are also remarkably similar and show a striking degree of overlap (see Plate 11.1). Thus, any differences between them in the studies completed over the years can be considered a direct view into the compensatory processes taking place in their brains.

One tempting hypothesis is that the brain's ability to compensate for this calcified area entails the selective recruitment of other brain regions. Our intention in this chapter is to identify the regions in which the twins seem to have compensated for the absence of an intact amygdala. In several instances, the twins differ in their individual results, indicating that the plasticity of the brain is not a standardized process and does not occur equally in all people. Additionally, this compensation has come at a price, and the twins do show several areas of cognitive and behavioral deficiencies.

Findings from Twins with UWD

In the following sections, findings from the twins A. M. and B. G. with UWD are presented. A summary of all findings can be seen in Table 11.1 at the end of the chapter.

Learning and Memory

As a part of the Papez circuit and the site where memories are coded, the hippocampus is arguably the most important region involved in the formation of new explicit (declarative) memories. However, anyone who has had an emotionally charged experience and learned from it has also recruited the amygdala in this memory. The amygdala acts as a type of filter, allocating resources to the hippocampus for emotional events, thus placing a higher priority on their encoding and consolidation in long-term declarative memory. Fundamental to this differential effect of the amygdala on emotional memory consolidation is, for one, an increased memory for emotional events following beta-adrenergic modulation (Cahill,

Prins, Weber, & McGaugh, 1994). For another, additional modulation via an amygdala–hippocampus interaction during emotional, but not non-emotional, memory occurs (Cahill, Babinsky, Markowitsch, & McGaugh, 1995). In terms of specific, intra-amygdalar pathways, noradrenaline (NA) release from the locus coeruleus (LC-NA) in the BLA during emotional memory consolidation has been found in animals (McGaugh, 2000, 2004), and an intra-amygdalar increase of LC-NA in humans (Strange & Dolan, 2004; van Stegeren et al., 2005). (See Box 11.2 for a more in-depth description of the amygdala's role in memory dysfunction disorders, such as posttraumatic stress disorder [PTSD].)

Against this background, we would expect to find that the absence of an amygdala, specifically the BLA, would impair privileged emotion-based declarative learning and memory, while purely hippocampus-based declarative memory would remain intact. In support of this, a block of NA modulation via the beta-noradrenergic receptor antagonist, as well as amygdala, similarly blocked enhanced declarative memory for emotional stimuli (Strange, Hurlemann, & Dolan, 2003). Additionally, both twins were both found to lack the typical anterograde and retrograde amnesia found in healthy controls following emotional stimuli. On the basis of this, we suggested that BLA dysfunction is a crucial inhibiting factor to arousal-based amygdala–hippocampal coupling, and that this coupling is a necessary condition for modulating valence-specific input from prefrontal brain regions during encoding of declarative memories (Hurlemann et al., 2007b).

In a further study showing support for impaired emotional processing in learning, the twins generally performed worse than healthy controls when given socially reinforced feedback in a learning paradigm, showing that the hippocampus, when free from the amygdala's modulatory influence, was unable to encode emotional declarative memories normally. The twins performed unimpaired, however, in non-socially reinforced feedback learning (Hurlemann et al., 2010a). In this task, participants were to decide whether the three-digit number shown alongside either a face or a circle belonged to category A or B. The participants were given visual feedback immediately following their decision. The membership of the number to either category A or B did not change over the six cycles, therefore testing participants' declarative learning.

In the social condition, the neutral face turned into a happy face following a correct response, or into an angry face following an incorrect response. Black circles changed to either green, following a correct response, or red, following an incorrect response. As mentioned above, results showed that the twins needed a significantly longer time and performed worse than healthy controls in only the social condition, not in the nonsocial condition (Hurlemann et al., 2010a).

BOX 11.2. Real-World Implications
of Amygdala-Modulated Memory in PTSD

In the course of the research amassed regarding the amygdala's modulation of emotional versus nonemotional memory, the fundamental question of why these findings are important can become foggy. Although amygdala dysfunction is a contributing factor to several psychiatric illnesses, its role in posttraumatic stress disorder (PTSD) is directly related to the findings listed in this chapter. The underlying mechanisms of PTSD have yet to be fully illuminated, but there is strong evidence that it is first and foremost based on dysfunction of emotional memory circuits, including both hyperamnesia for emotional stimuli and periemotional amnesia, or amnesia for other events surrounding the emotional stimulus, based on findings from emotional oddball paradigms (Hurlemann et al., 2005, 2007a, 2007b; Strange, Hurlemann, & Dolan, 2003).

Moreover, coactivation of cortisol and NE during emotional events appears to relate directly to the intensity of periemotional amnesia (Hurlemann et al., 2007a). The pathogenesis of peritraumatic amnesia and PTSD can be explained in a neurochemical model based on a harmful interaction of noradrenergic and cortisol signaling disinhibition, contributing to a peritraumatic amnesia and PTSD.

Under normal conditions, the medial prefrontal cortex (mPCF) directly modulates the BLA and the anterior hippocampus, as well as indirectly via inhibitory regulation of the hypothalamic–pituitary–adrenal (HPA) axis and locus coeruleus (LC), which in turn send input to the BLA. The HPA supplies cortisol; the LC supplies noradrenalin (NA). In the face of a lack of top-down inhibition in traumatic events, NA and cortisol signaling from the LC and HPA could be increased and might result in increased memory for the core emotional event, as well as peritraumatic amnesia and increased symptoms of PTSD, by deleting contextual information and increasing the salience of cues to activate recollections. Given an absence of or insufficient regulation from the mPFC in traumatic events, the uninhibited BLA could increase its input to the hippocampus (Hurlemann, 2008; Hurlemann et al., 2007a). By understanding this complex interaction between the amygdala and the hippocampus on the one hand, and NA and cortisol signaling on the other, important steps might be made toward finding a treatment for PTSD.

This means that although the twins and the controls had equal difficulty learning without social feedback, social feedback facilitated healthy individuals' learning but not that of the twins. Whereas healthy controls decided more quickly which answer was correct than when given nonsocial feedback, the twins did not make such a distinction. This indicates a more laborious cognitive process by the twins than by the controls, and that the amygdala is crucial to evaluating such feedback as being facilitative to learning. In short, there was not a great difference between social versus nonsocial feedback in the absence of a functional amygdala (Hurlemann et al., 2010a).

Interestingly, however, when presented with aversive words and asked to remember them in a facilitative recall task, both A. M. and B. G. are able to do so at the level of healthy controls, suggesting either that both twins have compensated in this specific aspect of emotional memory or that this particular aspect may not be directly related to the amygdala (Bach, Talmi, Hurlemann, Patin, & Dolan, 2011).

Reward and Risk Taking

The desire to gamble is based on the desire to take risks in the face of varying potential gains or losses. In an instance of irrationality, healthy individuals usually show an increased desire to gamble when the reward is framed in terms of a loss than when the same amount of money is framed as a win (Tversky & Kahneman, 1981). The amygdala's alarm goes off in response to the potential loss, thus causing the decision to be based on the emotional scare of a loss rather than the hard logic that the win or loss represents the same amount of money. When presented with this test, the twins gamble more frequently, regardless of the context, compared to controls, thus showing a lack of the moderation apparently stemming from the amygdala. However, compensation for the amygdala lesions was apparent in other aspects of the task; most notably, their framing effect was normal (Talmi, Hurlemann, Patin, & Dolan, 2010).

When comparing the twins to each other, A. M. was similar to the controls in terms of reaction time patterns. She and the controls thought longer and harder when they did decide to gamble than when they passed on the risk. B. G., on the other hand, showed the opposite effect: She took longer to decide to pass on a gamble and take a safe bet. This opposite reaction pattern is interesting because whereas both twins gambled more, the decision was apparently made following completely opposite thought processes. A. M., being similar to controls, appeared to show compensation of the amygdala, because she reflected the healthy controls' decision to take the safe route when faced with risk. The decision to gamble despite risk was cognitively laborious, and both A. M. and controls showed a hesitancy to take the risk. They seemed to employ the heuristic: Don't risk it, unless the payoff is deemed to be worth it. For controls, this heuristic was apparently based in the amygdala; for A. M., it was based in a compensatory network. B. G., on the other hand, seemed to employ the opposite heuristic: Risk it, unless the risk is too great. Thus, we can see that A. M. seems to show a greater level of compensation, because the heuristic she seems to use is close to what most healthy people would regard as the rational thing to do (Talmi et al., 2010).

Autonomic Response

The amygdala is also connected to autonomic response networks that control physiological responses to certain stimuli. Skin conductance, one such response, measures the activity of the sympathetic nervous system based on the amount of sweat a person produces. Because fluctuations in sweat production are minute and can change over a very short time span, they are a sensitive way of measuring sympathetic nervous system arousal, or emotional response. When A. M.'s skin conductance was tested, she and healthy controls showed a similar response while looking at faces showing fear, happiness, anger, and sadness (Becker et al., 2012). Interestingly, her response differed when shown a disgusted face, indicating that her compensatory response to this emotion was less developed than other emotions. Compensation of the amygdala thus appears to extend to autonomic effector structures such as the brainstem, thereby influencing brainstem activities the way the amygdala normally does.

Future studies would predict that conducting functional MRI (fMRI) in the UWD twins would show intact activation of the hypothalamus and brainstem structures normally activated by interoceptive panic. The latter is suggested by a behavioral experiment, during which the twins were presented with a mixture of 35% CO_2 (Feinstein et al., 2013; also see Feinstein, Adolphs, & Tranel, Chapter 1, this volume). In some healthy individuals and in most patients with panic disorder, this gaseous solution can induce a panic attack. Interestingly, both twins also showed a panic response when inhaling the CO_2 mixture. In a healthy population, the number of individuals exhibiting the same panic response is far lower, indicating that the amygdala may actually temper the panic response. However, the anticipatory anxiety prior to inhalation normally found in healthy controls was not present in the twins. Compensation for the amygdala's typical alert system seemed to be missing and the twins displayed no anticipatory physiological responses while waiting for the noxious stimulus to arrive (Feinstein et al., 2013).

Another physiological response, the acoustic startle reflex, involves the reticular formation in the brainstem and "protects animals from blows or predatory attacks by quickly stiffening the limbs, body wall and dorsal neck in the brief time period before directed evasive or defensive action can be performed" (Yeomans & Frankland, 1995, p. 301). This response, however, is modulated by the amygdala when combined with emotional stimuli (Buchanan, Tranel, & Adolphs, 2004), with the presentation of unpleasant foreground stimuli potentiating and pleasant ones diminishing the startle magnitude, respectively. Whereas A. M. showed a normal startle response to aversive scenes, B. G. showed a dampened response. Therefore, there is an indication of compensation for the amygdala-induced startle potentiation in A. M. but not B. G., and that the compensation covers top-down control over physiological fear responses (see Figure 11.2) (Becker et al., 2012).

It is conceivable that these experiments show a kind of step-like hierarchy of compensation based on what the twins have confronted more often in their lives, as well as what presents the most acute danger for the brain at the time. An aversive scene could present less danger than a lack of oxygen (or abundance of CO_2). Furthermore, a threatening scene could require a more complex evaluation than the direct lack of oxygen, thus involving recruitment of more areas of the brain to induce a flight response.

These archaic responses involve phylogenetically old, primal areas of the brain. The brainstem, for instance, is the oldest part of the brain responsible for the most basic of vital functions (e.g., breathing, defecation, and urination). In case of a missing (and uncompensated for) amygdala, these functions are completely independent of emotional modulation, although other brain regions may normally contribute to the modulation of these functions (e.g., the hypothalamus, insular cortex,

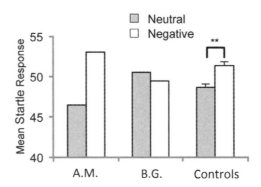

FIGURE 11.2. Results from an acoustic startle response-modulation task. Startle responses (*T*-scores) while viewing neutral and negative images are represented by the bars. Mean error rates ± *SEM* are shown for control data, **$p < .1$. It is apparent that the modulation of acoustic startle responses by fear-eliciting images is intact in A. M. but not in B. G. Reprinted with permission of Elsevier from Becker et al. (2012). Copyright 2012 by the Society of Biological Psychiatry.

and orbitofrontal cortex, to name a few). Emotional modulation of these functions extends the ability of the brain to react not only to the presence of CO_2 in the atmosphere or the pressure of urine on the bladder wall, but also to potentially threatening or dangerous stimuli in the external environment. Thus, compensation of the amygdala must extend to the furthest parts of the brain to preserve this instinct.

In a positron emission tomography (PET) study of the serotonergic (serotonin, 5-HT) receptor system, A. M. was found to have a 70% global decrease in 5-HT$_{2A}$ receptor binding potential (see Plate 11.3 on color insert) (Hurlemann et al., 2009). In animal studies, a knockout of the 5-HT$_{2A}$ gene shows reduced anxiety in mice (Weisstaub et al., 2006), thus providing for a plausible groundwork for the lowered anxiety in the twins. In healthy individuals, the amygdala and brainstem, including the serotonin-producing raphe nuclei, share a reciprocal relationship. Top-down control of the brainstem by the amygdala, combined with a bottom-up influence of the brainstem, appear to be crucial to the early stages of 5-HT development.

Questions about anxiety-inducing behavior indicated that A. M. seemed to have a higher threshold for anxiety: "She did not appear to have a normal sense of danger and would skydive from a plane without hesitation, if given the opportunity" (Hurlemann et al., 2009, p. 80). Any functional compensation present in A. M. does not, therefore, appear to extend to a normalized 5-HT receptor expression.

Emotional Processing

The picture of compensation in emotional processing is not entirely cut and dried: Whereas A. M. and B. G. both show similarities to healthy controls in some paradigms, indicating compensation in these areas in both twins, they also show differences in other areas, quintessentially suggesting that only one of the twins has compensated for the loss of an amygdala. For example, both twins showed the ability to discern fear and anger in a voice, suggesting a healthy compensation in amygdala-dependent auditory processing. A. M. even outperformed healthy individuals when identifying fear. Based on these findings, it appears that A. M. has been able to compensate for a missing amygdala more than her sister in this area, and even to overcompensate when listening to fear-filled voices (Bach, Hurlemann, & Dolan, 2013). In an attentional blink paradigm, which tests the amygdala's ability to process and judge stimuli rapidly depending on their relevancy, and consequently to allocate resources based on this judgment, both twins also showed an intact relevance detection, suggesting compensation (Bach, Talmi, Hurlemann, Patin, & Dolan, 2011).

In terms of the ability to discern emotions based on stimuli such as facial mimicry or another person's voice is one of the amygdala's most explored domains. In the event that the amygdala is compromised, the expectation is that this ability is also lowered. In reality, A. M. and B. G. show a mixed picture in terms of being similar to controls in some areas, but in other areas, they differed from controls and from each other. Both women show an intact theory of mind and can identify emotions based on facial expression (Hurlemann et al., 2010a). When this is separated among emotions, B. G. shows deficiencies when recognizing anger and fear compared to A. M., who is similar to healthy participants (Becker et al., 2012). When confronted with angry or happy faces in a crowd, the twins have difficulty picking out an angry face, even though they can identify this face without trouble as being angry (Bach, Hurlemann, & Dolan, 2015). These findings appear to be relatively specific to faces and human-related photos. When asked to rate a variety of emotional scenes from IAPS images (Lang, Bradley, & Cuthbert, 2008), B. G. was unable to detect the valence on most images, rating them instead as neutral (Scheele et al., 2012).

In both the laboratory and in everyday life, both twins exhibit evidence of hypoarousal to emotional events. For instance, they reported significantly lower arousal levels to IAPS images than did healthy individuals (Scheele et al., 2012), as well as to photos of emotional faces (Becker et al., 2012) (See Plate 11.4 on color insert.)

Likewise, during a research visit to the University of Iowa in 2011, the twins were exposed to a number of novel experiences but displayed essentially no excitement during any of these experiences. For example, it was their first time visiting America, and upon exiting the plane, both twins appeared somewhat apathetic, whereas their husbands were extremely excited. The next day, we took the twins and their family to a professional baseball game (marking the first time they had ever been to a baseball game), and once again the twins were uninterested and showed very little emotion, including after the game, during a firework show and concert. In stark contrast, their husbands were exuberant with joy and tried on numerous occasions to share this happy experience by laughing, smiling, and showing the twins affection. Neither twin reciprocated, and the disconnect between husband and wife (both in terms of overall arousal and emotionality, as well as displays of affection) was patently obvious.

Consistent with this observed real-life behavior, both twins reported feeling less empathy for people pictured in emotional photographs (Hurlemann et al., 2010a). In both categories (arousal and empathy), A. M. lay closer to controls than her sister, who showed far less reaction to the emotional stimuli. Additionally, A. M. showed an insignificant but moderate above-average ability to identify negatively valenced faces (Hurlemann et al., 2010a). This supports the idea of overcompensation by A. M. in emotional processing, at least of negative emotions. (See Box 11.3 for a discussion of the amygdala's role in empathy and theory of mind.)

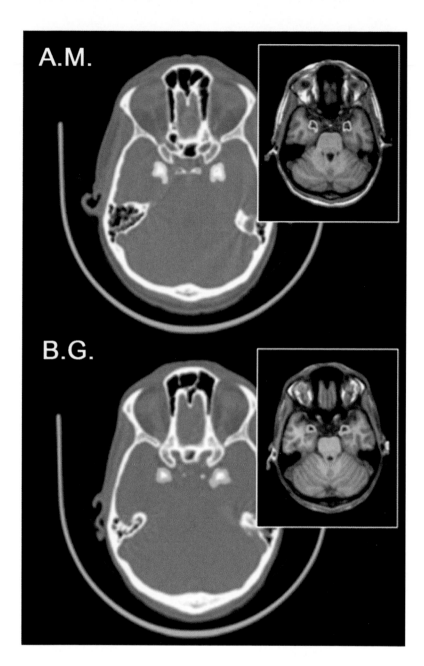

PLATE 11.1. Lesion imaging of patients A. M. and B. G. Both twins exhibit selective bilateral amygdala calcification lesions as a result of UWD. Displayed in the top row for each patient are X-ray computed tomography (CT) images placed onto high-resolution magnetic resonance imaging (MRI) scans. The larger image shows the CT image, with the outline of the lesion, which is then placed onto the smaller image of the MRI sections of the anterior medial temporal lobes. Remarkably equivalent and extensive bilateral amygdala damage is seen in both twins. Reprinted with permission of Elsevier from Becker et al. (2012). Copyright 2012 by the Society of Biological Psychiatry.

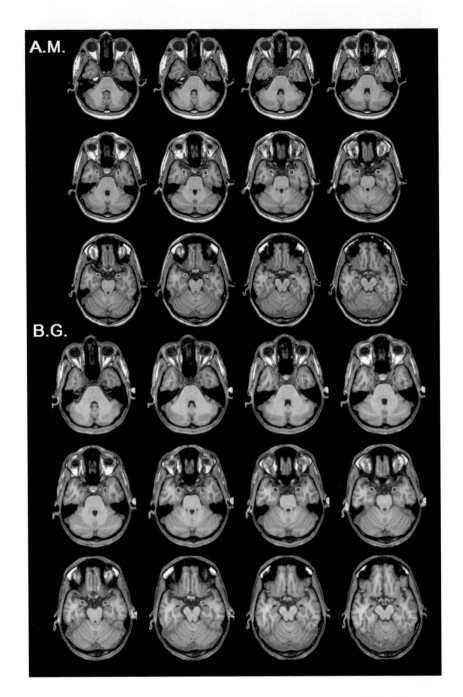

PLATE 11.2. MRI scans of A. M. and B. G., showing outlines of the lesions progressing from inferior (starting top left) to superior (ending bottom right). It is apparent that the amygdala is affected throughout multiple levels in both twins.

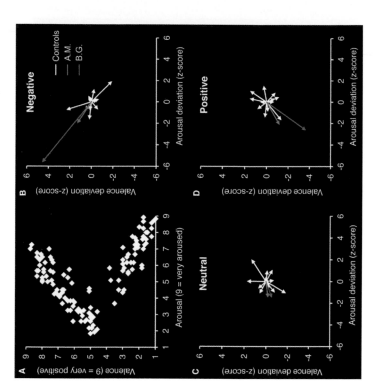

PLATE 11.4. (A) The arousal and valence ratings by healthy controls of 129 images from the International Affective Picture System (IAPS). (B, C, and D) Vector maps for the negative, neutral, and positive IAPS stimuli, respectively, illustrating abnormal arousal ratings in both A. M. and B. G., as well as abnormal valence ratings in A. M. Reprinted with permission of Elsevier from Scheele et al. (2012). Copyright 2012 by the Society of Biological Psychiatry.

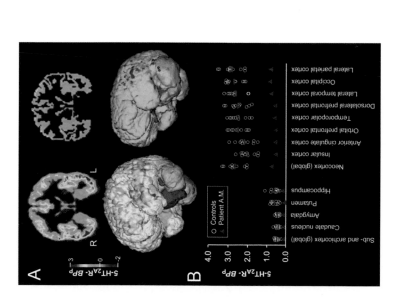

PLATE 11.3. MRI and [18F]altanserin PET data from A. M. (A) Parametric maps reveal a 70% global reduction of 5-HT$_{2A}$R BP$_P$ in A. M. compared to healthy controls. (B) A scatter plot of global and regional 5-HT$_{2A}$R BP$_P$ values in A. M. compared to controls (averaged across hemispheres). From Hurlemann et al. (2009). Copyright 2009 by Oxford University Press. Reprinted by permission.

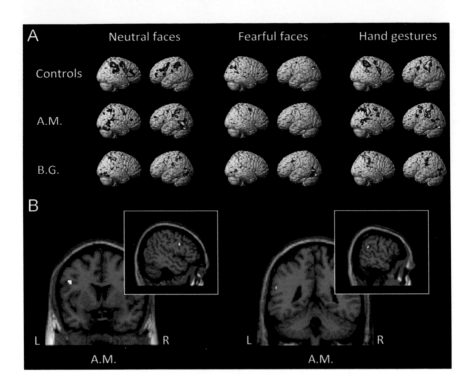

PLATE 11.5. (A) A widely distributed mirror neuron network (MNN) in response to gestures based on MRI results in healthy controls compared to A. M. and B. G. MNN activity was also found in response to dynamic face stimuli, but not hand movements, in the insula and anterior cingulum. (B) The larger MNN response in A. M. compared to B. G. is seen in the left inferior frontal operculum and superior temporal gyrus in response to viewing fearful faces. Reprinted with permission of Elsevier from Mihov et al. (2013). Copyright 2013 by the Society of Biological Psychiatry.

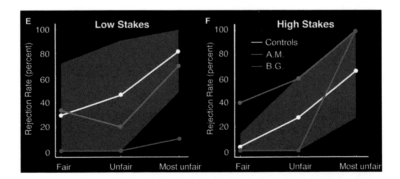

PLATE 11.6. A. M. and B. G. show deviant altruistic punishment during an ultimatum game, as seen by abnormal rejection rates (mean ± 1 *SD* as indicated by the gray area for controls) of unfair offers in both low- (E) and high-stakes (F) conditions. Reprinted with permission of Elsevier from Scheele et al. (2012). Copyright 2012 by the Society of Biologcal Psychiatry.

BOX 11.3. Empathy and Theory Of Mind

Although empathy as a notion of emotional processing has long since made it into everyday use, its academic definition is a highly complex, multifaceted concept. One highly prevalent definition of empathy includes the subcategories cognitive empathy (theory of mind) and emotional empathy (Baron-Cohen & Wheelwright, 2004). The definition of two different aspects of empathy as a whole is based in both behavioral and fMRI differences.

"Cognitive empathy" pertains to the identification of another person's emotion based on the ability to take his or her perspective or, more generally, understanding what the person is feeling, as well as the resulting inference of this person's intentions or actions (Baron-Cohen & Wheelwright, 2004; Kohler, 1929). In a meta-analysis, cognitive–evaluative forms of empathy were found to activate the dorsal left anterior midcingulate cortex, left orbitofrontal cortex, and left dorsal medial thalamus (Fan, Duncan, de Greck, & Northoff, 2011).

"Emotional empathy" pertains to the depth of feeling for the other person, the experience of a visceral or emotional reaction to another person's situation (Baron-Cohen & Wheelwright, 2004; Mehrabian & Epstein, 1972; Stotland, 1969). Relevant regions found in fMRI studies are the right anterior insula extending to the right inferior frontal gyrus, the ventral anterior midcingulate cortex extending to the right anterior cingulate cortex, the midbrain, and the right dorsal medial thalamus (Fan et al., 2011).

Findings in the monozygotic twins A. M. and B. G. with UWD have shed additional light on the different aspects of empathy: Although we found that both twins were unimpaired in cognitive empathy, self-reported emotional empathy ratings were far below those of healthy controls, indicating an amygdala component to emotional empathy (Hurlemann et al., 2010a). These findings could have important implications for the treatment of psychiatric illnesses characterized by a lack of empathy, including, but not limited to, cognitive empathy deficits in autism spectrum disorders and a lack of emotional empathy in antisocial personality disorders, both of which make up a significant portion of psychiatric illness.

In both B. G. and A. M., the mirror neuron network has shown a similar overall response when compared to healthy controls while observing fearful faces and hand gestures, lending support for a close reciprocal interplay between these regions and the potential for compensation through hyperactivity. Moreover, the twins have no trouble reproducing fearful facial expressions, showing intact mirror neuron network connections to motor components, which could support compensation when evaluating fearful faces. When the sisters' blood oxygen level-dependent (BOLD) responses while viewing fearful faces are compared with each other, A. M. shows additional response in the left inferior frontal operculum and superior temporal gyrus. Because A. M. appears to show a greater level of compensation than B. G. in emotional processing, this greater activation indicates that the operculum and superior temporal gyrus are involved in compensating for the amygdala as part of the mirror neuron network (see Plate 11.5 on color insert; Mihov et al., 2013). (See Box 11.4 for background on the mirror neuron network.)

Altogether, given that the twins have shown some compensation, the question becomes where this compensation is taking place. Is it between brain regions (e.g., specifically within the mirror neuron system) or are the parts that make up the conglomerate of the amygdala working together to pick up the slack left by damaged regions? In a study of five patients with UWD, the basolateral region was shown to be an inhibiting force on processing of fearful faces by the amygdala (Terburg et al., 2012). The central medial amygdala and superficial amygdala were intact in either all or most patients included in the study, and could therefore represent pathways for compensation, such as via the central medial nucleus (Gozzi et al., 2010; Terburg et al., 2012; Tye et al., 2011).

Another complicated question is raised by the twins' abilities when cognitively evaluating a stimulus versus feeling emotional arousal toward it: If the brain compensates for the most important roles lost by the calcified amygdala, then why is the cognitive ability to recognize fear given priority over the actual arousal, which would most likely be more effective in a threatening situation? The answer may lie in the capacity of the brain to compensate. The amygdala is a highly relevant site for the fight-or-flight response, alongside the brainstem, which recently has been shown to be crucial to a panic response (Feinstein et al., 2013). Therefore, any compensation for the dysfunctional amygdala can only be a shadow of what its ability is in a healthy individual. On the other hand, the cognitive ability to recognize an emotional stimulus and react to it appropriately may be modulated by the amygdala but require the interaction of other areas, such as the prefrontal cortex, hippocampus, and perhaps the brainstem, among others. Because these areas interact with each other in close relation in a healthy individual, the amygdala presumably shares more of the brunt of responsibility and can be more easily compensated. The degree

BOX 11.4. The Mirror Neuron Network

In the 1990s, researchers discovered for the first time a set of neurons in the premotor cortex of monkeys that fired not only when the monkey performed hand movement but also when simply watching the experimenter perform the movement (di Pellegrino, Fadiga, Fogassi, Gallese, & Rizzolatti, 1992; Gallese, Fadiga, Fogassi, & Rizzolatti, 1996). The researchers gave these neurons the name "mirror neurons" (Gallese et al., 1996), giving way to an entirely new field of study in neuroscience. In total, they recorded the activity of 92 such neurons that fired according to how the hand interacted with the object, such as whether it was placed or held in the left or the right hand, or moved from left to right or the other way around; in some categories, the researchers recorded the activity of a single neuron responsible for transmitting the information to other areas of the then-unknown mirror neuron network (Gallese et al., 1996).

Further early studies reported mounting evidence for an extensive mirror neuron network comprising the ventral premotor cortex (vPMC) and the inferior parietal lobule (inferior PL) in primates (Fogassi et al., 2005; Keysers & Gazzola, 2010; Keysers et al., 2003). Unfortunately, this seemingly clear evidence proved to be a red herring: As Keysers and Gazzola (2010) point out, over 90% of the neurons in the vPMC and inferior PL are unrelated to mirror neurons, and many researchers proclaim to have found mirror neuron activity in these areas regardless of whether mirror neurons were actually involved (Gallese et al., 1996; Keysers & Gazzola, 2010; Keysers et al., 2003).

In 2010, almost 15 years after the first mirror neurons were described in monkeys, mirror neurons were definitively reported in humans in the medial frontal lobe and medial temporal lobe, including the hippocampus, parahippocampal gyrus, and entorhinal cortex (Mukamel, Ekstrom, Kaplan, Iacoboni, & Fried, 2010). To date, hundreds of studies of mirror neurons have been conducted. In a recent meta-analysis, mirror neuron locations common to several studies were found in the left and right inferior frontal gyrus; vPMC; inferior PL; superior PL; dorsal PMC; insula; inferior, middle, and superior temporal gyri; cerebellum; and Brodmann areas 40, 6, 9, 7, and 44 (Molenberghs, Cunnington, & Mattingley, 2012). When broken down along task lines, the authors found that by watching and mimicking facial expressions, mirror neurons were activated in subjects' posterior inferior frontal gyrus, adjacent vPMC, amygdala, insula, and cingulate gyrus (Molenberghs et al., 2012), indicating that these areas are additionally integrated in the mirror neuron network. Importantly, the concept of mirror neurons is not cut and dried: There is still much debate surrounding the functionality of mirror neurons, and the findings regarding their role are to be viewed in this light.

of how closely coupled cognitive evaluation of emotion versus the rapid response to emotional stimuli is in a healthy individual is likely to show large differences. Furthermore, the question is raised whether observing and identifying an emotion such as fear is uncoupled from the amygdala or very well compensated. In both cases, the twins would show intact ability to recognize emotions. A complete uncoupling would be difficult to combine with the apparent overcompensation by A. M., as well as with the findings that indicate social feedback is either not evaluated as such or is evaluated correctly but does not influence learning. Therefore, it may be that the amygdala plays a small enough role to be easily compensated for. On the other hand, it might be that because of compensation, the other parts of A. M.'s brain have suffered from allocation of resources to a role they normally would not play (see Adolphs, Chapter 10, this volume). In fact, an exaggerated response to fearful faces has been found in some patients with UWD (Terburg et al., 2012). This suggests that at least some individuals with UWD actually overcompensated for the absence of a BLA (see van Honk, Terburg, Thornton, Stein, & Morgan, Chapter 12, this volume).

Altruistic Punishment

Unlike any other species, humans exhibit a tremendous propensity toward cooperation. Interestingly, such cooperation is not guided by rational imperatives alone but is strongly susceptible to and framed by the influence of emotion. An exquisite example is altruistic punishment, which "means that individuals punish, although the punishment is costly for them and yields no material gain" (Fehr & Gächter, 2002, p. 137). Mounting evidence suggests that negative emotion toward those who do not cooperate are the "proximate mechanism behind altruistic punishment" (Fehr & Gächter, 2002, p. 137), hence implicating a potentially pivotal role of the amygdala in the maintenance of human cooperation.

Experimentally, altruistic punishment has often been operationalized using the ultimatum game, in which the desire to punish others, even at a cost to oneself, is tested in terms of monetary losses and gains. Two players are given an amount of money that Player 1 divides up as he or she chooses. If Player 2 decides the amount given to him or her by Player 1 is too little and rejects the offer, then neither player receives any money. If Player 2 accepts the offer, the money is divided up accordingly. When tested with this paradigm, the twins showed very different strategies, indicating very different cognitive processes during these emotional decisions (Scheele et al., 2012; see Plate 11.6 on color insert). On the one hand, A. M. showed excessive rejection rates during high-stakes rounds, even when confronted with fair offers. Compared to healthy controls, she also took longer to decide whether to accept an offer. A. M. appeared, once again, to overcompensate compared with healthy individuals by presenting such extreme forms of behavior (Scheele et al., 2012).

B. G., on the other hand, performed similarly to controls on most rounds except during the most unfair offers. During low monetary stakes, she accepted nearly every unfair offer, whereas during the high monetary stakes, she rejected 100% of the offers. Thus, she appeared to employ an all-or-none rule-based strategy to compensate for her lack of arousal to unfair offers. However, an alternative explanation is that she did actually experience emotional arousal in response to unfairness, but it took higher monetary stakes to induce it (Scheele et al., 2012).

Collectively, the twins' behavioral abnormalities in the ultimatum game indicate a central role of the amygdala in contributing to the maintenance of human cooperation, and "corroborate the notion of altruistic punishment being an emotion-driven and impulsive act of retaliation" (Scheele et al., 2012, p. e5).

Discussion of Compensation

The potential for compensation when the amygdala is destroyed from an early enough stage in life is complex. This is in part because of its extraordinary integration in the brain and its relationship to a plethora of other neural regions. As Kennedy and Adolphs (2012, p. 563) write, "The amygdala, by itself, does nothing; instead, it is important to begin asking questions about the networks within which the amygdala participates— and of these there are many." Thus, the question of compensation turns from whether it is even possible to which other neural regions can take on some of the amygdala's roles in light of the brain's plastic nature (see Adolphs, Chapter 10, this volume).

Taken as a whole, the primate amygdala consists of approximately 13 nuclei (Amaral, Price, Pitkanen, & Carmichael, 1992; Holland & Gallagher, 1999; Pitkanen, Savander, & LeDoux, 1997), each of which has its own input and output from other neural regions (LeDoux, 2007). This classification on the level of nuclei serves to divide the amygdala not only structurally but also functionally. The temporal cortex delivers input regarding faces, the basal forebrain and sensory cortex areas receive output from the amygdala related to attention and perception, and output regarding emotional response is sent to the hypothalamus and brainstem (Kennedy & Adolphs, 2012).

One of the amygdala's most important roles for an organism's survival is the process of learning fear and/or learning what stimuli are fearful (Hitchcock & Davis, 1986; LeDoux, Cicchetti, Xagoraris, & Romanski, 1990; Slotnick, 1973). One region that shows great potential for being crucial to this learning is the medial prefrontal cortex (mPFC), which is highly functionally connected to the amygdala during fear conditioning and fear extinction (Sotres-Bayon & Quirk, 2010) and could therefore comprise a main route to compensate for missing evaluation of fear (Cho, Deisseroth, & Bolshakov, 2013). Whereas the amygdala is mainly responsible for the learning component of fear conditioning (Falls, Miserendino, & Davis, 1992), the mPFC appears to be crucial to the consolidation of extinction memories (for a review, see also Marek, Strobel, Bredy, & Sah, 2013; Morgan, Romanski, & LeDoux, 1993). Thus, the two regions are intricately involved in the fear conditioning process and could serve to compensate for each other's deficiencies. A further important region is the hippocampus, which likewise shares rich reciprocal connectivity with the amygdala. The hippocampus is also involved in fear learning (Maren, 2001) and is therefore also a possible route of compensation.

An interesting observation when examining these studies is that the twins differ from each other in several instances, but in every case, A. M. shows a greater level of compensation than B. G. A possible exception to this is during the gambling task, in which B. G., for the most part, was closer to healthy controls than A. M. However, even in this case, A. M. was most likely overcompensating and could be considered to have a greater level of compensation despite showing worse results.

These differences have apparent consequences for patients with amygdala lesions in everyday life. For instance, amygdala volume has been found to positively correlate with the Social Network Index (SNI), which measures both the size and the complexity of social networks (Bickart, Wright, Dautoff, Dickerson, & Barrett, 2011; Cohen, Doyle, Skoner, Rabin, & Gwaltney, 1997). The fact that A. M. was shown to have a higher score on the SNI than B. G., yet their lesions are extremely similar, could point to the twins showing different levels of compensation (Becker et al., 2012).

The idea of compensation is important, because it could be one of the most influential factors in successful treatment following an amygdala lesion, such as following a stroke or infection. However, it can also mean important progress in research on amygdala disorders, which, analogous to structural amygdala lesions, show a functional deficit and require the brain to make up for lost neurons. Mood and anxiety disorders such as major depression, PTSD, and illnesses such as autism or psychopathy, have all been linked to an amygdala dysfunction. Thus, the ability to recover from such a loss of amygdalar input, either following a structural lesion or because of a functional disruption, could have vast therapeutic consequences for a variety of patient groups. The twins A. M. and B. G. currently provide the only reliable and stable model of amygdala compensation in the world, and their participation in the growing number of studies provides a unique look at the way the mind works when faced with such a massive challenge of long-term amygdala dysfunction.

TABLE 11.1. Findings from UWD Twins A. M. and B. G. Compared to Healthy Controls

Study	Parameter	Both normal[a]	Both pathological[a]	Differences between twins
		Learning and Memory		
Strange, Hurlemann, & Dolan (2003)	Emotion-induced memory impairment		X[a]	
Hurlemann et al. (2010a)	Socially reinforced feedback learning		X	
Hurlemann et al. (2010a)	Nonsocially reinforced feedback learning	X		
Hurlemann et al. (2010a)	Response times for socially reinforced feedback learning		X	
Hurlemann et al. (2007b)	Episodic memory (neutral condition)	X		
Hurlemann et al. (2007b)	Emotion-induced anterograde and retrograde memory effects		X	
		Reward and risk taking		
Talmi, Hurlemann, Patin, & Dolan (2010)	Framing effect: gambling frequency in loss frame	X		
Talmi et al. (2010)	Framing effect: gambling frequency overall		X	
Talmi et al. (2010)	Reaction times when deciding whether to gamble	X		
		Emotional processing		
Mihov et al. (2013)	Response to observing fear			A. M. showed activation in left frontal operculum and superior temporal gyrus.

(continued)

TABLE 11.1. *(continued)*

Study	Parameter	Both normal[a]	Both pathological[a]	Differences between twins
Bach, Talmi, Hurlemann, Patin, & Dolan (2011)	Attentional blink: recall facilitation for aversive words	X		
Hurlemann et al. (2010a)	Cognitive empathy judgments	X		
Becker et al. (2012)	Fear recognition			A. M. showed normal ability; B. G. had lowered ability.
Becker et al. (2012)	Anger recognition			A. M. showed normal ability, B. G. had lowered ability.
Bach, Hurlemann, & Dolan (2013)	Emotion discrimination: fear vs. neutral prosody	X		
Bach et al. (2013)	Emotion discrimination: anger vs. neutral prosody	X		
Bach et al. (2013)	Multinomial classification of fear, sadness, anger, disgust, happiness, and neutral emotions	X		
Scheele et al. (2012)	Arousal judgments of emotional stimuli		X	
Scheele et al. (2012)	Valence judgments of emotional stimuli			B. G. rated most stimuli as neutral; A. M. comparable to controls.
Scheele et al. (2012)	Ultimatum game			A. M. showed excessive rejection rates for fair offers during high stakes, and reaction times were longer. B. G. played at the level of controls, except for the most unfair offers.
Hurlemann et al. (2010a)	Direct and indirect emotional empathy		X	A. M. showed moderate impairment; B. G. showed severe impairment.

(continued)

TABLE 11.1. *(continued)*

Study	Parameter	Both normal[a]	Both pathological[a]	Differences between twins
Bach et al. (in press)	Threat detection		X	

Autonomic, extraneural responses

Study	Parameter	Both normal[a]	Both pathological[a]	Differences between twins
Becker et al. (2012)	Skin conductance response to fearful faces	X[a]		
Becker et al. (2012)	Acoustic startle response			A. M. was comparable to controls; B. G. showed lowered response.

Neural parameters related to emotion

Study	Parameter	Both normal[a]	Both pathological[a]	Differences between twins
Feinstein et al. (2013)	Brainstem panic reflex (35% CO_2)	X		
Feinstein et al. (2013)	Anticipatory anxiety		X	
Hurlemann et al. (2009)	Global spatial distribution of 5-HT_{2A} receptor		X[a]	

Mirror neurons

Study	Parameter	Both normal[a]	Both pathological[a]	Differences between twins
Mihov et al. (2013)	Overall mirror neuron network response (fMRI)	X		
Mihov et al. (2013)	Fear imitation	X		

Social networks

Study	Parameter	Both normal[a]	Both pathological[a]	Differences between twins
Becker et al. (2012)	Social Network Index (SNI; size and complexity of social network)			A. M. showed a normal SNI; B. G. was found to be at the lower end of controls. A. M.'s scores were double those of B. G. for both size and complexity.

In three studies[a], only A. M. was tested. The results are then listed as either "Both normal" or "Both pathological" to simplify the table, but it should be clear that B. G. did not take part.

REFERENCES

Afifi, A., & Bergman, R. A. (2005). *Functional neuroanatomy: Text and atlas* (2nd ed.). New York: McGraw-Hill Education.

Aggleton, J. P. (2000). *The amygdala: A functional analysis.* Oxford, UK: Oxford University Press.

Altman, J. (1963). Autoradiographic investigation of cell proliferation in the brains of rats and cats. *Anatomical Record, 145*, 573–591.

Altman, J., & Das, G. D. (1965). Autoradiographic and histological evidence of postnatal hippocampal neurogenesis in rats. *Journal of Comparative Neurology, 124*(3), 319–335.

Amaral, D., Price, J., Pitkanen, A., & Carmichael, S. (1992). Anatomical organization of the primate amygdaloid complex. In J. Aggleton (Ed.), *The amygdala: Neurobiological aspects of emotion, memory, and mental dysfunction* (pp. 1–66). New York: Wiley-Liss.

Amunts, K., Kedo, O., Kindler, M., Pieperhoff, P., Mohlberg, H., Shah, N. J., et al. (2005). Cytoarchitectonic mapping of the human amygdala, hippocampal region and entorhinal cortex: intersubject variability and probability maps. *Anatomy and Embryology (Berlin), 210*(5–6), 343–352.

Appenzeller, S., Chaloult, E., Velho, P., de Souza, E. M., Araujo, V. Z., Cendes, F., et al. (2006). Amygdalae calcifications associated with disease duration in lipoid proteinosis. *Journal of Neuroimaging, 16*(2), 154–156.

Arvidsson, A., Collin, T., Kirik, D., Kokaia, Z., & Lindvall, O. (2002). Neuronal replacement from endogenous precursors in the adult brain after stroke. *Nature Medicine, 8*(9), 963–970.

Bach, D. R., Hurlemann, R., & Dolan, R. J. (2013). Unimpaired discrimination of fearful prosody after amygdala lesion. *Neuropsychologia, 51*(11), 2070–2074.

Bach, D. R., Hurlemann, R., & Dolan, R. J. (2015). Impaired implicit threat processing after selective bilateral amygdala lesions. *Cortex, 63*, 206–213.

Bach, D. R., Talmi, D., Hurlemann, R., Patin, A., & Dolan, R. J. (2011). Automatic relevance detection in the absence of a functional amygdala. *Neuropsychologia, 49*(5), 1302–1305.

Barbas, H. (1995). Anatomic basis of cognitive–emotional interactions in the primate prefrontal cortex. *Neuroscience and Biobehavioral Reviews, 19*(3), 499–510.

Baron-Cohen, S., & Wheelwright, S. (2004). The empathy quotient: An investigation of adults with Asperger syndrome or high functioning autism, and normal sex differences. *Journal of Autism and Developmental Disorders, 34*(2), 163–175.

Bauer, E. A., Santa-Cruz, D. J., & Eisen, A. Z. (1981). Lipoid proteinosis: *In vivo* and *in vitro* evidence for a lysosomal storage disease. *Journal of Investigative Dermatology, 76*(2), 119–125.

Becker, B., Mihov, Y., Scheele, D., Kendrick, K. M., Feinstein, J. S., Matusch, A., et al. (2012). Fear processing and social networking in the absence of a functional amygdala. *Biological Psychiatry, 72*(1), 70–77.

Bickart, K. C., Wright, C. I., Dautoff, R. J., Dickerson, B. C., & Barrett, L. F. (2011). Amygdala volume and social network size in humans. *Nature Neuroscience, 14*(2), 163–164.

Brantigan, C. O., Brantigan, T. A., & Joseph, N. (1982). Effect of beta blockade and beta stimulation on stage fright. *American Journal of Medicine, 72*(1), 88–94.

Brockhaus, H. (1938). Zur normalen und pathologischen Anatomie des Mandelkerngebiets [On the normal and pathological anatomy of the amygdala region]. *Journal für Psychologie und Neurologie, 49*, 1–136.

Brockhaus, H. (1940). Die Cyto-und Myeloarchitektonik des Cortex claustralis und des Claustrum beim Menschen [The cyto- and myeloarchitecture of the claustral cortex and the claustrum in humans]. *Journal für Psychologie und Neurologie, 49*, 249–348.

Buchanan, T. W., Tranel, D., & Adolphs, R. (2004). Anteromedial temporal lobe damage blocks startle modulation by fear and disgust. *Behavioral Neuroscience, 118*(2), 429–437.

Cahill, L., Babinsky, R., Markowitsch, H. J., & McGaugh, J. L. (1995). The amygdala and emotional memory. *Nature, 377*(6547), 295–296.

Cahill, L., Prins, B., Weber, M., & McGaugh, J. L. (1994). [beta]-Adrenergic activation and memory for emotional events. *Nature, 371*(6499), 702–704.

Caro, I. (1978). Lipoid proteinosis. *International Journal of Dermatology, 17*(5), 388–393.

Chan, I., Liu, L., Hamada, T., Sethuraman, G., & McGrath, J. A. (2007). The molecular basis of lipoid proteinosis: Mutations in extracellular matrix protein 1. *Experimental Dermatology, 16*(11), 881–890.

Cho, J. H., Deisseroth, K., & Bolshakov, V. Y. (2013). Synaptic encoding of fear extinction in mPFC–amygdala circuits. *Neuron, 80*(6), 1491–1507.

Cohen, S., Doyle, W. J., Skoner, D. P., Rabin, B. S., & Gwaltney, J. M., Jr. (1997). Social ties and susceptibility to the common cold. *Journal of the American Medical Association, 277*(24), 1940–1944.

Colucci-D'Amato, L., Bonavita, V., & di Porzio, U. (2006). The end of the central dogma of neurobiology: Stem cells and neurogenesis in adult CNS. *Neurological Sciences, 27*(4), 266–270.

di Giandomenico, S., Masi, R., Cassandrini, D., El-Hachem, M., De Vito, R., Bruno, C., et al. (2006). Lipoid proteinosis: Case report and review of the literature. *Acta Otorhinolaryngologica Italica, 26*(3), 162–167.

di Pellegrino, G., Fadiga, L., Fogassi, L., Gallese, V., & Rizzolatti, G. (1992). Understanding motor events: A neurophysiological study. *Experimental Brain Research, 91*(1), 176–180.

Doetsch, F., Garcia-Verdugo, J. M., & Alvarez-Buylla, A. (1999). Regeneration of a germinal layer in the adult mammalian brain. *Proceedings of the National Academy of Sciences USA, 96*(20), 11619–11624.

Ernst, A., Alkass, K., Bernard, S., Salehpour, M., Perl, S., Tisdale, J., et al. (2014). Neurogenesis in the striatum of the adult human brain. *Cell, 156*(5), 1072–1083.

Falls, W. A., Miserendino, M. J., & Davis, M. (1992). Extinction of fear-potentiated startle: blockade by infusion of an NMDA antagonist into the amygdala. *Journal of Neuroscience, 12*(3), 854–863.

Fan, Y., Duncan, N. W., de Greck, M., & Northoff, G. (2011). Is there a core neural network in empathy?: An fMRI based quantitative meta-analysis. *Neuroscience and Biobehavioral Reviews, 35*(3), 903–911.

Fehr, E., & Gächter, S. (2002). Altruistic punishment in humans. *Nature*, *415*(6868), 137–140.

Feinstein, J. S., Buzza, C., Hurlemann, R., Follmer, R. L., Dahdaleh, N. S., Coryell, W. H., et al. (2013). Fear and panic in humans with bilateral amygdala damage. *Nature Neuroscience*, *16*(3), 270–272.

Fogassi, L., Ferrari, P. F., Gesierich, B., Rozzi, S., Chersi, F., & Rizzolatti, G. (2005). Parietal lobe: From action organization to intention understanding. *Science*, *308*(5722), 662–667.

Gallese, V., Fadiga, L., Fogassi, L., & Rizzolatti, G. (1996). Action recognition in the premotor cortex. *Brain*, *119*(2), 593–609.

Gordon, H., Gordon, W., & Botha, V. (1969). Lipoid proteinosis in an inbred Namaqualand community. *Lancet*, *1*(7604), 1032–1035.

Gozzi, A., Jain, A., Giovannelli, A., Bertollini, C., Crestan, V., Schwarz, A. J., et al. (2010). A neural switch for active and passive fear. *Neuron*, *67*(4), 656–666.

Hamada, T. (2002). Lipoid proteinosis. *Clinical and Experimental Dermatology*, *27*(8), 624–629.

Hamada, T., McLean, W. H., Ramsay, M., Ashton, G. H., Nanda, A., Jenkins, T., et al. (2002). Lipoid proteinosis maps to 1q21 and is caused by mutations in the extracellular matrix protein 1 gene (*ECM1*). *Human Molecular Genetetics*, *11*(7), 833–840.

Hamada, T., Wessagowit, V., South, A. P., Ashton, G. H., Chan, I., Oyama, N., et al. (2003). Extracellular matrix protein 1 gene (*ECM1*) mutations in lipoid proteinosis and genotype–phenotype correlation. *Journal of Investigative Dermatology*, *120*(3), 345–350.

Heimer, L., de Olmos, J. S., Alheid, G. F., Pearson, J., Sakamoto, N., Shinoda, K., et al. (1999). *The human basal forebrain: Part II. The primate nervous system.* New York: Elsevier.

Hitchcock, J., & Davis, M. (1986). Lesions of the amygdala, but not of the cerebellum or red nucleus, block conditioned fear as measured with the potentiated startle paradigm. *Behavioral Neuroscience*, *100*(1), 11–22.

Holland, P. C., & Gallagher, M. (1999). Amygdala circuitry in attentional and representational processes. *Trends in Cognitive Sciences*, *3*(2), 65–73.

Hurlemann, R. (2006). Noradrenergic control of emotion-induced amnesia and hypermnesia. *Reviews in the Neurosciences*, *17*(5), 525–532.

Hurlemann, R. (2008). Noradrenergic–glucocorticoid mechanisms in emotion-induced amnesia: From adaptation to disease. *Psychopharmacology*, *197*(1), 13–23.

Hurlemann, R., Hawellek, B., Matusch, A., Kolsch, H., Wollersen, H., Madea, B., et al. (2005). Noradrenergic modulation of emotion-induced forgetting and remembering. *Journal of Neuroscience*, *25*(27), 6343–6349.

Hurlemann, R., Matusch, A., Hawellek, B., Klingmuller, D., Kolsch, H., Maier, W., et al. (2007a). Emotion-induced retrograde amnesia varies as a function of noradrenergic-glucocorticoid activity. *Psychopharmacology*, *194*(2), 261–269.

Hurlemann, R., Patin, A., Onur, O. A., Cohen, M. X., Baumgartner, T., Metzler, S., et al. (2010a). Oxytocin enhances amygdala-dependent, socially reinforced learning and emotional empathy in humans. *Journal of Neuroscience*, *30*(14), 4999–5007.

Hurlemann, R., Schlaepfer, T. E., Matusch, A., Reich, H., Shah, N. J., Zilles, K., et al. (2009). Reduced 5-HT$_{2A}$ receptor signaling following selective bilateral amygdala damage. *Social Cognitive and Affective Neuroscience, 4,* 79–84.

Hurlemann, R., Wagner, M., Hawellek, B., Reich, H., Pieperhoff, P., Amunts, K., et al. (2007b). Amygdala control of emotion-induced forgetting and remembering: Evidence from Urbach–Wiethe disease. *Neuropsychologia, 45*(5), 877–884.

Hurlemann, R., Walter, H., Rehme, A. K., Kukolja, J., Santoro, S. C., Schmidt, C., et al. (2010b). Human amygdala reactivity is diminished by the beta-noradrenergic antagonist propranolol. *Psychological Medicine, 40*(11), 1839–1848.

Kempermann, G. (2014). Off the beaten track: new neurons in the adult human striatum. *Cell, 156*(5), 870–871.

Kennedy, D. P., & Adolphs, R. (2012). The social brain in psychiatric and neurological disorders. *Trends in Cognitive Sciences, 16*(11), 559–572.

Keysers, C., & Gazzola, V. (2010). Social neuroscience: Mirror neurons recorded in humans. *Current Biology, 20*(8), R353–R354.

Keysers, C., Kohler, E., Umilta, M. A., Nanetti, L., Fogassi, L., & Gallese, V. (2003). Audiovisual mirror neurons and action recognition. *Experimental Brain Research, 153*(4), 628–636.

Kohler, W. (1929). *Gestalt psychology.* New York: Liveright.

Lang, P., Bradley, M., & Cuthbert, B. (2008). International Affective Picture System (IAPS): Affective ratings of pictures and instruction manual (Technical Report A-8). Gainesville, FL: University of Florida.

LeDoux, J. (2007). The amygdala. *Current Biology, 17*(20), R868–R874.

LeDoux, J. E., Cicchetti, P., Xagoraris, A., & Romanski, L. M. (1990). The lateral amygdaloid nucleus: Sensory interface of the amygdala in fear conditioning. *Journal of Neuroscience, 10*(4), 1062–1069.

Marek, R., Strobel, C., Bredy, T. W., & Sah, P. (2013). The amygdala and medial prefrontal cortex: partners in the fear circuit. *Journal of Physiology, 591*(10), 2381–2391.

Maren, S. (2001). Neurobiology of Pavlovian fear conditioning. *Annual Review of Neuroscience, 24,* 897–931.

McGaugh, J. L. (2000). Memory—A century of consolidation. *Science, 287*(5451), 248–251.

McGaugh, J. L. (2004). The amygdala modulates the consolidation of memories of emotionally arousing experiences. *Annual Review of Neuroscience, 27*(1), 1–28.

Mehrabian, A., & Epstein, N. (1972). A measure of emotional empathy1. *Journal of Personality, 40*(4), 525–543.

Mihov, Y., Kendrick, K. M., Becker, B., Zschernack, J., Reich, H., Maier, W., et al. (2013). Mirroring fear in the absence of a functional amygdala. *Biological Psychiatry, 73*(7), e9–e11.

Molenberghs, P., Cunnington, R., & Mattingley, J. B. (2012). Brain regions with mirror properties: A meta-analysis of 125 human fMRI studies. *Neuroscience and Biobehavioral Reviews, 36*(1), 341–349.

Morgan, M. A., Romanski, L. M., & LeDoux, J. E. (1993). Extinction of emotional learning: contribution of medial prefrontal cortex. *Neuroscience Letters, 163*(1), 109–113.

Moynahan, E. J. (1966). Hyalinosis cutis et mucosae (lipoid proteinosis): Demonstration of a new disorder of mucopolysaccharide metabolism. *Prococeedings of the Royal Society of Medicine, 59*(11, Pt. 1), 1125–1126.

Mukamel, R., Ekstrom, A. D., Kaplan, J., Iacoboni, M., & Fried, I. (2010). Single-neuron responses in humans during execution and observation of actions. *Current Biology, 20*(8), 750–756.

Onur, O. A., Walter, H., Schlaepfer, T. E., Rehme, A. K., Schmidt, C., Keysers, C., et al. (2009). Noradrenergic enhancement of amygdala responses to fear. *Social Cognitive and Affective Neuroscience, 4*(2), 119–126.

Ozawa, H., Sasaki, M., Sugai, K., Hashimoto, T., Matsuda, H., Takashima, S., et al. (1997). Single-photon emission CT and MR findings in Klüver–Bucy syndrome after Reye syndrome. *American Journal of Neuroradiology, 18*(3), 540–542.

Patin, A., & Hurlemann, R. (2011). Modulating amygdala responses to emotion: Evidence from pharmacological fMRI. *Neuropsychologia, 49*(4), 706–717.

Pessoa, L. (2008). On the relationship between emotion and cognition. *Nature Reviews Neuroscience, 9*(2), 148–158.

Phelps, E. A. (2004). Human emotion and memory: interactions of the amygdala and hippocampal complex. *Current Opinion in Neurobiology, 14*(2), 198–202.

Pitkanen, A., Savander, V., & LeDoux, J. E. (1997). Organization of intra-amygdaloid circuitries in the rat: An emerging framework for understanding functions of the amygdala. *Trends in Neuroscience, 20*(11), 517–523.

Ramón y Cajál, S. (1913–1914). *Estudios sobre la degeneración del sistema nervioso* [Degeneration and regeneration of the nervous system]. Madrid: Moya.

Rosenthal, A. R., & Duke, J. R. (1967). Lipoid proteinosis: Case report of direct lincal transmission. *American Journal of Ophthalmology, 64*(6), 1120–1125.

Salloway, S., Malloy, P., & Cummings, J. L. (1997). *The neuropsychiatry of limbic and subcortical disorders*. Washington, DC: American Psychiatric Press.

Scheele, D., Mihov, Y., Kendrick, K. M., Feinstein, J. S., Reich, H., Maier, W., et al. (2012). Amygdala lesion profoundly alters altruistic punishment. *Biological Psychiatry, 72*(3), e5–e7.

Seri, B., Garcia-Verdugo, J. M., McEwen, B. S., & Alvarez-Buylla, A. (2001). Astrocytes give rise to new neurons in the adult mammalian hippocampus. *Journal of Neuroscience, 21*(18), 7153–7160.

Seymour, B., & Dolan, R. (2008). Emotion, decision making, and the amygdala. *Neuron, 58*(5), 662–671.

Slotnick, B. M. (1973). Fear behavior and passive avoidance deficits in mice with amygdala lesions. *Physiology and Behavior, 11*(5), 717–720.

Sotres-Bayon, F., & Quirk, G. J. (2010). Prefrontal control of fear: More than just extinction. *Current Opinion in Neurobiology, 20*(2), 231–235.

Stine, O. C., & Smith, K. D. (1990). The estimation of selection coefficients in Afrikaners: Huntington disease, porphyria variegata, and lipoid proteinosis. *American Journal of Human Genetics, 46*(3), 452–458.

Stotland, E. (1969). Exploratory investigations of empathy. *Advances in Experimental Social Psychology, 4*, 271–314.

Strange, B., & Dolan, R. (2004). β-Adrenergic modulation of emotional memory-evoked human amygdala and hippocampal responses. *Proceedings of the National Academy of Sciences USA, 101*(31), 11454–11458.

Strange, B. A., Hurlemann, R., & Dolan, R. J. (2003). An emotion-induced retrograde amnesia in humans is amygdala- and beta-adrenergic-dependent. *Proceedings of the National Academy of Sciences USA, 100*(23), 13626–13631.

Swanson, L. W. (2003). The amygdala and its place in the cerebral hemisphere. *Annals of the New York Academy of Sciences, 985*, 174–184.

Swanson, L. W., & Petrovich, G. D. (1998). What is the amygdala? *Trends in Neurosciences, 21*(8), 323–331.

Talmi, D., Hurlemann, R., Patin, A., & Dolan, R. J. (2010). Framing effect following bilateral amygdala lesion. *Neuropsychologia, 48*(6), 1823–1827.

Terburg, D., Morgan, B. E., Montoya, E. R., Hooge, I. T., Thornton, H. B., Hariri, A. R., et al. (2012). Hypervigilance for fear after basolateral amygdala damage in humans. [Original Article]. *Translational Psychiatry, 2*, e115.

Tversky, A., & Kahneman, D. (1981). The framing of decisions and the psychology of choice. *Science, 211*(4481), 453–458.

Tye, K. M., Prakash, R., Kim, S. Y., Fenno, L. E., Grosenick, L., Zarabi, H., et al. (2011). Amygdala circuitry mediating reversible and bidirectional control of anxiety. *Nature, 471*(7338), 358–362.

Tyrer, P. (1988). Current status of beta-blocking drugs in the treatment of anxiety disorders. *Drugs, 36*(6), 773–783.

Urbach, E., & Wiethe, C. (1929). Lipoidosis cutis et mucosae [Lipoid proteinosis].*Virchows Archiv für Pathologische Anatomie und Physiologie und für klinische Medizin, 273*, 285–319.

van Stegeren, A. H., Goekoop, R., Everaerd, W., Scheltens, P., Barkhof, F., Kuijer, J., et al. (2005). Noradrenaline mediates amygdala activation in men and women during encoding of emotional material. *NeuroImage, 24*(3), 898–909.

Weisstaub, N. V., Zhou, M., Lira, A., Lambe, E., Gonzalez-Maeso, J., Hornung, J. P., et al. (2006). Cortical 5-HT$_{2A}$ receptor signaling modulates anxiety-like behaviors in mice. *Science, 313*(5786), 536–540.

Yeomans, J. S., & Frankland, P. W. (1995). The acoustic startle reflex: Neurons and connections. *Brain Research: Brain Research Reviews, 21*(3), 301–314.

CHAPTER 12

Consequences of Selective Bilateral Lesions to the Basolateral Amygdala in Humans

Jack van Honk
David Terburg
Helena Thornton
Dan J. Stein
Barak Morgan

Urbach–Wiethe disease (UWD) is rare genetic disorder characterized by developmental brain calcification with selective damage to the bilateral amygdala in some cases. Research on these subjects with UWD has contributed significantly to our understanding of the roles of the human amygdala in social and emotional behavior. In rodents, there is a wealth of research with multiple techniques (e.g., lesion, neuroimaging, pharmacological) investigating the role of the amygdala in social and emotional behavior, but a drawback is that these data are often not translatable to humans. Rodent research typically uses an amygdala subregion model with a focus on the basolateral amygdala (BLA) and the central–medial amygdala (CMA). The BLA and CMA in rodent research unmistakably have different and even antagonist social and emotional functions. In human research, however the amygdala is still mostly considered and researched as a unified structure. Recently, a group of subjects with UWD, identified in the Northern Cape mountain deserts of South Africa, arguably have provided a Rosetta Stone for the translation of rodent to human data. In this chapter, we discuss the remarkable history behind the relatively large population of South African subjects with UWD. Furthermore, we review our first findings from these subjects, focusing in particular on their fear processing, socioeconomic behavior, and emotional conflict processing. These new data not only seem to stand in stark contrast to the seminal findings on subjects with UWD with full amygdala damage, but also importantly are consistent with findings in rodents with BLA lesions. Further brain and behavioral research on this group, especially combined with research on subjects with full amygdala lesions, as well as with animal research, provides an important opportunity to better understand the function of the human amygdala.

Among the Rarest of Diseases

In 1929 two medical researchers from Austria, Erich Urbach and Camillo Wiethe, reported a rare genetic syndrome marked at birth by hoarseness of voice (Urbach & Wiethe, 1929) that came to bear the name Urbach–Wiethe disease (UWD). (UWD is known in the medical literature as lipoid proteinosis [LP].) Later in childhood, many, though not all, subjects with UWD suffer from easily damaged skin and poor wound healing. Nevertheless, UWD is not a life-threatening disease and does not seem to decrease lifespan. In 2002, Hamada and coworkers at the University of Witwatersrand in South Africa characterized the genetic bases of UWD. These involve very rare loss of function mutations within the extracellular matrix protein 1 gene (*ECM1*), leading to a recessive condition (Hamada et al., 2002). With a known world population of less than 100 subjects, UWD is among the rarest of genetic diseases. However, even more captivating and more rare are the manifestations of selective bilateral amygdala damage, first studied extensively in case SM046 and more recently in some other cases, especially in Germany (Markowitsch et al., 1994; Tranel & Hyman, 1990; Hurlemann et al., 2007). A further remarkable phenomenon is that nearly 50% of the identified individuals suffering from UWD live in South Africa. There is an interesting history behind this statistic. UWD was most likely introduced into South Africa with the arrival of the first European settlers in 1652. The *ECM1* mutation in UWD affects both sexes equally, but its infrequency and recessive nature make the disease very rare. However, when the first settlers arrived in South Africa, this population was a very small, closed community wherein rare mutations stand a much better chance to survive. Jacob Cloete and his sister Else from Cologne, Germany, were among the initial settlers of the South African Cape colony in 1652. They joined with and married into a colony of Dutch settlers, and Jacob is believed to be the progenitor of a relatively large number of Cloete families that still live in South Africa, especially in the Northern Cape province. Jacob and Else Cloete are thought to be the progenator of the disease in this extended set of relatives (Stine & Smith, 1990; Van Hougenhouck-Tulleken et al., 2004).

For nearly 150 years, the mutation remained in the white population, but in 1790 the Cloete family rejected Jasper Cloete because he was of mixed race. Jasper left the family, but he and his offspring are thought to be responsible for the widespread dissemination of the *ECM1* mutation into the mixed-race population of Namaqualand (Van Hougenhouck-Tulleken et al., 2004). There are early records of hundreds of UWD cases in this population but, as of 2014, only approximately 30 cases are known. Nonetheless, Namaqualand still contains the largest known UWD population in the world (Thornton et al., 2008). The mutation was also carried by a small population of white South Africans who left Namaqualand, possibly as part of the Gold Rush of 1886, which led to the establishment of sub-Saharan Africa's largest city, Johannesburg, on the Witwatersrand in what is now known as Gauteng province of South Africa. Originally there must have been more UWD cases in Gauteng also, but currently there are only a dozen identified cases distributed over the city of Johannesburg. This smaller UWD population in the urbanized Johannesburg environment might in coming generations completely disappear. Figure 12.1 shows the areas in which the white and mixed-race UWD groups live in South Africa.

The *ECM1* mutation in UWD is not uniform: It presents in variant forms, and the variants may well define the distribution of damage in the brain, and in the amygdala in particular. The mutation responsible for UWD in South Africa has been identified as the Q276X mutation in exon 7 of the *ECM1* gene, a mutation not yet described in any other UWD population. Focal bilateral damage to the amygdala is not present in all subjects with UWD; there are several reports of subjects with UWD having different and more extensive brain calcifications (Goncalves, de Melo, de L. Matos, Barra, & Figueroa, 2010) that sometimes do not even involve the amygdala. Behavioral manifestations of selective bilateral damage to

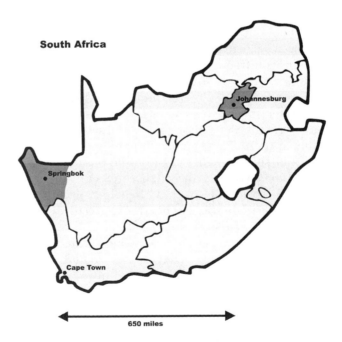

FIGURE 12.1. UWD group locations; Namaqualand, which is the area around Springbok and part of the Northern Cape province; Gauteng province, which is the area around Johannesburg.

the amygdala were first reported in UWD case SM046 (Tranel & Hyman, 1990), an adult female and currently the world's most famous living neurological patient.

Many important insights into the functions of the human amygdala have been gained from SM046, especially in the recognition, experience, and expression of fear (Adolphs, 2003; Adolphs et al., 2005; Adolphs, Tranel, Damasio, & Damasio, 1994; Feinstein, Adolphs, Damasio, & Tranel, 2011; see Feinstein, Adolphs, & Tranel, Chapter 1, this volume). Other key insights stemming from research with SM046 involve the role of the amygdala in social judgment (Adolphs, Tranel, & Damasio, 1998) and in the regulation of personal space (Kennedy, Glascher, Tyszka, & Adolphs, 2009; see Adolphs, Chapter 10, this volume). These single-case studies have greatly influenced the fields of social and affective neuroscience. However, there have also been noteworthy findings in other subjects with UWD. Hans Markowitsch, Larry Cahill, and colleagues investigated two German UWD cases (a male and a female), and provided key insights into the role of the human amygdala in emotional memory (Cahill, Babinsky, Markowitsch, & McGaugh, 1995; Markowitsch et al., 1994).

René Hurlemann and colleagues have a very productive line of research with two female patients (twins with UWD) from Germany, with focal amygdala damage. Their research provided further evidence on the role of the amygdala in emotion and memory, specifically, the interaction between episodic memory and emotion encoding that appears to depend on the amygdala (Hurlemann et al., 2007). Furthermore, the UWD twins showed deficits in emotional empathy but not in cognitive empathy (Hurlemann et al., 2010). Fear-processing deficits similar to those in SM046 were observed in only one of these twins with UWD. Fascinatingly, however, a recent neuroimaging study indicates that neuroplasticity in the cortical mirror neuron system may underly preserved fear processing in the other twin (Becker et al., 2012; see Patin & Hurlemann, Chapter 11, this volume). Finally, in a recent experiment, CO_2 inhalation was used to provoke panic and fear internally in both SM046 and the German twins with UWD. CO_2 did evoke slightly higher levels of fear and panic in these three amygdala-damaged subjects. Considering earlier findings with SM046, this suggests that the role of the amygdala may differ for externally and internally triggered fear (Feinstein et al., 2011, 2013; see Feinstein et al., Chapter 1, this volume).

Taken together, the data from mainly single and dual UWD case reports discussed earlier have been, and are, highly influential in the social and affective neurosciences. The main reasons for that impact is that these human natural lesion studies, unlike neuroimaging research, allow stronger causal inferences about the role of the amygdala, which otherwise are uncommon in research on human subjects, and the lesions are also relatively selective to the bilateral amygdala, with sparing of other structures. Case reports, of course, have their own limitation; see the editorial "When Once Is Enough" (2004) in *Nature Neuroscience* on this issue. But in the absence of causal evidence, human neuroscience is lost in correlation, and definitive conclusions are difficult to draw. Research on the South African UWD population may allow for larger sample sizes and substantiate earlier findings in UWD case reports, as well as provide for new insights into the workings of the human amygdala.

Namaqualand UWD Population

Helena Thornton performed the largest neuropsychological study to date on UWD in South Africa from 2002 to 2006 (Thornton et al., 2008). She researched both the Namaqualand and a part of the Gauteng population, and tested an impressive 34 subjects with UWD, mostly using standardized neuropsychological and psychiatric measures. Her scientific data and statistical analyses, however, focus on the Namaqualand group of 27 subjects that was matched with 47 controls from the same environment. Considering data from case SM046 demonstrating her pronounced deficiency in experiencing and expressing fear (Feinstein et al., 2011; see Feinstein et al., Chapter 1, this volume), it is remarkable that there is a high incidence of clinical and subclinical manifestation of anxiety disorders in the Namaqualand UWD population (Thornton et al., 2008). Furthermore, these subjects with UWD, compared to Namaqualand controls, performed poorly on several neuropsychological IQ measures, particularly memory and executive function, and they showed a decreased ability to recognize emotional expressions that was, however, not specific to fear.

These data deviate importantly from the findings in SM046, but brain measures had not yet been taken from the Namaqualand population. Thus, it has remained unclear whether there are brain calcifications in these subjects. The research performed by Thornton in Namaqualand nonetheless has been invaluable, mapping the distribution of a large number of hard-to-find subjects with UWD over the vast mountain desert areas of Namaqualand. In the same period of time, a group led by Hans Markowitsch from the University of Bielefeld in Germany, and Peter Bartel from the University of Pretoria in South Africa, started research on the smaller Gauteng UWD population, in which they did use brain measures (Siebert, Markowitsch, & Bartel, 2003).

Gauteng UWD Population

The project led by Markowitsch and Bartel is, to our knowledge, the largest UWD study to date using brain measures. Although no structural or functional magnetic resonance imaging (fMRI) was used, computed tomography (CT) and single-photon emission computerized tomography (SPECT) were used to investigate eight subjects with UWD from Gauteng. A single brain-damaged subject with UWD from Austria, assessed by CT and positron emission tomography (PET) was also included. The major South African part of the study was performed at the academic hospital of the University of Pretoria in Gauteng (Siebert et al., 2003). Although MRI currently is the "gold standard" for determining structural brain damage and brain calcifications (Wu et al., 2009), the combination of CT and SPECT also provides an invaluable window into structural and functional cerebral irregularities.

In the Siebert et al. (2003) study, temporal lobe perfusion abnormalities were observed in all subjects with UWD. Complete bilateral amygdala calcification was apparent in more than half of the patients in this group. However, CT and SPECT pointed out other calcifications in individual UWD cases (e.g., in the temporal lobes beyond the amygdala, expanding into uncinate and parahippocampal gyri, bilaterally to the parietal lobe, to the pineal gland and the basal ganglia. In summary, amygdala processing abnormalities were confirmed in the Gauteng UWD group investigated by Siebert and coworkers, but in many cases, calcified brain tissue was not confined to the amygdala or even to the temporal lobe. Notably, despite calcification in significant brain regions, these subjects with UWD displayed no obvious secondary psychopathology, and little, if any, of the cognitive, IQ-related impairments reported by Thornton et al. (2008) for the Namaqualand UWD population.

The Gauteng subjects with UWD were more highly educated than the Namaqualand subjects, which may account for some of these differences. Remarkably, four Gauteng subjects with UWD and calcifications to the brain finished high school, and two of these had a university degree. All in all, these educational data stand in stark contrast to those of the Namaqualand subjects with UWD. Furthermore, apart from a general IQ difference between the Namaqualand and the Gauteng UWD groups, Thornton et al. (2008) reported IQ impairments in the Namaqualand UWD group compared to healthy control subjects. It is possible that the secondary psychopathology in the Namaqualand UWD population also contributed to these relative IQ impairments.

Siebert and coworkers (2003), however, did find subtle abnormalities in negative and positive emotional memory in the Gauteng UWD group that coincide with earlier findings of the Markowitsch group (1994) on emotional memory impairments following amygdala damage. Furthermore, the patients with UWD had difficulties in judging the intensity of facial expressions, although no specific impairments in fear recognition were observed. In summary, Siebert et al. (2003) found minor emotion-processing deficits in Gauteng UWD group, but these brain damaged "patients" apparently functioned perfectly normally in everyday life. In this volume, Adolphs (Chapters 10) and Patin and Hurlemann (Chapter 11) discuss developmental neuroplasticity, which is relevant for understanding this observation.

The UWD study involving neuroimaging performed by Siebert et al. (2003) constitutes an invaluable and unique contribution. Apart from being the largest neuroscientific UWD study to date, it is the sole neuroscientific investigation of this particular UWD population. Additionally, their educational and neuropsychological IQ data are of particular interest when compared with those reported by Thornton et al. (2008) for a Namaqualand UWD group that carries the same *ECM1* mutation as its Gauteng counterparts (Stine & Smith, 1990).

It is, however, important to note that the UWD subjects from Gauteng are Caucasian, or "white," and therefore, in South Africa generally from a higher socioeconomic class and that they are from an urban environment. On the other hand, the Namaqualand UWD group of mixed-race subjects inhabit an economically impoverished rural environment and belong to a population that has suffered centuries of racial oppression, including the intentionally suboptimal education that prevailed when subjects were school-age children. The Gauteng group was educated at private schools, where the level of education in South Africa is high. The subjects from Namaqualand attended public schools, and the level of education in such schools is among the poorest in the world. Thus, findings from these groups are not directly comparable.

Excluding Secondary Pathology in the Namaqualand UWD Population

To get further insights into the impact of amygdala lesions, we focused our follow-up research, which started in 2007 in Cape Town, on the otherwise healthy Namaqualand UWD population (including only subjects with absence of any secondary brain pathology). We also exclusively studied females for several reasons. The first and main reason is that there was apparently less secondary pathology in UWD females. The explanation for this is not clear, but it may partly be due to alcohol abuse in the male UWD Namaqualand population. The choice to focus exclusively on females also is an advantage in that we can compare our data better because the majority of publications related to UWD cases in human neuroscience involve female subjects, especially SM046 and the German twins of Hurlemann and colleagues (2007). Sex differences suggest that sex hormones might affect calcification processes, as well as subsequent neuroplasticity in the brain (van Honk, 2009; see Patin & Hurlemann, Chapter 11, this volume).

In 2007, we selected five otherwise healthy subjects with UWD and 12 healthy controls, all from Namaqualand. We genetically screened both the subjects and the controls, and as expected, subjects with UWD were homozygous for the *ECM1* mutation, whereas all controls proved homozygous for the normal variant of the gene. Furthermore, the Full Scale IQ, Performance IQ and Verbal IQ levels we found were similar to those measured 5 years earlier and reported by Thornton et al. (2008). However, at that time, there were no significant differences between subjects with UWD and controls on any of these IQ measures. Subjects with UWD even scored slightly higher on the Wechsler Adult Intelligence Scale–III (WAIS-III; Wechsler, 1997) than controls. These new data from the Namaqualand subjects with UWD seemed to agree with the findings on the subjects with UWD from Gauteng (Siebert et al., 2003), that is, with respect to the differences between UWD subject and healthy controls. Presumably, our preselection of a criterion of absence of secondary pathology removed the earlier observed IQ differences between UWD and control subjects.

Nonetheless, several of our subjects with UWD and controls still scored in the low borderline range. The WAIS-III, however, was developed according to Western norms, and its use in other cultural settings is problematic. This reflects the WEIRD (Western, Educated, Industrialized, Rich and Democratic) discussion, which is currently transforming psychology and neuroscience (Henrich, Heine, & Norenzayan, 2010a, 2010b; Jones, 2010). Most of the data from psychology and human neuroscience are drawn from WEIRD populations, especially from college students. Data from this relatively unrepresentative sample of students is recorded in standard psychology textbooks as normative, but in the world at large the behaviors of this group are literally weird, in the sense of being unrepresentative (Henrich et al., 2010a, 2010b; Jones, 2010).

Our subjects clearly are non-WEIRD and therefore have a great cultural and educational disadvantage in performing on the WAIS-III. In an attempt to get a more objective picture, we made changes to the way the tests were administered and tested everyone again in the period 2010–2012. First, our subjects with UWD and controls were tested in their local environment, by a local psychologist who speaks their dialect. We furthermore used an abbreviated test, the Wechsler Abbreviated Scale of Intelligence (WASI; which provides for a reliable IQ estimate [Wechsler, 1999]), because the subjects were overwhelmed by the hours of WAIS-III testing in 2007. Finally, the Verbal IQ tests were carefully translated into the language spoken in Namaqualand.

The 2010–2012 IQ scores showed a global increase of approximately 10%, with all participants with UWD now falling into the normal range. We attribute the IQ improvement to the fact that in 2007, participants were tested in a strange environment by a person of a different race, culture, and language group. The 2010–2012 IQ scores we currently use nonetheless are likely an underestimate of the intellectual capabilities of this population, because we obviously cannot overcome all cultural, language, and educational biases inherent in the WASI (Nell, 2000).

The next critical issue for our research was to find out the extent of damage to the brain in these subjects with UWD from Namaqualand, and especially to see whether they had selective and bilateral calcifications to the amygdala.

Structural and Functional Neuroimaging in the Namaqualand UWD Population

UWD often leads to calcifications in the brain, but these calcifications are not uniform; they vary from subject to subject and are often not selective to the amygdala. The reason for the variation in brain calcification is not clear, but it might depend on the type of *ECM1* mutation. To get firm insights into the neurological status in the Namaqualand subjects with UWD, we carried out structural MRIs (sMRIs) and functional MRIs (fMRIs) in our five (otherwise healthy) female subjects with UWD. sMRI and lesion overlap techniques were used to establish amygdala subregion damage, and fMRI was used to establish remaining amygdala subregion functionality. High-resolution MRI scans were made to produce three-dimensional (3D) structural images, which is the most common methodology for inspecting amygdala calcifications in UWD (Adolphs et al., 2005; Hurlemann et al., 2007), together with functional measurements of brain activity in response to emotional stimuli (Terburg et al., 2012). After the structural MRI scan was obtained, subjects with UWD performed an "emotion-matching task" during fMRI scanning. The emotion-matching task, a highly validated and widely used paradigm, can provide an index of amygdala activation when the participant is comparing the emotional expressions of multiple faces (Hariri et al., 2002). This task has the advantage that it simultaneously recruits both those parts of the amygdala that automatically respond to emotional faces and the parts involved in the more complex process of recognizing and comparing different emotions. As such, this task recruits the full amygdala, which makes it very suitable for the identification of healthy and functional amygdala tissue.

Figure 12.2 shows a selected brain slice for each of the five women we examined. It can be seen that the calcifications occur symmetrically within both hemispheres, and seem to increase with age. Our comparisons of these scans with so-called "cytoarchitectonic probability maps" of the amygdala and the adjacent hippocampus (Amunts et al., 2005) clearly showed that the calcifications are located almost exclusively within the basolateral amygdala (BLA) and spare other regions of the amygdala, such as the central and superficial nuclei. Quantification confirmed that

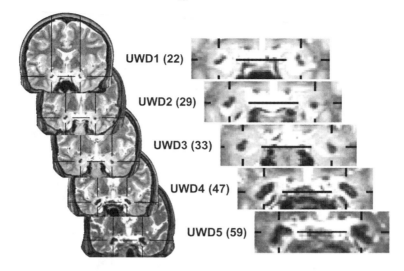

FIGURE 12.2. T2-weighted magnetic resonance images (coronal view) of the five subjects with UWD, with age at the time of scanning and crosshairs indicating the calcified brain damage.

the other subregions are spared from calcification; indeed, the central–medial and superficial regions of the amygdala were significantly activated during the emotion-matching task (Terburg et al., 2012).

In summary, the main results of our combined structural–functional MRI analyses in five subjects with UWD confirmed bilateral damage that was restricted to the BLA. On the basis of visual inspection, together with probability analyses of high-resolution structural MRI lesion overlap and of fMRI activations, we can conclude that these five women have calcifications on both sides of their brain, that these calcifications are localized within the BLA, and that the other areas of the amygdala are spared and functional.

When comparing these findings with what is known of the amygdala damage in SM046 and the German twins with UWD, also taking into account age, there is substantially less extensive amygdala damage in our subjects with UWD, and notably no damage to the central–medial amygdala (CMA). Partial to complete CMA calcifications were observed in the German twins and SM046. Reasons for these differences might be that the calcification process is slower in subjects with UWD from Namaqualand, or has a later onset. The BLA comprises a cortical type of neuronal tissue, whereas the CMA has a striatal type of neuronal tissue, and calcification in the Namaqualand subjects with UWD might for yet unknown reasons not progress into striatal-type CMA tissue. Different *ECM1* mutations, or perhaps gene × environment interactions may play a role.

Why might it be relevant that damage to the amygdala is completely or selectively restricted to the BLA? To start with, there is abundant research showing different behavioral effects after lesions to, or pharmacological manipulation of, the BLA or the CMA (Balleine & Killcross, 2006). We can therefore anticipate that behavioral effects of lesions to the BLA may also differ from those seen after lesions to both BLA and CMA. Stalnaker, Franz, Singh, and Schoenbaum (2007) even suggest that complete amygdala lesions (lesions to both BLA and CMA) may negate the behavioral effects of lesions to the BLA. The BLA receives basic, as well as highly processed, sensory information from especially the thalamus and the prefrontal cortex (PFC), and projects to the CMA. The CMA projects to hypothalamic and brainstem target areas that directly mediate fear, and the CMA underlies the execution of a fear response. There is mounting evidence that the rodent BLA also implements regulation of acute fear responses and responses to unconditioned innate fear stimuli. Pharmacological manipulation or selective inactivation of the BLA in rodents produces fear hypervigilance (Graeff & Del-Ben, 2008; Macedo, Cuadra, Molina, & Brandao, 2005; Macedo, Martinez, Albrechet-Souza, Molina, & Brandao, 2007; Macedo, Martinez, & Brandao, 2006; Martinez, Ribeiro de Oliveira, & Brandao, 2007). Moreover, Tye et al., (2011) demonstrated that optogenetic activation of a BLA–CMA pathway can reduce innate fear behaviors, which implies that the regulation of fear behaviors by the BLA is directly via the CMA. However, the BLA can also regulate the behavioral output functions of the CMA via the PFC, that is, especially the orbitofrontal cortex (OFC; Barbas, Saha, Rempel-Clower, & Ghashghaei, 2003).

On the basis of these findings in rodents, it may be hypothesized that selective damage to the BLA in our subjects with UWD should result in increased fear responses to innate danger cues (fear hypervigilance). Damage to BLA and CMA (or complete amygdala) should, however, hinder the execution of fear response, and produce the fear hypovigilance observed in SM046 (Feinstein et al., 2011). The crucial hypothesis now is to test whether our subjects with UWD and bilateral calcifications limited to the BLA show increased behavioral response to innate fear stimuli. However, first we address another hypothesis about the essential sensory role of the BLA, that is, its presumed role as the brain's salience detector, continuously on the lookout for dangers and rewards in the environment (Sander, Grafman, & Zalla, 2003).

The Working Memory Paradox

Within the amygdala, the BLA is the central structure for processing sensory information. The vast majority of incoming thalamic and cortical signals converge in the BLA, and most of the fibers projecting from the amygdala to the cortex stem from the BLA. The BLA has bidirectional connections with sensory association cortices, and extremely rich bidirectional connections with the main sensory system of the PFC, the OFC (Davis & Whalen, 2001). The BLA, also by interacting with and regulating the OFC, acts as a central hub orchestrating the activity of multifarious cortical and subcortical networks to ensure continual detection, evaluation, and regulation of salient information. The BLA is the sensory amygdala, the salience detector of the brain, constantly on the lookout for rewarding and threatening stimuli in the environment (Sander et al., 2003).

fMRI studies on working memory that measure amygdala activity indeed suggest that salience detection is a continuous process that consumes brain resources at the expense of PFC executive systems; that is, amygdala activity is inversely correlated with working memory (WM) performance (Anticevic, Repovs, & Barch, 2010). The dorsolateral prefrontal cortex (DLPFC) controls working memory, and failure to suppress amygdala activation under increasing WM load hampers performance (Yun, Krystal, & Mathalon, 2010). Hypothetically, the BLA takes away resources from the DLPFC, via its connections with the OFC, and this in turn impairs WM. Indeed, to perform properly on working memory, progressively less amygdala activation and more DLPFC activation is necessary with increasing load. And amygdala activity impairs WM performance not only during negative affect but also when nothing salient is happening (Anticevic et al., 2010). This suggests that the amygdala (or perhaps more accurately the BLA) operates automatically as a surveillance mechanism, continuously consuming processing resources. If the BLA automatically consumes resources at the expense of the PFC executive systems, selective damage to the BLA in our subjects with UWD might lead to WM improvement.

We investigated this hypothesis in young adult subjects with UWD (UWD 1, 2, and 3) and a matched (age, education, and IQ) healthy control group (n = 10), also from Namaqualand (Morgan, Terburg, Thornton, Stein, & van Honk, 2012). IQ and WM generally are positively correlated; thus, the matching on IQ is a conservative approach and reduces the chance for finding differences in WM between UWD and control subjects. For WM, the WAIS-III (Wechsler, 1997) Digit Span Forward (DSF) task was used and administered to all subjects. In this task, a sequence of digits is read aloud to the participant, who must then verbally repeat the sequence. The first item comprises a sequence of only two digits; the second item, three digits; the third item, four digits; and so on. There are two trials per item (e.g., the third item comprises two separate four-digit sequence trials). Subjects score one point for each correct trial. The task continues until the subject fails both trials of any item.

To exclude alternative explanations in terms of possible emotional differences between UWD and control subjects, the Spielberger State–Trait Anxiety Inventory (STAI-T; Spielberger, Gorusch, & Lushene, 1970) was administered. Furthermore, the researchers controlled for differences in mood during the WM task by asking subjects to rate their subjective feelings of stress and tension on a scale from 1 to 100 after performing the WM task. Figure 12.3 shows the results with significantly enhanced WM in BLA-damaged subjects with UWD compared to controls. Self-reported measures of trait anxiety, stress, and tension showed no group differences.

This enhanced WM performance following BLA damage can be defined as "paradoxical functional facilitation" (Kapur, 1996), a phenomenon resulting from reduced interference caused by dysfunction of a part of the brain. In the present context, the BLA's salience surveillance via especially the OFC normally interferes with the WM functions of the DLPFC, and damage to the BLA in our subjects with UWD reduced or removed this interference and allowed the DLPFC to perform better than normal on WM. In summary, our data from these BLA-damaged subjects provide evidence for a tonic regulatory function of the BLA, that is, surveillance for salient stimuli or threat in the environment, at a cost for PFC executive networks with which the BLA competes for resources (Figure 12.3).

More research, however, is necessary to confirm these findings and interpretations. The next steps are to investigate WM in these subjects with UWD under high-load and changing threat conditions, and to perform neuroimaging experiments with validated WM designs (Yun et al., 2010; Anticevic et al., 2010) in both UWD and healthy subjects using BLA and CMA as regions of interest (ROIs). Neuroimaging of functional connectivity in these patients could confirm whether the salience network of the human brain (e.g., anterior insula, dorsal anterior cingulate cortex, and midbrain; Craig, 2009; Seeley et al., 2007), is indeed hypoactive under nonthreatening and resting-state conditions.

Innate and Acute Fear

The human BLA is constantly scanning the environment for salient and especially threatening stimuli. What happens in case the BLA detects a threat? Different scenarios are possible because threats may be mild or severe (e.g., distant or nearby; Mobbs et al., 2007). The BLA is best capable, positioned and connected, to estimate the severity and the distance of threat and to regulate the brain depending on this threat imminence. Indeed, as described earlier, rodent research suggests that the BLA directly and indirectly, by way of the OFC, exerts regulatory control

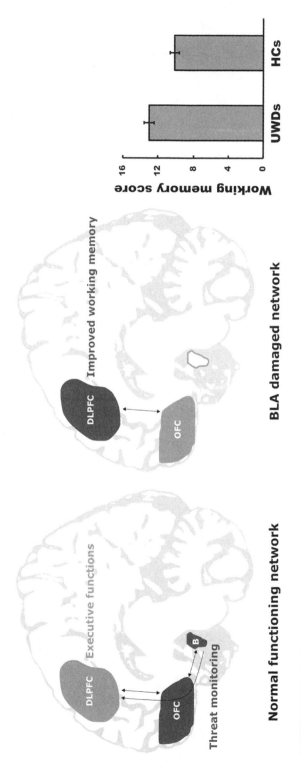

FIGURE 12.3. Safe environment model and improved working memory performance in UWD. The basolateral amygdala, together with the orbitofrontal cortex (OFC), continuously scan the environment for threat, which takes resources from prefrontal executive functioning. Basolateral amygdala (B) damage therefore results in improved working memory. DLPFC, dorsolateral prefrontal cortex.

of the fear response at the level of the CMA and the brainstem (Graeff & Del-Ben, 2008; Macedo et al., 2005, 2006; Macedo, Martinez, Albrechet-Souza, Molina, & Brandao, 2007; Martinez et al., 2007; Tye et al., 2011).

An important human neuroimaging study (Mobbs et al., 2007) compared such regulation in response to distant and close threat. The study suggests that regulation might be inhibitory in the case of mild, distant, and avoidable threat. That is, hypothetically, mild threat cues and distant dangers recruit BLA and OFC to increase evaluation of the situation and may also exert inhibitory control, because activation of the fear response is not yet warranted. However, when threat becomes imminent and cannot be avoided, the BLA (and therefore the OFC) switches off its inhibition, resulting in activation of the CMA and the brainstem periaqueductal gray (PAG): The fear response is activated (Mobbs et al., 2007). The BLA in this model functions as a switchboard, regulating the inhibition and the activation of the fear response directly and indirectly by the OFC at the CMA level (Graeff & Del-Ben, 2008; Macedo et al., 2005, 2006, 2007; Martinez et al., 2007; Tye et al., 2011).

However, no research has directly addressed the question of whether the human BLA inhibits the fear response to mild, innate threat cues. The key innate threat cue in humans is the fearful facial expression, which provides us with a silent salience signal that warns the onlooker of impending threats of an ambiguous nature (van Honk, Peper, & Schutter, 2005). UWD subject SM042, who has damage to the BLA and the CMA, is impaired in the recognition of facial fear (Adolphs et al., 1994). This impairment is caused by her inability to direct her attention automatically to the defining fearful eyes of these expressions (Adolphs et al., 2005). SM046 demonstrates lack of fear in behavior and experience when confronted with other (even nearby and nonambiguous) innate threat cues (i.e., spiders and snakes; (Feinstein et al., 2011; see Adolphs, Chapter 10, this volume). Remarkably, members of the Namaqualand UWD population seem predisposed for fear: They have an abnormally high prevalence of anxiety disorders (Thornton et al., 2008). To critically address this apparent discrepancy we investigated the processing of innate fear stimuli in this UWD population in five subjects with UWD (see Figure 12.2).

The conscious recognition of fear, as measured by emotion recognition tasks, is not an emotional response. However, our first experiment was designed in line with the seminal reports on SM042 (Adolphs et al., 1994, 2005) to test facial emotion recognition and visual attention using infrared eye tracking. The five BLA-damaged subjects with UWD and a group of 12 healthy women from the same mountain desert villages in Namaqualand, of the same age and with similar IQs, watched short video clips of neutral faces changing in increments of 10% into full-blown angry, disgusted, fearful, happy, sad, and surprised expressions. Subjects had to identify the emotion of the face, which, over the course of the task, therefore became gradually easier to identify. This is a highly sensitive measure of emotion recognition, with the added value that we could record eye movements over a substantial number of trials of varying difficulty. The five BLA-damaged subjects with UWD compared to the control group performed better in the recognition of full-blown facial fear. Furthermore, they looked equally often to the eyes of the faces but, crucially, when looking at fearful eyes, they did so for a longer period of time. This is a completely opposite pattern of fear recognition and eye tracking behavior than that observed for SM046, but our findings nonetheless confirm the relation between visual attention to the eyes and fear recognition (Adolphs et al., 2005). SM042 does not automatically look at fearful eyes and is therefore impaired in recognizing fear, whereas our subjects with UWD looked longer than did control subjects at the fearful eyes and therefore demonstrated above-normal fear recognition (Terburg et al., 2012).

The next important question is why there is this hyperattention to the fearful eyes in our BLA-damaged subjects. One hypothesis is that these subjects with UWD are simply hypervigilant for fear. A successful research paradigm for investigating fear hypervigilance in humans is the emotional Stroop task. Attentional biases in terms of increased color-naming reaction times to threat stimuli observed in the emotional Stroop task are observed in subjects with subclinical fear and fear disorders, and point at fear hypervigilance (Williams, Mathews, & MacLeod, 1996). The most reliable findings with the emotional Stroop task occur on subliminal (i.e., unconscious) processing levels, that is, when using backwardly masked stimuli (van Honk et al., 2005; van Honk, Schutter, d'Alfonso, Kessels, & de Haan, 2002). We used this subliminal emotional Stroop task to assess whether BLA-damaged subjects with UWD were hypervigilant to unseen fearful faces (van Honk et al., 2005). This task exploits subtle interference caused by unconsciously processed emotional stimuli on performance of a reaction time task, in this case, color naming. The participants see nonsense images that are blue, green, or red, and are instructed to name the color as fast as possible. What they do not know is that just before these images are presented, a happy, fearful, or neutral face is presented. This face is presented for only 14 milliseconds and is not consciously visible. Nonetheless, the emotional content of the face automatically captures attention, revealed by a slowdown in the naming of the color of the nonsense image, which serves as the backward mask.

We convincingly demonstrate unconscious fear hypervigilance in our BLA-damaged subjects with UWD (see Figure 12.4). Thus, fearful eyes not only attract more attention consciously in the emotion recognition task, but apparently also do so nonconsciously (Whalen et al., 2004) in the BLA-damaged subjects compared to control subjects. These findings correspond to data from rodent research that indicate the BLA exerts regulatory control over innate and acute fear responses. Inhibitory regulation

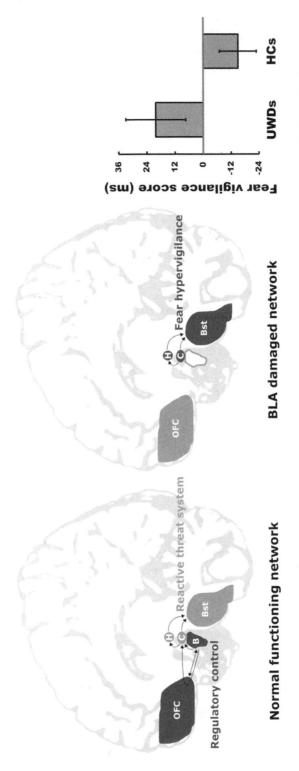

FIGURE 12.4. Innate threat model and fear hypervigilance in UWD. The basolateral amygdala (B), together with the orbitofrontal cortex (OFC), act out inhibitory control on the central–medial amygdala (C) when threat cues are mild or when danger is distant. Basolateral amygdala damage therefore results in hypervigilant responses to innate fear cues. Bst, brainstem; H, hypothalamus.

by the BLA of the fear response to the mild threat cues (e.g., facial fear) prevents unwarranted hypervigilant fear responses from being executed by the CMA (Graeff & Del-Ben, 2008; Macedo et al., 2005, 2006, 2007; Martinez et al., 2007; Tye et al., 2011), but this mechanism is not fully functional in our BLA-damaged subjects.

The BLA subserves fear behaviors in calculated, instrumental, and goal-directed ways, and, as noted, it has the sensory inputs and the regulatory outputs to do that. The CMA, on the other hand, acts reflexively and on impulse in fear behaviors, and without proper regulation by the BLA, the CMA may execute uncalled-for fear responses (Macedo et al., 2005; Tye et al., 2011; see Figure 12.4).

These are the fundamentals of the serial amygdala processing model, in which the BLA directly and indirectly, by way of the OFC, regulates acute and innate fear responses on the level of the CMA, while the CMA executes the fear response at hypothalamic and brainstem levels (Macedo et al., 2005; Terburg et al., 2012; Tye et al., 2011). In the light of this model, our data suggest that unless restrained by the BLA, the CMA executes hypervigilant responses to mild threat cues in the Namaqualand subjects with UWD (Terburg et al., 2012). A shortcoming of this interpretation is that the CMA is considered to be dependent on the BLA's sensory input for producing the innate fear response.

The question is how that sensory input can reach the CMA in our BLA-damaged subjects and produce the hypervigilant fear response. First, the OFC and the superficial amygdala (SFA) are regions that are also involved in sensory processing, and act upon the CMA, and the sensory transfer of fear information might have shifted to OFC and SFA as a result of plasticity (see Patin & Hurlemann, Chapter 11, this volume). Second, the brain calcifications in our subjects with UWD are focal and bilateral, and increase with age, but do not cover the complete BLA. Since the BLA has various subregions with different functions, it might be speculated that the calcifications have especially damaged regions involved in fear regulation, with less damage to those regions involved in BLA–CMA sensory transfer. However, Macedo et al. (2006) showed that BLA inactivation in rodents resulted in increased unconditioned fear, suggesting that the BLA's sensory input is not indispensable for the fear response. Future research in the South African UWD population is necessary to for more definitive insights into humans.

Nonetheless, after damage to both BLA and CMA in SM046, the fear response logically cannot be executed. Accordingly, SM046 is hypovigilant for innate threat cues, even when danger is clear and present (Feinstein et al., 2011). In summary, on the basis of the combined data in SM046 and the Namaqualand subjects with UWD, the rodent serial amygdala processing model appears to translate seamlessly to the human case.

When Conflict Arises

Evidence for improved fear recognition, enhanced attentional capture of fearful eyes, and unconscious fear hypervigilance in the Namaqualand subjects with UWD (Terburg et al., 2012) provides novel insights into the function of the human BLA in innate and acute fear processing. However, one might wonder, given improved WM in this group (Morgan et al., 2012), whether selective damage to the BLA would not lead to more impairment in information processing on the behavioral level. To investigate this matter, we focused on conflict in the processing of emotional faces and emotional body language. Increased reactivity to threat (fear hypervigilance) may be beneficial in truly dangerous situations, but unwarranted hypervigilant responses to mildly threatening facial expressions may lead to behavioral impairment in the case of conflicting tasks. We found that in nonthreatening conditions, WM is improved in BLA-damaged subjects with UWD (Morgan et al., 2012), but when a mild threat is introduced, advantage may turn to disadvantage because, theoretically, when unrestrained, the CMA executes unwarranted hypervigilant fear responses to mild threat cues, as seen in emotional Stroop interference in response to masked facial fear (Terburg et al., 2012). We tested this idea further on the perceptual level using the so-called "face–body compound task," which exploits the fact that a person can send emotionally conflicting information when the facial expression does not fit the body language (Meeren, van Heijnsbergen, & de Gelder, 2005). For instance, a person with an angry face who holds up his fists sends a clear signal of aggression, but when the upraised fists are accompanied by a fearful face, it is hard to judge the person's intentions.

BLA damage in subjects with UWD was therefore expected to result in greater difficulty in dealing with emotionally conflicting information. In the face–body compound task, participants need to identify the facial emotion (angry or fearful) of a person who simultaneously expresses the same or a different (again, angry or fearful) emotion. In these experiments, we again used eye tracking to make sure objectively that the participants actually looked at the face when identifying its emotion, and not at the body. The three youngest subjects with UWD were tested (see Figure 12.2), and we first confirmed in a control experiment that they, as well as the healthy control group, were able to identify bodily emotions correctly (de Gelder et al., 2014).

The results on the face–body compound task support our notion that subjects with UWD have greater difficulty with emotionally conflicting information. Both groups performed very well on recognizing the facial emotions that were accompanied by a body expressing the same emotion. As expected, performance of the healthy control group dropped when the bodily emotion did not match the facial emotion, but in the UWD group, this drop was much more dramatic. Importantly, the eye tracking data indicated that all subjects looked predominantly at the faces, which confirms that they did try to identify the facial emotion as instructed. Note that there were no differences in fear recognition. This, however, is not surprising, because the emotion recognition task in which differences in fear recognition were observed is a more sensitive recognition paradigm, employing a gradual expression morphing technique (Terburg et al., 2012). BLA-damaged subjects were perfectly capable of identifying the facial emotions, but they crucially failed when the bodily emotion provided conflicting information. In other words, BLA-damaged subjects are behaviorally impaired in situations in which different emotions need to be processed that provide for conflicting information. We argue that this is caused by the lack of inhibitory regulation on the level of the CMA as a result of BLA dysfunction. Inappropriate fear activation resources were distributed to processing mildly threating emotional stimuli that should have been ignored.

Generous Economic Investments

In classical economic models, humans are rational and instrumental, and their decisions are based on cost–benefit analyses. Contemporary views, however, propose that human decisions can also be affective–impulsive, and noninstrumental ("economically irrational") in nature. This dichotomy is observed in trust interactions between an investor and a trustee in the trust game. When investors perceive potential partners as trustworthy, high investments can be instrumental, because high returns are anticipated. However, with affective–impulsive decisions, high investments may occur for noninstrumental reasons in the absence of expectations for high profits (van Honk, Eisenegger, Terburg, Stein, & Morgan, 2013).

Economic behaviors in both rodents and humans involve the brain's reward system and especially the nucleus accumbens (NAc) (Floresco, St Onge, Ghods-Sharifi, & Winstanley, 2008; Knutson, Rick, Wimmer, Prelec, & Loewenstein, 2007). And recent human neuroimaging data suggest that the question of whether economic decisions will be selfish or prosocial is decided on the levels of the NAc and amygdala (Haruno, Kimura, & Frith, 2014). Indeed, parallel processing models of the rodent amygdala imply that the BLA subserves (selfish) calculative–instrumental economic choice behaviors by directly acting on the NAc, and by its indirect regulatory actions via the OFC on the NAc. The CMA separately by its actions on the NAc contrariwise subserves impulsive–affective economic choice behaviors (Balleine & Killcross, 2006; Phillips, Ahn, & Howland, 2003), and these might be prosocial in nature.

We performed neuroeconomic research in Namaqualand to investigate whether the parallel amygdala model of economic behavior might be applicable to the human case. Crucially, the leading dual-perspective view of economics claims that humans correspondingly are instrumental and impulsive in their economic decisions (Camerer, Loewenstein, & Prelec, 2005; Fehr & Camerer, 2007). We used the Trust Game, wherein low and high investments can be rational (calculative) and goal-directed (instrumental) when done in the expectation of subsequently low or high returns. Materialistic, egoistic concerns underlie such economic choices. However, low and high investments in the Trust Game can also be impulsive–affective in nature when they are done for noninstrumental reasons in the absence of any expectations of return. Low investments might be driven by an aggressive impulse, whereas high investments suggest prosocial, altruistic motives (van Honk et al., 2013).

BLA-damage on the basis of the parallel processing amygdala model for economic behavior, might impair subjects in behaving in calculative–instrumental ways in socioeconomic situations. A one-shot Trust Game (Kosfeld, Heinrichs, Zak, Fischbacher, & Fehr, 2005) was used to address this question. Three young adult subjects with UWD participated (see Figure 12.2) and were compared to 12 healthy controls matched for age, intelligence, environment, and economic income. To understand the motivations underlying the behavior in the Trust Game, we also investigated general risk-taking behaviors, expectations about back-transfers of the trustees, and trustworthiness ratings of unfamiliar faces.

The results showed that our BLA-damaged subjects transfer nearly 100% more money to the anonymous trustees than do control subjects. In the risk task, a lottery using the exact monetary properties as the Trust Game, there were no significant differences. BLA-damaged subjects even took slightly less risk than did control subjects. In summary, the social nature of the Trust Game caused the different investments in BLA-damaged subjects and controls (see Figure 12.5).

One "social" reason might be that BLA-damaged subjects are simply socially naive and have overly optimistic expectations about the trustees´ monetary returns. Accordingly, we measured subjects' expectations about the trustees' back-transfers, but there were no differences between BLA-damaged subjects and control subjects in expected return. Both the BLA-damaged and the control subjects expected no fair sharing by the trustees; the overall expected return was very low. This is in keeping with the fact that all these subjects belong to the mixed-race Namaqualand population that endured long-term social and economic abuse during Apartheid. The low levels of *psychological* trust were substantiated by follow-up interview. However, whereas control subjects suggested that their investments in the Trust Game were low because they did not expect fair sharing by trustees (a calculative–instrumental decision), BLA-damaged

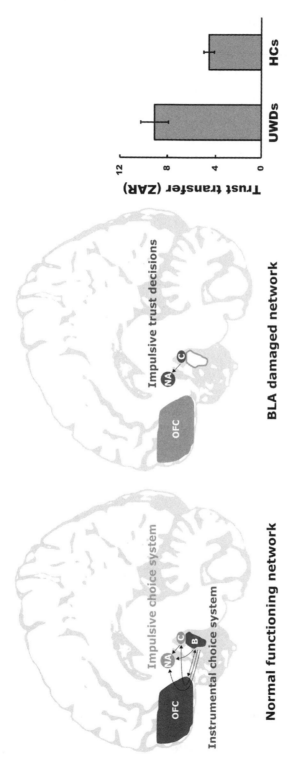

FIGURE 12.5. Parallel socioeconomic choice model and increased generosity in UWD. The parallel outputs of the basolateral (B) and central–medial amygdala (C) to the nucleus accumbens (NA), respectively, subserve calculative–instrumental and affective–impulsive economic choice behaviors. Basolateral amygdala damage therefore results in the impulse-driven decision to contribute generously in the Trust Game. OFC, orbitofrontal cortex.

subjects could not provide a rationale for their irrational generosity in the Trust Game, which suggests that it is based on impulsive–affective choice. We argued, therefore, that their generous investments are altruistic in nature (van Honk et al., 2013).

Low levels of psychological trust in BLA-damaged subjects seem remarkable in light of findings in subjects with extensive amygdala damage (Adolphs et al., 1998), who show heightened trustworthiness ratings of unfamiliar faces. However, as noted, damage to the BLA produces different and perhaps even opposite effects than damage to both the BLA and CMA (Stalnaker et al., 2007). We also tested the BLA-damaged subjects and matched controls with an adapted version of Adolphs et al.'s (1998) facial trustworthiness task (see Bos, Terburg, & van Honk, 2010). Corresponding to results on back-transfer expectations, trustworthiness ratings in BLA-damaged and control subjects were low, and there were no group differences.

In summary, our economic data indicate that three young adult subjects with UWD and focal bilateral damage to the BLA invested generously in unfamiliar others in the Trust Game. Furthermore, this generosity is not based on risk-taking abnormalities or social naivete. Selective damage to the human BLA thus impairs instrumental choice behavior; that is, the irrational large investments of our BLA-damaged subjects in the Trust Game are affective–impulsive behaviors, which are hypothetically driven by the CMA (Balleine & Killcross, 2006; Phillips et al., 2003; Terburg et al., 2012; Tye et al., 2011; see Figure 12.5). Follow-up behavioral and neuroimaging research in these BLA-damaged subjects with learning paradigms in a social context, such as repeated Trust Games, is necessary for more definitive insights into this matter.

Conclusions, Prospects, and Priorities

In rodents and humans there is a wealth of research with multiple techniques (e.g., lesion, neuroimaging, pharmacological) investigating the role of the amygdala in social and affective behavior. Many important insights have been gained from these lines of human and animal research, but a drawback is that the data are often not readily translatable to humans. The data presented in this chapter on Namaqualand subjects with UWD and selective bilateral damage to the BLA, on the other hand, are consistent with prominent rodent models of the function of the BLA and CMA in fear and economic behaviors.

The reasons for this good match, in our view, is because the Namaqualand UWD group provided an opportunity to investigate the BLA selectively, and it is by far the most studied subregion in rodents. Rodent research focuses often on not only the BLA but also the CMA and has established that these amygdala substructures have separate, and even antagonistic, functions on a wide variety of behaviors. Structural and functional neuroimaging techniques in humans currently allow analyses of these amygdala subnuclei, but most researchers still investigate and discuss the human amygdala as a single unit.

This undifferentiated amygdala model used in humans has been very influential in both neuroimaging research and lesions studies. High-impact research studies of subjects with UWD and complete and nearly complete amygdala lesions have in the last two decades importantly contributed to our understanding of the role of the human amygdala in social and affective behavior (Adolphs et al., 1994, 1998, 2005; Becker et al., 2012; Feinstein et al., 2011, 2013; Hurlemann et al., 2010; Siebert et al., 2003; Strange, Hurlemann, & Dolan, 2003). The unprecedentedly large cohort of still largely unexplored South African UWD subjects provides further and new opportunities, especially for better understanding the function of amygdala subregions in humans, and for investigating parallels between the rodent and human BLA.

International collaborations with researchers from animal and human neuroscience are currently under way to exploit these opportunities. Further in-depth insights into the roles of the human BLA and CMA in innate fear processing might be gained by comparative behavioral and neuroimaging research on the Namaqualand UWD subjects with selective damage to the BLA, and UWD subjects with damage to BLA and CMA (Feinstein et al., 2013). Our key hypothesis is that fear hypervigilance in BLA-damaged subjects turns to hypovigilance when the damage includes the BLA and CMA. There is convergent evidence supporting this assumption, both from our own work reviewed in this chapter and from studies in rodents, but further brain–behavior research is necessary for definitive insights.

Another priority is to gain a better understanding on the role of the human amygdala in development, as also discussed by Ralph Adolphs (Chapter 10, this volume). We are currently surveying the South African UWD population, both from Namaqualand and Gauteng, to see whether there are young patients who can be studied longitudinally. Calcification of the amygdala in UWD seems to start early in childhood and possibly even at birth, although this may depend on the type of *ECM1* mutation. Figure 12.6 shows considerable damage to the BLA in the 8-year old Namaqualand male with UWD. The grayish tone, when compared to the dark tone of the skull, suggests that the damaged amygdala tissue is not yet fully calcified. In the light of the very slow course of calcification extrapolated from Figure 12.2, the onset of BLA calcification in the Namaqualand subjects with UWD likely occurs close to birth.

From that perspective, the amygdala lesions in UWD subjects from Namaqualand may be similar to the neonatal amygdala lesion in rhesus

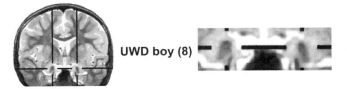

FIGURE 12.6. T2-weighted magnetic resonance image (coronal view) of an 8-year-old boy with UWD, showing starting calcifications in the amygdala (indicated with crosshairs).

monkeys (see Bliss-Moreau, Moadab, & Amaral, Chapter 6, this volume). The UWD amygdala lesion, of course, differs from the neonatal amygdala lesion in monkeys in that it is progressive and very small at the start, and it may for that reason allow for more neuroplasticity (see Patin & Hurlemann, Chapter 11, this volume). Nonetheless, comparative research targeting the biobehavioral effects of experimental developmental neonatal animal lesions and natural developmental human amygdala lesions is of the essence.

A Translational Framework for Human Amygdala Function

In conclusion, we have framed our findings in terms of a BLA–DLPFC resource competition model, and an adapted serial and parallel amygdala (BLA–CMA) processing model based on rodent research. We propose that on the basis of our data, the human BLA subserves unceasing threat surveillance, competing with the DLPFC for resources. The human BLA furthermore subserves instrumental behaviors that are calculative and goal-directed in fine-tuning unconditioned fear responses and acquiring economic (food, monetary) resources. The BLA can act serially on the CMA to regulate the unconditioned fear response, and in parallel restricts impulsive economic decisions driven by the CMA on the level of the NAc in economic decision making. Absence of threat surveillance in safe conditions in subjects with UWD and selective BLA damage results in more DLPFC resources and improves WM. Unwarranted fear hypervigilance in mildly threatening conditions in our BLA-damaged subjects reflects an inability to down-regulate the CMA, directly or via the OFC. As a result, the system for implementing fear responses, CMA–hypothalamus–PAG, responds with fear hypervigilance when the conditions do not call for this. The BLA and CMA also act in parallel on the NAc, differentially influencing economic choice behaviors. The BLA acts on the NAc directly, and by way of the OFC, triggering calculative–instrumental economic choice

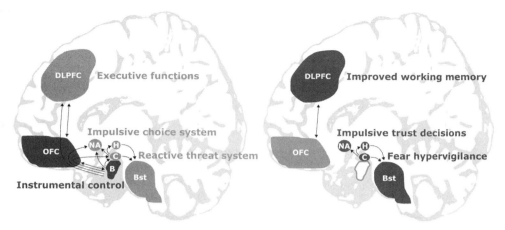

Normal functioning network   **BLA damaged network**

FIGURE 12.7. Overall model. Basolateral amygdala (B) damage decouples sub-cortical threat and reward systems from goal-directed instrumental control by the basolateral amygdala and orbitofrontal cortex (OFC), and also decouples other cortical executive systems (dorsolateral prefrontal cortex [DLPFC]). This results in not only unwarranted fear hypervigilance and irrationally generous economic investments but also improved working memory. C, central–medial amygdala; Bst, brainstem; H, hypothalamus; NA, nucleus accumbens.

behaviors. The CMA, on the other hand, acts on the NAc to trigger the affective–economic choice behaviors seen in our subjects with UWD, again, in more extreme forms (Balleine & Killcross, 2006; Phillips et al., 2003; van Honk et al., 2013). Figure 12.7 illustrates our findings in the Namaqualand subjects with UWD according to resource competition, serial, and parallel models of the amygdala.

ACKNOWLEDGMENTS

This work was funded by grants from the South African National Research Foundation (NRF), and the Netherlands Society of Scientific Research (NWO). Dan J. Stein is funded by the Medical Research Council of South Africa.

REFERENCES

Adolphs, R. (2003). Amygdala damage impairs emotion recognition from scenes only when they contain facial expressions. *Neuropsychologia, 41*(10), 1281–1289.

Adolphs, R., Gosselin, F., Buchanan, T. W., Tranel, D., Schyns, P., & Damasio, A.

R. (2005). A mechanism for impaired fear recognition after amygdala damage. *Nature, 433*(7021), 68–72.

Adolphs, R., Tranel, D., & Damasio, A. R. (1998). The human amygdala in social judgment. *Nature, 393*(6684), 470–474.

Adolphs, R., Tranel, D., Damasio, H., & Damasio, A. R. (1994). Impaired recognition of emotion in facial expressions following bilateral damage to the human amygdala. *Nature, 372*(6507), 669–672.

Amunts, K., Kedo, O., Kindler, M., Pieperhoff, P., Mohlberg, H., Shah, N. J., et al. (2005). Cytoarchitectonic mapping of the human amygdala, hippocampal region and entorhinal cortex: Intersubject variability and probability maps. *Anatomy and Embryology, 210*(5–6), 343–352.

Anticevic, A., Repovs, G., & Barch, D. M. (2010). Resisting emotional interference: Brain regions facilitating working memory performance during negative distraction. *Cognitive Affective and Behavioral Neuroscience, 10*(2), 159–173.

Balleine, B. W., & Killcross, S. (2006). Parallel incentive processing: An integrated view of amygdala function. *Trends in Neurosciences, 29*(5), 272–279.

Barbas, H., Saha, S., Rempel-Clower, N., & Ghashghaei, T. (2003). Serial pathways from primate prefrontal cortex to autonomic areas may influence emotional expression. *BMC Neuroscience, 4,* 25.

Becker, B., Mihov, Y., Scheele, D., Kendrick, K. M., Feinstein, J. S., Matusch, A., et al. (2012). Fear processing and social networking in the absence of a functional amygdala. *Biological Psychiatry, 72*(1), 70–77.

Bos, P. A., Terburg, D., & van Honk, J. (2010). Testosterone decreases trust in socially naive humans. *Proceedings of the National Academy of Sciences USA, 107*(22), 9991–9995.

Cahill, L., Babinsky, R., Markowitsch, H. J., & McGaugh, J. L. (1995). The amygdala and emotional memory. *Nature, 377*(6547), 295–296.

Camerer, C., Loewenstein, G., & Prelec, D. (2005). Neuroeconomics: How neuroscience can inform economics. *Journal of Economic Literature, 43*(1), 9–64.

Craig, A. D. (2009). How do you feel—now? The anterior insula and human awareness. *Nature Reviews Neuroscience, 10*(1), 59–70.

Davis, M., & Whalen, P. J. (2001). The amygdala: Vigilance and emotion. *Molecular Psychiatry, 6*(1), 13–34.

de Gelder, B., Terburg, D., Morgan, B., Hortensius, R., Stein, D. J., & van Honk, J. (2014). The role of human basolateral amygdala in ambiguous social threat perception. *Cortex, 52,* 28–34.

Fehr, E., & Camerer, C. F. (2007). Social neuroeconomics: The neural circuitry of social preferences. *Trends in Cognitive Sciences, 11*(10), 419–427.

Feinstein, J. S., Adolphs, R., Damasio, A., & Tranel, D. (2011). The human amygdala and the induction and experience of fear. *Current Biology, 21*(1), 34–38.

Feinstein, J. S., Buzza, C., Hurlemann, R., Follmer, R. L., Dahdaleh, N. S., Coryell, W. H., et al. (2013). Fear and panic in humans with bilateral amygdala damage. *Nature Neuroscience, 16*(3), 270–272.

Floresco, S. B., St. Onge, J. R., Ghods-Sharifi, S., & Winstanley, C. A. (2008). Cortico–limbic–striatal circuits subserving different forms of cost–benefit decision making. *Cognitive Affective and Behavioral Neuroscience, 8*(4), 375–389.

Goncalves, F. G., de Melo, M. B., de L. Matos, V., Barra, F. R., & Figueroa, R. E.

(2010). Amygdalae and striatum calcification in lipoid proteinosis. *American Journal of Neuroradiology, 31*(1), 88–90.

Graeff, F. G., & Del-Ben, C. M. (2008). Neurobiology of panic disorder: From animal models to brain neuroimaging. *Neuroscience and Biobehavioral Reviews, 32*(7), 1326–1335.

Hamada, T., McLean, W. H., Ramsay, M., Ashton, G. H., Nanda, A., Jenkins, T., et al. (2002). Lipoid proteinosis maps to 1q21 and is caused by mutations in the extracellular matrix protein 1 gene (*ECM1*). *Human Molecular Genetics, 11*(7), 833–840.

Hariri, A. R., Mattay, V. S., Tessitore, A., Kolachana, B., Fera, F., Goldman, D., et al. (2002). Serotonin transporter genetic variation and the response of the human amygdala. *Science, 297*(5580), 400–403.

Haruno, M., Kimura, M., & Frith, C. D. (2014). Activity in the nucleus accumbens and amygdala underlies individual differences in prosocial and individualistic economic choices. *Journal of Cognitive Neuroscience, 26*(8), 1861–1870.

Henrich, J., Heine, S. J., & Norenzayan, A. (2010a). Most people are not WEIRD. *Nature, 466*(7302), 29.

Henrich, J., Heine, S. J., & Norenzayan, A. (2010b). The weirdest people in the world? *Behavioral and Brain Sciences, 33*(2–3), 61–83.

Hurlemann, R., Patin, A., Onur, O. A., Cohen, M. X., Baumgartner, T., Metzler, S., et al. (2010). Oxytocin enhances amygdala-dependent, socially reinforced learning and emotional empathy in humans. *Journal of Neuroscience, 30*(14), 4999–5007.

Hurlemann, R., Wagner, M., Hawellek, B., Reich, H., Pieperhoff, P., Amunts, K., et al. (2007). Amygdala control of emotion-induced forgetting and remembering: Evidence from Urbach–Wiethe disease. *Neuropsychologia, 45*(5), 877–884.

Jones, D. (2010). A WEIRD view of human nature skews psychologists' studies. *Science, 328*(5986), 1627.

Kapur, N. (1996). Paradoxical functional facilitation in brain–behaviour research. A critical review. *Brain, 119*, 1775–1790.

Kennedy, D. P., Glascher, J., Tyszka, J. M., & Adolphs, R. (2009). Personal space regulation by the human amygdala. *Nature Neuroscience, 12*(10), 1226–1227.

Knutson, B., Rick, S., Wimmer, G. E., Prelec, D., & Loewenstein, G. (2007). Neural predictors of purchases. *Neuron, 53*(1), 147–156.

Kosfeld, M., Heinrichs, M., Zak, P. J., Fischbacher, U., & Fehr, E. (2005). Oxytocin increases trust in humans. *Nature, 435*(7042), 673–676.

Macedo, C. E., Cuadra, G., Molina, V., & Brandao, M. L. (2005). Aversive stimulation of the inferior colliculus changes dopamine and serotonin extracellular levels in the frontal cortex: Modulation by the basolateral nucleus of amygdala. *Synapse, 55*(1), 58–66.

Macedo, C. E., Martinez, R. C., Albrechet-Souza, L., Molina, V. A., & Brandao, M. L. (2007). 5-HT2- and D1-mechanisms of the basolateral nucleus of the amygdala enhance conditioned fear and impair unconditioned fear. *Behavioural Brain Research, 177*(1), 100–108.

Macedo, C. E., Martinez, R. C., & Brandao, M. L. (2006). Conditioned and unconditioned fear organized in the inferior colliculus are differentially sensitive to injections of muscimol into the basolateral nucleus of the amygdala. *Behavioral Neuroscience, 120*(3), 625–631.

Markowitsch, H. J., Calabrese, P., Wurker, M., Durwen, H. F., Kessler, J., Babinsky, R., et al. (1994). The amygdala's contribution to memory—A study on two patients with Urbach–Wiethe disease. *NeuroReport, 5*(11), 1349–1352.

Martinez, R. C., Ribeiro de Oliveira, A., & Brandao, M. L. (2007). Serotonergic mechanisms in the basolateral amygdala differentially regulate the conditioned and unconditioned fear organized in the periaqueductal gray. *European Neuropsychopharmacology, 17*(11), 717–724.

Meeren, H. K., van Heijnsbergen, C. C., & de Gelder, B. (2005). Rapid perceptual integration of facial expression and emotional body language. *Proceedings of the National Academy of Sciences USA, 102*(45), 16518–16523.

Mobbs, D., Petrovic, P., Marchant, J. L., Hassabis, D., Weiskopf, N., Seymour, B., et al. (2007). When fear is near: Threat imminence elicits prefrontal-periaqueductal gray shifts in humans. *Science, 317*(5841), 1079–1083.

Morgan, B., Terburg, D., Thornton, H. B., Stein, D. J., & van Honk, J. (2012). Paradoxical facilitation of working memory after basolateral amygdala damage. *PloS ONE, 7*(6), e38116.

Nell, V. (2000). *Cross-cultural neuropsychological assessment: Theory and practice.* Mahwah, NJ: Erlbaum.

Phillips, A. G., Ahn, S., & Howland, J. G. (2003). Amygdalar control of the mesocorticolimbic dopamine system: Parallel pathways to motivated behavior. *Neuroscience and Biobehavioral Reviews, 27*(6), 543–554.

Sander, D., Grafman, J., & Zalla, T. (2003). The human amygdala: An evolved system for relevance detection. *Reviews in the Neurosciences, 14*(4), 303–316.

Seeley, W. W., Menon, V., Schatzberg, A. F., Keller, J., Glover, G. H., Kenna, H., et al. (2007). Dissociable intrinsic connectivity networks for salience processing and executive control. *Journal of Neuroscience, 27*(9), 2349–2356.

Siebert, M., Markowitsch, H. J., & Bartel, P. (2003). Amygdala, affect and cognition: Evidence from 10 patients with Urbach–Wiethe disease. *Brain, 126*(12), 2627–2637.

Spielberger, C. D., Gorusch, R. L., & Lushene, R. E. (1970). *State–Trait Anxiety Inventory.* Palo Alto, CA: Consulting Psychologists Press.

Stalnaker, T. A., Franz, T. M., Singh, T., & Schoenbaum, G. (2007). Basolateral amygdala lesions abolish orbitofrontal-dependent reversal impairments. *Neuron, 54*(1), 51–58.

Stine, O. C., & Smith, K. D. (1990). The estimation of selection coefficients in Afrikaners: Huntington disease, porphyria variegata, and lipoid proteinosis. *American Journal of Human Genetics, 46*(3), 452–458.

Strange, B. A., Hurlemann, R., & Dolan, R. J. (2003). An emotion-induced retrograde amnesia in humans is amygdala- and beta-adrenergic-dependent. *Proceedings of the National Academy of Sciences USA, 100*(23), 13626–13631.

Terburg, D., Morgan, B. E., Montoya, E. R., Hooge, I. T., Thornton, H. B., Hariri, A. R., et al. (2012). Hypervigilance for fear after basolateral amygdala damage in humans. *Translational Psychiatry, 2,* e115.

Thornton, H. B., Nel, D., Thornton, D., van Honk, J., Baker, G. A., & Stein, D. J. (2008). The neuropsychiatry and neuropsychology of lipoid proteinosis. *Journal of Neuropsychiatry and Clinical Neurosciences, 20*(1), 86–92.

Tranel, D., & Hyman, B. T. (1990). Neuropsychological correlates of bilateral amygdala damage. *Archives of Neurology, 47*(3), 349–355.

Tye, K. M., Prakash, R., Kim, S. Y., Fenno, L. E., Grosenick, L., Zarabi, H., et al. (2011). Amygdala circuitry mediating reversible and bidirectional control of anxiety. *Nature, 471*(7338), 358–362.

Urbach, E., & Wiethe, C. (1929). Lipoidosis cutis et mucosae [lipoid proteinosis]. *Virchows Archiv für Pathologische Anatomie und Physiologie und für Klinische Medizin, 273,* 285–319.

van Honk, J. (2009). Neuroendocrine manipulation of the sexually dimorphic human social brain. In E. Harmon-Jones & J. S. Beer (Eds.), *Methods in social neuroscience* (pp. 45–69). New York: Guilford Press.

van Honk, J., Eisenegger, C., Terburg, D., Stein, D. J., & Morgan, B. (2013). Generous economic investments after basolateral amygdala damage. *Proceedings of the National Academy of Sciences USA, 110*(7), 2506–2510.

van Honk, J., Peper, J. S., & Schutter, D. J. (2005). Testosterone reduces unconscious fear but not consciously experienced anxiety: Implications for the disorders of fear and anxiety. *Biological Psychiatry, 58*(3), 218–225.

van Honk, J., Schutter, D. J., d'Alfonso, A. A., Kessels, R. P., & de Haan, E. H. (2002). 1 hz rTMS over the right prefrontal cortex reduces vigilant attention to unmasked but not to masked fearful faces. *Biological Psychiatry, 52*(4), 312–317.

Van Hougenhouck-Tulleken, W., Chan, I., Hamada, T., Thornton, H., Jenkins, T., McLean, W. H., et al. (2004). Clinical and molecular characterization of lipoid proteinosis in Namaqualand, South Africa. *British Journal of Dermatology, 151*(2), 413–423.

Wechsler, D. (1997). *Wechsler Adult Intelligence Scale–III.* San Antonio, TX: Psychological Corporation.

Wechsler, D. (1999). *Wechsler Abbreviated Scale of Intelligence.* San Antonio, TX: Psychological Corporation.

Whalen, P. J., Kagan, J., Cook, R. G., Davis, F. C., Kim, H., Polis, S., et al. (2004). Human amygdala responsivity to masked fearful eye whites. *Science, 306*(5704), 2061.

When once is enough. (2004). *Nature Neuroscience, 7*(2), 93.

Williams, J. M., Mathews, A., & MacLeod, C. (1996). The emotional Stroop task and psychopathology. *Psychological Bulletin, 120*(1), 3–24.

Wu, Z., Mittal, S., Kish, K., Yu, Y., Hu, J., & Haacke, E. M. (2009). Identification of calcification with MRI using susceptibility-weighted imaging: A case study. *Journal of Magnetic Resonance Imaging, 29*(1), 177–182.

Yun, R. J., Krystal, J. H., & Mathalon, D. H. (2010). Working memory overload: Fronto-limbic interactions and effects on subsequent working memory function. *Brain Imaging and Behavior, 4*(1), 96–108.

CHAPTER 13

Attending to the World without an Amygdala

REBECCA M. TODD
ADAM K. ANDERSON
ELIZABETH A. PHELPS

In normally developing humans, selective tuning to emotionally important aspects of the world relies on activity in the amygdala. Here we review studies conducted with patient S. P., who suffered from gliosis throughout her left amygdala, and had her right amygdala and surrounding anterior temporal lobe regions surgically removed at age 48 due to severe epilepsy. Studies with S. P. suggest that amygdala loss can result in reduction of both affective learning and memory, and "affect-biased attention," which is the capacity to rapidly and reflexively perceive what is most emotionally relevant in the environment. Combined with subsequent neuroimaging studies in healthy adults, these results suggest that the amygdala's sensitivity to emotional aspects of the world may in turn be linked to the vividness of emotional memories. In contrast, S. P.'s capacity to rate the emotional significance of stimuli was relatively intact and her daily subjective emotional experience was normal, suggesting that the amygdala is not required for fluctuations of subjective emotion experienced from day to day. Impairments of affect-biased attention observed in S. P. have not been consistently observed in patients who have lost amygdala function due to other disorders, suggesting that the nature of life without an amygdala may depend on when and precisely where the damage occurred.

The Role of the Amygdala in Tuning Attention

It is well known that as we go about our days, we constantly filter the information that comes into contact with our senses, selectively paying attention to what is important to us and ignoring distracting or irrelevant information, which we often do not even see. This process is known as "selective attention." And for most of us, emotionally compelling, or affectively salient, objects in the environment capture the eye as we navigate the world, often so seamlessly that we are not even aware of it. For example, in a crowded street scene, we are more likely to notice a face that is strikingly beautiful or ugly, or emotionally expressive; a bright bunch of daffodils; a tempting cake in a bakery window; a dangerously fast approaching vehicle; or a suspicious or potentially deranged person. This is a form of selective attention we have called "affect-biased attention," and we have argued that it is tuned by our experience with a particular type of object or event in a given situation (Markovic, Anderson, & Todd, 2014; Todd, Cunningham, Anderson, & Thompson, 2012a); that is, it is based on emotional learning. An example is how a particular facial expression means that good or bad things are going to happen to us, and the emotional arousal that those consequences of pain or pleasure evoke. And clearly, under many circumstances, this is a useful function, tuning us to the world in a way that maximizes our ability to notice and respond to events that have consequences for our well-being.

In normally developing humans, this capacity for affect-biased attention relies on the activity in the amygdala. Numerous brain imaging studies in humans have found amygdala activity to be greater for emotionally salient than for more mundane pictures (e.g., Pourtois, Schettino, & Vuilleumier, 2013). Amygdala activity is also linked to the subjective experience of affectively salient images as being more vivid (Todd, Talmi, Schmitz, Susskind, & Anderson, 2012b). This activation in the amygdala also predicts the vividness of memory for emotional events later on (Todd, Schmitz, Susskind, & Anderson, 2013b), and the amygdala is also active when one recalls an emotionally important memory (LaBar & Cabeza, 2006).

The sensitivity of the amygdala to what is emotionally relevant often depends on the process of emotional learning, which also depends on the amygdala. We can think about the process of Pavlovian conditioning in terms of the creation and tuning of affective control settings that track stimuli that have proved to be a significant source of punishment and reward. Human conditioning studies have revealed that associative learning mechanisms play a key role in acquisition of affect-biased attention. For example, the human amygdala has been found to be active during aversive conditioning studies, in which a neutral stimulus (e.g., a colored square) is paired with a naturally unpleasant stimulus (e.g., a shock or an unpleasant smell or taste or puff of air; LaBar, Gatenby, Gore, LeDoux, & Phelps, 1998; Phelps, 2006; Sehlmeyer et al., 2009). Patients who have had regions of the temporal lobe, including the amygdala, removed are less susceptible to this conditioning, which indicates that these regions are necessary for aversive Pavlovian conditioning (LaBar, LeDoux, Spencer, &

Phelps, 1995). The amygdala also plays a role in "appetitive conditioning," in which a neutral stimulus is paired with a pleasurable event (Belova, Paton, Morrison, & Salzman, 2007; Prevost, McNamee, Jessup, Bossaerts, & O'Doherty, 2013). What is more, it is active during more indirect or socioemotional learning, when participants watch another person experiencing fear conditioning (Olsson & Phelps, 2007).

Introducing Patient S. P.

So what happens if you lose your amygdala in adulthood, after decades of learning that certain things or events are associated with pleasure and pain? One challenge to answering this question is that in many cases it is difficult to determine the precise onset of amygdala pathology. Studies of one patient, S. P., who had gliotic changes throughout her left amygdala and had her right amygdala and surrounding temporal lobe tissues removed at age 48 due to severe epilepsy, suggest that one loses the capacity for affect-biased attention—the capacity to notice rapidly, and without having to think about it, what in a given environment is most important for one's ongoing goals of maximizing pleasure and avoiding pain.

S. P. has been described as a "funny," and "likable" woman who is divorced, with grown children, an average IQ, a high school degree, and some college (Phelps et al., 1998). She ran a successful business before her epilepsy got too severe. After surgery S. P. no longer suffered from seizures, and she began working again part time. Her basic memory and intelligence are in the normal range. In her spare time she enjoys painting and writing poetry. However, S. P. exhibits many of the hallmarks of amygdala dysfunction, including impaired Pavlovian aversive conditioning and altered emotional modulation of memory (Phelps et al., 1998), and upon initial testing revealed selective impairments in emotional expression recognition. S. P. revealed a differential impairment in understanding expressions of fear, despite intact cognitive appraisals of the larger meaning of fear and other emotions (Anderson & Phelps, 2000). At the time of the studies described here, she was between 54 and 58 years old.

S. P.'s Medical History

S. P.'s medical history indicates that she first showed signs of neurological impairment as young as age 4 years. She was later diagnosed with epilepsy, which became more severe over time. The origin of her seizures was localized to the right medial temporal lobe, but postsurgery magnetic resonance imaging (MRI) indicated damage to the left amygdala. A biopsy of the left amygdala revealed gliosis, or scar tissue (Figure 13.1).

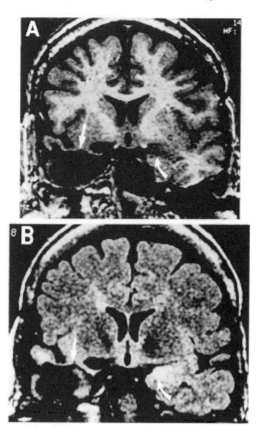

FIGURE 13.1. Coronal T1-weighted (A) and fluid-attenuated inversion recovery (FLAIR) T2-weighted (B) images at the level of the amygdala. There is abnormal signal intensity in the left amygdala secondary to gliosis (curved arrows). There is some indication of the left amygdala abnormality in the standard inversion time (T1) image (A), but it is clearly apparent in the more sensitive FLAIR imaging sequence (B). The absence of the right amygdala secondary to surgery (straight arrows) is also portrayed. The right hemisphere is depicted on the left side of each image. From Phelps, LaBar, Anderson, O'Connor, Fulbright, and Spencer (1998). Copyright 1998 by Taylor & Francis, Ltd. Reprinted by permission.

The origin of the gliosis is unknown (Phelps et al., 1998). There are no data regarding her behavior in the years before the surgical resection of her right anterior temporal lobe, and her left amygdala was already damaged. Although her standard neuropsychological profile was normal both before and after surgery, all we know about S. P.s behavior on more selective affective tasks was after her surgery (Phelps et al., 1998). For this reason, while we discuss S. P. as a potential example of amygdala loss later in life, it is important to remember that due to her extensive neurological history, it is not possible to know whether S. P. developed with two normally functioning amygdalae, with the first indication of some dysfunction appearing in childhood.

S. P. and Affect-Biased Attention

A key series of studies investigated S. P.'s capacity for affect-biased attention, measuring the influence of affective salience on her capacity to report stimuli under conditions of limited attention using a variation of a commonly used experiment known as the *attentional blink* (AB). In classic AB experiments, two "target" stimuli (e.g., numbers or words) are presented among a series of "distractor" words that follow each other, one after the other very quickly—at the rate of roughly a 10th of a second (Figure 13.2). Participants are told they have to remember the two target stimuli and report them after the end of each rapid series of words. When the second target (T2) appears too soon (up to roughly half a second) after the first target (T1), participants typically cannot report seeing T2.

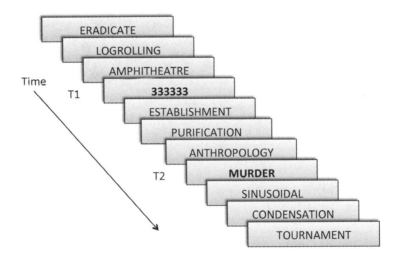

FIGURE 13.2. The attentional blink task. Two targets were presented among a series of distractors: the first target (T1) was a string of numbers, and the second (T2) was an emotionally arousing or neutral word. T2 followed T1 after one of four possible lags, with 0 (lag 1), 1 (lag 2), 3 (lag 4), or 6 (lag 7) distractor words in between. Words in each category were matched for average word length, written frequency, and neighborhood frequency. At the end of each trial, participants had to report both targets. From Markovic, Anderson, and Todd (2014). Copyright 2014 by Elsevier. Reprinted by permission.

This is the AB effect, so named because it is as if one's mind blinks and cannot perceive the target, even though it passes right before one's eyes. There are many theories about why the AB occurs, but nearly all agree that it is due to limitations in the attentional resources that are available. According to one interpretation of the AB, limited resources result in a failure rapidly to switch attentional sets, or mental templates, from those tuning one's attention to the T1 stimulus to those tuned to the T2 stimulus if it appears too quickly after T1, resulting in impaired perceptual awareness (Di Lollo, Kawahara, Shahab Ghorashi, & Enns, 2005).

A series of studies used a variation of the AB experiment to manipulate the affective salience of T2 stimuli. The goal was to examine whether emotionally salient T2 stimuli are less subject to the AB blink than neutral stimuli in healthy participants (Anderson, 2005). One study compared the AB for negative high-arousal words (e.g., "rape"), negative low-arousal words (e.g., "hurt"), and neutral words (e.g., "rule"). Results showed that high-arousal words had a significantly smaller blink effect than low-arousal words, which themselves had a smaller AB effect than neutral words. Thus, the more arousing the negative words, the easier they were to detect during the time window in which the blink is observed. Or, as we like to describe it, there was an emotional "sparing" of the blink for such words. A second study showed that this effect applied to positive emotionally arousing target words as well, implying that what is important for detection of the stimuli is emotional arousal rather than valence (whether the word is good or bad). These experiments revealed that when attentional resources are limited, emotionally salient stimuli are perceived more easily than neutral stimuli—a finding that may reflect more resilient attentional filters for affectively salient stimuli. One way of looking at this is that when one has a healthy functioning amygdala, one carries a habitual affective attentional set for things that are emotionally important.

But if one loses his or her amygdala, he or she should lose the capacity to maintain these affective attentional sets based on previously acquired emotional associations. After surgery, S. P. was impaired in her capacity for emotional learning. A conditioning study revealed that she could not acquire associations between a shock and a colored square (Phelps et al., 1998). Thus, she had difficulty acquiring new emotional associations. Using an AB task with S. P. provided the opportunity to see whether emotional associations she would have to have learned before her surgery would still bias her attention. This gave us the chance to test the hypothesis that the amygdala plays a critical role in prioritizing perception of affectively salient stimuli and maintenance of affective attentional sets.

One study measured AB performance in S. P. and a group of healthy controls. S. P. showed a normal AB effect for neutral targets: She was as bad as anyone else at reporting neutral T2 words when they were shown too soon after T1. Yet, unlike the controls, she did not show the pattern of

AB sparing for negatively arousing emotional words. To rule out the possibility that S. P. was just poor at perception in general, the visual similarity of targets and distractors was manipulated, so that the targets would stand out from distractors to a greater or lesser degree. Like controls, S. P. showed AB sparing for words that were visually easier to perceive in contrast to impaired AB sparing for emotional words. The conclusion was that the amygdala influences perceptual awareness of affective salience but not perceptual salience.

The amygdala, of course, is not just one brain structure but instead is two separate clusters of nuclei (some researchers refer to it by its plural form, "amygdalae"), one in each hemisphere of the brain. The next study explored whether, given the importance of the left hemisphere in visual word representation, emotional sparing of the AB specifically required the left amygdala. In this study, participants comprised a group of five patients with right amygdala damage and five patients with left amygdala damage. Results showed that patients with right amygdala lesions performed like controls, and showed affective AB sparing, whereas patients with left amygdala lesions, like S. P., showed no sparing for emotionally arousing words. This suggested that it was specifically S. P.'s selective amygdala damage in her language-dominant left hemisphere that was responsible for failure of affect-biased attention and resulting enhanced awareness. Activity in the amygdala may be influencing the processing of written words, specifically in the left temporal lobe, to boost their access to awareness. Since the amygdala is not part of brain systems that are key for understanding the meaning of words, it must act in concert with the left temporal cortex to extract meaning and emotional value from the written word forms themselves.

A further study investigated whether the lack of AB sparing for negative words was linked to lack of overall comprehension of the emotional value of words. This was done by asking S. P. and the group of left amygdala patients to rate the valence (how good or bad) and arousal levels (how emotionally arousing) of the T2 words. Just like normal controls, participants with amygdala lesions rated the negative stimuli as more negative and more arousing than neutral words. This indicates that the impaired influence of affective salience on perceptual awareness was not related to overall differences in comprehension of the emotional value of the words. We conclude that, if one loses his or her left amygdala, as S. P. did through gliotic changes, and other patients did through surgical resection, one understands that emotionally important words are more emotionally important. They just do not have the same capacity to influence attention and awareness.

The AB studies with S. P. suggest that a key function of the amygdala may be to segregate neural representations of the significant from the mundane by shaping perceptual experience directly. Amygdala tuning of perceptual efficiency may be the mechanism underlying affective attentional sets, and thus the advantage of emotionally important stimuli in reaching awareness even under conditions of limited attention. Thus, the amygdala can help to keep the parts of the brain required for seeing tuned to what is emotionally important, even when one's mind is occupied with other tasks.

We have suggested that the finding that S. P. failed to show typical emotional sparing suggests that amygdala lesions result in an inability to influence the *efficiency* of perceptual processing for emotionally important items in other brain regions, particularly the visual cortex (Anderson & Phelps, 2001). Signals from the amygdala may enhance sensitivity in these perceptual regions of the brain, because the amygdala trains the visual system to respond with lower levels of information. We suggest that the importance of the amygdala for affect-biased attention comes from its broad connectivity. The amygdala not only receives visual information from the visual cortex (Amaral, Behniea, & Kelly, 2003) but its connections to the cortex also include links to medial, orbital, and lateral regions of the prefrontal cortex (Ghashghaei, Hilgetag, & Barbas, 2007) which in turn influence visual cortex activity, as well as direct projections to visual cortex as early as V1 (Amaral et al., 2003; Amaral & Price, 1984).

Neuroimaging Studies of the Role of the Amygdala in Affect-Biased Attention

Since the studies of S. P. and patients with anterior temporal lobectomy were conducted, neuroimaging studies have probed brain activity underlying emotional sparing of the AB in healthy participants. One study used aversive conditioning, so that participants first learned that previously neutral stimuli were emotionally important (Lim, Padmala, & Pessoa, 2009). The aim of this study was to investigate directly the links between amygdala activation, enhanced visual processing, and the AB advantage for emotionally salient stimuli. Here, T1 was a face, and T2 was either a scene (a house or a building) or a non-scene. In the learning phase of the study, for each participant, either the house or the building was paired with shock on 50% of trials (CS+) versus no shock in any trials (CS–).

As predicted, there was an AB advantage for CS+ trials, with greater accuracy for identifying T2s in emotionally salient (CS+) than for neutral (CS–) trials. Functional magnetic resonance imaging (fMRI) results showed greater activation in both in the parahippocampal place area (PPA), which is a region of the visual cortex that responds preferentially to scenes, and in the amygdala for CS+ trials than for CS– trials. Additionally, PPA and amygdala activation predicted greater accuracy in identifying T2 more strongly for CS+ trials, suggesting that emotional learning strengthens the neural representation of a scene, making it more likely to reach awareness. As suggested by the studies of S. P., this finding indicated that affect-biased attention as indexed by an AB task relies on representations in the visual cortex. Furthermore, as amygdala activation increased, the link between visual cortex activation and behavior became stronger. Finally, amygdala and visual cortex connections with prefrontal regions also played an important role in emotional sparing. The authors concluded that emotional salience provides an emotional AB advantage via enhanced visual processing that is modulated by the amygdala. Building on previous research, this study demonstrated that a key function of the amygdala is to segregate neural representations of the "significant from the mundane," playing a role in filtering what we see by shaping perceptual experience directly. Importantly, the emotional salience of the houses was learned at the time of the study, underlining the importance of the amygdala in affect-biased attention to associations between objects/events and emotional arousal that is learned through experience. Thus, if one lose one's amygdala, one may lose access to the influence of a lifetime of emotional learning on one's habits of paying attention.

Another study used magnetic encephalography (MEG), a form of brain imaging that is highly sensitive to changes in brain activation over time, to investigate the timing and sequence of brain activity linked to emotional sparing of the AB (Todd et al., 2014b). This study, again using negative arousing and neutral words as T2 stimuli in healthy adults, found that very rapid (145 milliseconds) amygdala activity first discriminated emotionally important from neutral T2 stimuli. This quick amygdala activity was followed by a large and long-lasting pattern of greater activity for salient T2s in prefrontal regions of the brain linked to more explicit evaluative processing. Prefrontal activity occurred within a time window during which brain activity was linked to conscious awareness of the stimuli. This finding suggests the amygdala may play a role in rapidly sorting the significant from the mundane before frontal regions are active in processes associated with conscious awareness of stimuli. However, it is important to note that the speed at which amygdala activation discriminates emotional stimuli is controversial, as is the question of how accurately we can measure amygdala activity with MEG.

Finally, another brain region that plays a role in amygdala involvement in affect-biased attention is the locus coeruleus (LC) in the brainstem, which is an evolutionarily old brain region that influences visual cortex activity and works in close tandem with the amygdala. It is a small nucleus that produces the neurochemical norepinephrine (NE) and sends projections that distribute NE all over the brain, including the amygdala, which has many NE receptors. Although it is hard to use imaging methods to measure LC activity in humans, because the LC is so small and deep in the brain, a large body of nonhuman animal research has demonstrated that the LC is important for both learning what is salient in a given situation and developing associations between events (Sara, 2009). The LC–NE system may work with the amygdala to modulate specific mechanisms of selective attention in the visual cortex (Markovic et al., 2014).

Some research in humans indicates that NE plays an important role in emotional sparing of the AB. Increasing levels of NE by administering the NE reuptake inhibitor reboxetine improves emotional sparing of the AB (De Martino, Strange, & Dolan, 2008). This suggests that if one loses one's amygdala, then the loss of affect-biased attention may be due specifically to the role of NE in the amygdala. This is consistent with findings of the importance of NE in the emotional enhancement of memory, and the amygdala's role in modulating memory formation (Cahill, Gorski, & Le, 2003; Cahill et al., 1996; Roozendaal, McEwen, & Chattarji, 2009). Moreover, our research suggests that there is a genetic component to the role of NE in emotional sparing as well. Individuals who carry a common "deletion" variant of the *ADRA2B* gene (we have found this to be roughly half of our participants) are thought to have greater NE availability in the brain. Previous studies had shown that deletion carriers had greater capacity for emotional memory and were more vulnerable to traumatic memory than people who did not carry the deletion variant (noncarriers) (de Quervain et al., 2007). They also showed greater amygdala activation for negative emotional scenes than did noncarriers (Rasch et al., 2009). To investigate whether this genetic variation also influences affect-biased attention, we collected DNA samples from 207 healthy young adults and had them perform a version of the AB task with negative arousing, positive arousing, and neutral T2 words. We found that participants consistently showed emotional sparing of positive and negative over neutral words. However deletion variant carriers showed a strong additional emotional sparing for negative over positive words (Todd et al., 2013a). Moreover, these same deletion carriers rated emotionally salient images as more arousing than did noncarriers, and showed a stronger relation between how arousing they rated images to be at the time of encoding and how well they remembered them 1 week later (Todd et al., 2014a). This suggests that common genetic differences influencing NE availability enhance memory by enhancing encoding, and that the relation between encoding and memory is heightened in deletion carriers.

One interpretation is that the genetic variation tunes the amygdala to bias attention to threat. But the LC is responsive to both positive and negative salient events, and we have already seen the role of learning in tuning emotional sparing of the AB. Furthermore, our previous research has found that although young adults in general tend to be biased toward the negative, young children, like older adults, show preferential amygdala activity for positive stimuli (Todd, Evans, Morris, Lewis, & Taylor, 2011). So another explanation is that young adults who carry the deletion variant are more exquisitely tuned to what is already emotionally salient to them. If we tested 6-year-olds, we might find deletion carriers to be more sensitive to positive stimuli, since at that phase of life amygdala tuning is biased in that direction. This suggests that there may be individual differences related to genetic influences in NE availability in the manner in which affect-biased attention is influenced with amygdala loss in adulthood. What the amygdala is tuned to varies across one's life, likely depending on one's experience. The amygdala represents the capacity for this selective tuning and resulting emotional salience. It is also possible that if one is born without an amygdala or loses it early in life the LC–NE system may develop with prefrontal cortex and other subcortical regions to compensate, creating an alternative system for affect-biased attention.

The Amygdala and the Vividness of Emotional Perception and Memory

Our research has also followed up on the findings with S. P. and other patients by investigating the role of the amygdala in the vividness of emotional perception and memory in healthy young adults. First, to investigate whether emotional salience influences the subjective experience of perceptual vividness, we used an emotional version of a classic magnitude estimation paradigm from psychophysics experiments of the 1950s (Stevens, 1956, 1957). In a classic magnitude estimation task, participants are presented with a stimulus (e.g., a light or a tone) and are asked to compare the magnitude of the stimulus to a standard presented at a constant magnitude. In our adaptation, emotionally salient and neutral images were overlaid with one of three levels of visual noise (like static on an old TV), and standards were created for each image by scrambling the image so that its contents were not recognizable, and overlaying a standard level of noise (Figure 13.3). Participants were asked to judge the proportion of noisiness of each image relative to the standard (Todd et al., 2012b). This design allowed us to look at the subjective vividness of affectively salient relative to neutral images measured as the signal of the underlying image relative to the overlaid noise. Results showed that participants were very accurate in estimating objective levels of noise. Crucially, both positive and negative arousing images were perceived as less noisy, or more perceptually vivid, than neutral images. Even after we controlled for the objective characteristics of each image, participants still rated positive and negative images as containing lower levels of noise, suggesting that affectively salient images are subjectively experienced as more vivid than mundane ones. Moreover, when we created a direct measure of perceptual vividness by calculating the inverse of the noise estimation ratings (NE^{-1}, a measure of how clearly or vividly the image signal underneath the

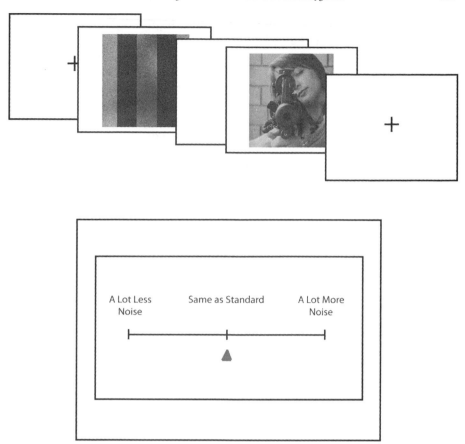

FIGURE 13.3. :Noise estimation (NE) task to assess perceptual vividness. A standard, overlaid with a constant level of noise, was given an arbitrary value of 100. Each standard was followed by a positive, negative, or neutral image overlaid with one of three levels of noise. In each trial, participants used a scale to indicate the degree to which the image had higher, equal, or lower levels of noise. From Markovic, Anderson, and Todd (2014). Copyright 2014 by Elsevier. Reprinted by permission.

noise was perceived), we found that, image by image, perceptual vividness predicted ratings of emotional salience (Figure 13.4). This relationship remained after we controlled for computational measures of objective visual salience, such as color, image complexity, and a composite measure of visual salience. We refer to this influence of emotional salience on perceptual vividness as emotionally enhanced vividness (EEV).

Several control studies were performed to rule out confounding explanations. Results indicated that EEV is not the result of differences in patterns of eye movements in response to emotionally salient images or image color or differential effects arising from repetition of emotional images; rather, it is due to the emotional content of the images themselves. To see whether the behavioral phenomenon of EEV reflected relatively rapid perceptual processes rather than later conceptual evaluative processes, we further examined the time course of event-related potential (ERP) activity following presentation of the images. Results showed that that EEV involves relatively rapid perceptual processing regions around 200–300 ms following stimulus onset, but still late enough to reflect extraction of the emotional meaning of the complex scenes. Furthermore, the neural signature of decreased noise in the perceptual cortices was similar to that of EEV, suggesting that an individual's brain represents emotional images as if they were presented with less noise. Images associated with emotional arousal were represented as being more vivid.

But what of the role of the amygdala? We employed fMRI to examine amygdala activation and patterns of relationship between amygdala and visual cortex activation linked to EEV. We found that activation in the left amygdala, as well as left lateral occipital cortex (LOC), a region of the visual cortex that plays an important role in perceiving objects, was greater for pictures rated higher in EEV (Figure 13.4). Further analyses found correlated activity between the amygdala and visual cortex for emotionally salient but not for neutral images. These findings can again be interpreted as reflecting the role of the amygdala in tagging emotional salience, which in turn may enhance the experience of seeing (reflected in LOC activation). In short, we found that emotional salience modulates the subjective visual experience of seeing an image. In this case, the amygdala accounted for enhanced visual cortex activation linked to EEV in a manner that is consistent with the role of the amygdala in tuning visual cortex activation for emotionally salient aspects of the world.

A second question concerned whether amygdala activation that modulated EEV was related to increased subsequent memory vividness. It is well known that the amygdala plays an important role in emotional enhancement of memory, and previous studies had shown that S. P. was impaired in recognition of previously viewed emotionally arousing stimuli. To test the relationship between EEV and memory vividness in healthy participants, we employed two memory tasks: a cued recall task and a recognition memory task (Todd et al., 2012b). The cued recall study was performed 45 minutes after the completion of the noise estimation task. Participants were given one-word cues that corresponded to one of the pictures seen in the noise estimation task and asked to provide a written description of the picture in as much detail as possible. Descriptions were rated for number of details recalled from correctly remembered images, including thoughts and emotions associated with the image. Participants recalled more details about affectively salient than about

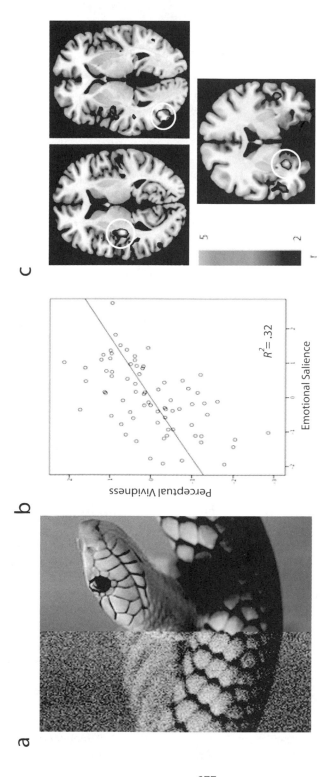

FIGURE 13.4. (a) Arousing images were subjectively perceived as containing lower levels of overlaid noise, despite equal levels of objective noise (i.e., were perceived as more perceptually vivid). The right side of the image illustrates a 15% decrement in noise level from the left. (b) Image by image, emotional salience predicted perceptual vividness after controlling for objective salience. (c) fMRI activation parametrically modulated by emotionally enhanced vividness in left insula (left), lateral occipital cortex (LOC; right), and amygdala (bottom). From Markovic, Anderson, and Todd (2014). Copyright 2014 by Elsevier. Reprinted by permission.

neutral images, and inverse noise estimation was correlated with number of details recalled, as well as associated thoughts and emotions. Thus, although participants were not more likely to recall an emotional image than a neutral one, it appears that the vividness with which we view emotionally salient images modulates memory vividness as well.

In the recognition memory task, participants returned 1 week after performing the noise estimation task. They were shown all of the images from the original task, as well as unfamiliar images matched for emotional salience, scene content, and objective image characteristics. Participants were asked to rate each image as old or new, and to rate the vividness of the memory. Again, perceptual vividness predicted memory vividness. fMRI findings further revealed that the same regions of amygdala and LOC that were linked to EEV also influenced later ratings of recognition memory vividness (Todd et al., 2013b). However, memory vividness was uniquely influenced by additional activity in the hippocampus and other regions important for memory. These findings suggest shared neural substrates for the influence of emotional salience on perception and memory vividness, with amygdala and visual cortex activation at the time the events are encountered contributing to the experience of both perception and subsequent memory. Overall, these findings shed light on how a functioning amygdala may work with other key brain regions to influence emotional memory at the time of perception, as well as later processes that allow consolidation of the memories. Again, the amygdala's role in emotional learning suggests the hypothesis that losing the amygdala would result in loss of enhanced perception and memory for things one has learned are emotionally important.

Emotional Processes That Are Spared in S. P.

If the amygdala is key for affect-biased attention, emotional enhancement of perceptual vividness, and emotional enhancement of memory, what emotion-related processes may be spared by loss of the amygdala? Further studies with S. P. suggested that losing the amygdala did not influence the capacity to understand emotional meaning or produce emotional facial expressions (Anderson & Phelps, 2000). In one study, S. P. and 20 control subjects who were equivalent to S. P. in age, sex, and level of education, were asked to match an emotional word ("afraid," "angry," "disgusted," "happy," "sad," and "surprised") to a facial expression. They were also asked to match the same emotion words to written sentences describing emotional situations. Finally they were asked to produce the facial expression that went along with each of the words. Like Method actors, they were asked to think of an event that would make them feel each specific emotion, then show what the facial expression would look like. Then, four separate judges scored the appropriateness of the facial emotions posed. When rating the facial emotion, S. P. had difficulty rating expressions of fear, disgust, sadness and (to a lesser extent) happiness relative to controls, and she tended to confuse expressions of fear and sadness, consistent with the role of the amygdala in perception or appraisal of emotion. Yet she performed as well as control subjects at matching emotion terms to written descriptions of situations, suggesting that her difficulty in recognizing facial emotion was not due to a lack of understanding what the emotions meant. She also performed as well as control subjects in producing facial expressions of emotion and in some cases displayed even greater facial expressiveness.

Another study suggested that S. P.'s amygdala damage did not result in altered magnitude or frequency of emotional states (Anderson & Phelps, 2002). Here S. P. and two matched control subjects were asked to fill out the Positive and Negative Affect Schedule (PANAS), a mood questionnaire, to measure daily experience of positive (e.g., inspired, excited) and negative (e.g., afraid, nervous) emotional states over the course of a month. In terms of the magnitude or degree of emotional experience, on a 5-point scale ranging from *very slightly* to *extremely*, S. P.'s reports of the magnitude of and frequency of her emotional states were largely equal to or greater than that reported from controls: All reported overall more positive than negative emotions and equivalent levels of fear/anxiety. A principal components analysis was then performed on the correlations among the 20 independent PANAS emotion categories for each participant. This analysis of the fluctuations of daily emotion also revealed similar patterns for S. P. and for controls, indicating that positive and negative emotional states were relatively independent of each other. Thus, the structure of underlying affect experiences as falling into positive versus negative states appeared to remain intact. Like controls, S. P. appeared to experience the same type of daily fluctuations between emotions, with positive and negative emotion varying along independent dimensions.

This independence of positive and negative affect is not something S. P. knows about how emotions work, and it would be hard to fake. Nonetheless these self-reports are retrospective, occurring at the end of a day rather than online as the experiences took place. Interestingly, patient S. M., whose bilateral amygdala damage dated from earlier in life, did show abnormalities in experience of emotion, demonstrating blunted negative emotion in relation to highly emotional life experiences (Tranel, Gullickson, Koch, & Adolphs, 2006). It may be that altered emotional experience related to amygdala loss emerges only with regard to extreme emotion expressed in the moment, which was not captured in the record of daily experience. Therefore, while research done with S. P. indicates that amygdala loss need not influence the experience of daily emotional fluctuations, differences between S. P. and S. M. suggest that differences in the timing and other details of amygdala loss, which we discuss below, may influence the role the amygdala plays in affective experience.

What does research on S. P. tell us about the amygdala? The findings described earlier suggest that acquired amygdala damage does not necessarily decrease the experienced aspect of emotion, or understanding of the overall significance of arousing stimuli. One interpretation of these findings is that the amygdala is not necessary for the subjective experience of an emotional state, which in humans may be more tied to internal emotional representations than to direct perceptual experience. Rather, our studies suggest that amygdala lesions impair the enhanced perceptual processing of emotionally arousing stimuli, as well as the prominence of emotionally salient events in memory. This suggests that in normal adults the amygdala plays a key role tuning us to what is important in the external world, and influencing the sensitivity of other brain regions, in order to enhance perception and memory for what is important. These effects may yet have important implications for subjective experience of emotions in the moment and potentially long-term consequences for recollection of past emotions.

Yet, as other chapters in this volume attest, those who experience damage to amygdala early in development due to progressive disorders show different patterns of behavior. For example studies of patient S. M. have found that she is spared emotional influences on early perceptual processes and her deficit lies in later evaluation of emotional stimuli and in understanding social cues (Kennedy, Gläscher, Tyszka, & Adolphs, 2009; Tsuchiya, Moradi, Felsen, Yamazaki, & Adolphs, 2009). Other studies suggest that patients in whom loss of amygdala function is evident early in life show modulation of attention by affectively salient stimuli equivalent to control subjects (Bach, Talmi, Hurlemann, Patin, & Dolan, 2011). These findings suggest that over development, other systems may wire themselves in such a way as to compensate for the amygdala's role in affect-biased attention, while later-developing links between frontal regions and the amygdala that allow later socioemotional evaluation are not developed. In contrast, in S. P., connections in amygdala and prefrontal regions linked to evaluation of socioemotional processes may have been able to develop into adulthood. For S. P., other regions, such as the orbitofrontal cortex, may allow her to perform those functions, potentially working with other regions sensitive to affective salience such as the LC or regions of the thalamus, in the absence of the amygdala. Finally, congenital amygdala damage centered on the basolateral region of the amygdala in a cluster of South African women has been linked to *increased* affect-biased attention to threat-related cues such as fearful faces and ambiguous body cues (de Gelder et al., 2014; Terburg et al., 2012). These authors suggest that the basolateral region may play a role in inhibiting arousal responses linked to activity of the central nucleus. Yet, at the same time, because they may have been unable to learn aversive associations between trusting behavior and negative outcomes, these same subjects may show higher levels of trust when making socioeconomic decisions, despite "knowing better" (van Honk, Eisenegger, Terburg, Stein, & Morgan, 2013). However, it is important to stress that any conclusions about differences related to the onset of damage are qualified by the fact that we cannot make definitive claims without more precise information on the onset of amygdala pathology, and that precise localization of subnuclei are difficult to determine precisely in humans. Here animal models are key to providing information about the role of specific subnuclei.

Overall, the evidence suggests that damage to specific subregions of the amygdala, combined with different patterns of life experience, as well as different levels of compensatory brain reorganization, may produce very different behavioral patterns, suggesting that the nature of life without an amygdala depends on when and precisely where the damage occurred. If one develops with a functioning amygdala, one may have a deficit in affect-biased attention, which implicitly tunes one to emotionally relevant aspects of the world. As a result, features of the environment may stand out because they are brighter, moving quickly, or are unusual, just as they do for any other sighted person; however, they may not stand out because they are important to one's long-term emotional goals of avoiding pain and increasing pleasure. For example, one may be less likely to have one's attention rapidly captured by a stranger's hostile expression, and may need to be more vigilant in situations where there are potential hazards. On the other hand, one may be less vulnerable to being distracted by the seductive shoes or rewarding electronic gadgets that catch one's eye when hurrying by a shop window. The visual world may also be flatter, with less emotional enhancement of the vividness of what one sees. One may also lose enhancement of memory for emotionally important events that occur after the loss of the amygdala. Thus, while the memory of positive events may lose their sweetness and vividness, one may also be spared enhanced or intrusive memories of painful events. This may sound pretty good—but to paraphrase the famous quote from George Santayana, those who cannot remember painful events may fail to avoid them in the future.

REFERENCES

Amaral, D. G., Behniea, H., & Kelly, J. L. (2003). Topographic organization of projections from the amygdala to the visual cortex in the macaque monkey. *Neuroscience, 118*(4), 1099–1120.

Amaral, D. G., & Price, J. L. (1984). Amygdalo–cortical projections in the monkey (*Macaca fascicularis*). *Journal of Comparative Neurology, 230*(4), 465–496.

Anderson, A. K. (2005). Affective influences on the attentional dynamics support-ing awareness. *Journal of Experimental Psychology: General, 134*(2), 258–281.

Anderson, A. K., & Phelps, E. A. (2000). Expression without recognition: Contri-butions of the human amygdala to emotional communication. *Psychological Science, 11*(2), 106–111.

Anderson, A. K., & Phelps, E. A. (2001). Lesions of the human amygdala impair enhanced perception of emotionally salient events. *Nature, 411*(6835), 305–309.

Anderson, A. K., & Phelps, E. A. (2002). Is the human amygdala critical for the subjective experience of emotion?: Evidence of intact dispositional affect in patients with amygdala lesions. *Journal of Cognitive Neuroscience, 14*(5), 709–720.

Bach, D. R., Talmi, D., Hurlemann, R., Patin, A., & Dolan, R. J. (2011). Automatic relevance detection in the absence of a functional amygdala. *Neuropsycholo-gia, 49*(5), 1302–1305.

Belova, M. A., Paton, J. J., Morrison, S. E., & Salzman, C. D. (2007). Expecta-tion modulates neural responses to pleasant and aversive stimuli in primate amygdala. *Neuron, 55*(6), 970–984.

Cahill, L., Gorski, L., & Le, K. (2003). Enhanced human memory consolidation with post-learning stress: Interaction with the degree of arousal at encoding. *Learning and Memory, 10*(4), 270–274.

Cahill, L., Haier, R. J., Fallon, J., Alkire, M. T., Tang, C., Keator, D., et al. (1996). Amygdala activity at encoding correlated with long-term, free recall of emotional information. *Proceedings of the National Academy of Sciences USA, 93*(15), 8016–8021.

de Gelder, B., Terburg, D., Morgan, B., Hortensius, R., Stein, D. J., & van Honk, J. (2014). The role of human basolateral amygdala in ambiguous social threat perception. *Cortex, 52*, 28–34.

De Martino, B., Strange, B. A., & Dolan, R. J. (2008). Noradrenergic neuromodu-lation of human attention for emotional and neutral stimuli. *Psychopharma-cology (Berlin), 197*(1), 127–136.

de Quervain, D. J., Kolassa, I. T., Ertl, V., Onyut, P. L., Neuner, F., Elbert, T., et al. (2007). A deletion variant of the alpha2b-adrenoceptor is related to emotional memory in Europeans and Africans. *Nature Neuroscience, 10*(9), 1137–1139.

Di Lollo, V., Kawahara, J., Shahab Ghorashi, S. M., & Enns, J. T. (2005). The atten-tional blink: Resource depletion or temporary loss of control? *Psychological Research, 69*(3), 191–200.

Ghashghaei, H. T., Hilgetag, C. C., & Barbas, H. (2007). Sequence of information processing for emotions based on the anatomic dialogue between prefrontal cortex and amygdala. *NeuroImage, 34*(3), 905–923.

Kennedy, D. P., Gläscher, J., Tyszka, J. M., & Adolphs, R. (2009). Personal space regulation by the human amygdala. *Nature Neuroscience, 12*(10), 1226–1227.

LaBar, K. S., & Cabeza, R. (2006). Cognitive neuroscience of emotional memory. *Nature Reviews Neuroscience, 7*(1), 54–64.

LaBar, K. S., Gatenby, J. C., Gore, J. C., LeDoux, J. E., & Phelps, E. A. (1998). Human amygdala activation during conditioned fear acquisition and extinc-tion: A mixed-trial fMRI study. *Neuron, 20*(5), 937–945.

LaBar, K. S., LeDoux, J. E., Spencer, D. D., & Phelps, E. A. (1995). Impaired fear conditioning following unilateral temporal lobectomy in humans. *Journal of Neuroscience, 15*(10), 6846–6855.

Lim, S. L., Padmala, S., & Pessoa, L. (2009). Segregating the significant from the mundane on a moment-to-moment basis via direct and indirect amygdala contributions. *Proceedings of the National Academy of Sciences USA, 106*(39), 16841–16846.

Markovic, J., Anderson, A. K., & Todd, R. M. (2014). Tuning to the significant: Neural and genetic processes underlying affective enhancement of visual perception and memory. *Behavioural Brain Research, 259,* 229–241.

Olsson, A., & Phelps, E. A. (2007). Social learning of fear. *Nature Neuroscience, 10*(9), 1095–1102.

Phelps, E. A. (2006). Emotion and cognition: Insights from studies of the human amygdala. *Annual Review of Psychology, 57,* 27–53.

Phelps, E. A., LaBar, K. S., Anderson, A. K., O'Connor, K. J., Fulbright, R. K., & Spencer, D. D. (1998). Specifying the contributions of the human amygdala to emotional memory: A case study. *Neurocase, 4,* 527–540.

Pourtois, G., Schettino, A., & Vuilleumier, P. (2013). Brain mechanisms for emotional influences on perception and attention: What is magic and what is not. *Biological Psychology, 92*(3), 492–512.

Prevost, C., McNamee, D., Jessup, R. K., Bossaerts, P., & O'Doherty, J. P. (2013). Evidence for model-based computations in the human amygdala during Pavlovian conditioning. *PLoS Computational Biology, 9*(2), e1002918.

Rasch, B., Spalek, K., Buholzer, S., Luechinger, R., Boesiger, P., Papassotiropoulos, A., et al. (2009). A genetic variation of the noradrenergic system is related to differential amygdala activation during encoding of emotional memories. *Proceedings of the National Academy of Sciences USA, 106*(45), 19191–19196.

Roozendaal, B., McEwen, B. S., & Chattarji, S. (2009). Stress, memory and the amygdala. *Nature Reviews Neuroscience, 10*(6), 423–433.

Sara, S. J. (2009). The locus coeruleus and noradrenergic modulation of cognition. *Nature Reviews Neuroscience, 10*(3), 211–223.

Sehlmeyer, C., Schoning, S., Zwitserlood, P., Pfleiderer, B., Kircher, T., Arolt, V., et al. (2009). Human fear conditioning and extinction in neuroimaging: A systematic review. *PLoS ONE, 4*(6), e5865.

Stevens, S. S. (1956). The direct estimation of sensory magnitudes—Loudness. *American Journal of Psychology, 69,* 1–25.

Stevens, S. S. (1957). On the psychophysical law. *Psychological Review, 64*(3), 153–181.

Terburg, D., Morgan, B. E., Montoya, E. R., Hooge, I. T., Thornton, H. B., Hariri, A. R., et al. (2012). Hypervigilance for fear after basolateral amygdala damage in humans. *Translational Psychiatry, 2,* e115.

Todd, R. M., Cunningham, W. A., Anderson, A. K., & Thompson, E. (2012a). Affect-biased attention as emotion regulation. *Trends in Cognitive Sciences, 16*(7), 365–372.

Todd, R. M., Evans, J. W., Morris, D., Lewis, M. D., & Taylor, M. J. (2011). The changing face of emotion: Age-related patterns of amygdala activation to salient faces. *Social Cognitive and Affective Neuroscience, 6*(1), 12–23.

Todd, R. M., Muller, D. J., Lee, D. H., Robertson, A., Eaton, T., Freeman, N., et al.

(2013a). Genes for emotion-enhanced remembering are linked to enhanced perceiving. *Psychological Science, 24*(11), 2244–2253.

Todd, R. M., Muller, D. J., Palombo, D. J., Robertson, A., Eaton, T., Freeman, N., et al. (2014a). Deletion variant in the *ADRA2B* gene increases coupling between emotional responses at encoding and later retrieval of emotional memories. *Neurobiology of Learning and Memory, 112*, 222–229.

Todd, R. M., Schmitz, T. W., Susskind, J., & Anderson, A. K. (2013b). Shared neural substrates of emotionally enhanced perceptual and mnemonic vividness. *Frontiers in Behavioral Neuroscience, 7*, 40.

Todd, R. M., Talmi, D., Schmitz, T. W., Susskind, J., & Anderson, A. K. (2012b). Psychophysical and neural evidence for emotion-enhanced perceptual vividness. *Journal of Neuroscience, 32*(33), 11201–11212.

Todd, R. M., Taylor, M. J., Robertson, A., Cassel, D. B., Doesberg, S. M., Lee, D. H., et al. (2014b). Temporal–spatial neural activation patterns linked to perceptual encoding of emotional salience. *PLoS ONE, 9*(4), e93753.

Tranel, D., Gullickson, G., Koch, M., & Adolphs, R. (2006). Altered experience of emotion following bilateral amygdala damage. *Cognitive Neuropsychiatry, 11*(3), 219–232.

Tsuchiya, N., Moradi, F., Felsen, C., Yamazaki, M., & Adolphs, R. (2009). Intact rapid detection of fearful faces in the absence of the amygdala. *Nature Neuroscience, 12*(10), 1224–1225.

van Honk, J., Eisenegger, C., Terburg, D., Stein, D. J., & Morgan, B. (2013). Generous economic investments after basolateral amygdala damage. *Proceedings of the National Academy of Sciences USA, 110*(7), 2506–2510.

CHAPTER 14

Implications for Understanding Amygdala Function in Mental Disorders

CHRISTOPHER S. MONK
DANIEL S. PINE

From the earliest days when neuroimaging data were acquired from psychiatric patients, the amygdala has been a source of intense focus. Such a focus was well founded. As articulated in other chapters in this book, the amygdala is crucial to emotional function. Given that many psychiatric disorders involve disturbances in emotion, brain imaging investigations have extensively examined amygdala activation across a range of mental conditions. In this chapter, we focus on functional MRI (fMRI) studies of three disorders: anxiety, depression, and autism. Each condition has a rich literature that has begun to identify more precisely how the amygdala contributes to the symptoms. In addition, the chapter also focuses on amygdala functioning during development, particularly child and adolescent development, and, where possible, describes data on developmental changes in amygdala function. Anxiety, depression, and autism each exhibit different development trajectories in terms of onset and course. By characterizing amygdala function for disorders with three important but distinct developmental components, this chapter illustrates the diverse ways in which amygdala dysfunction may evolve in a developmental context.

The amygdala, directly and indirectly via ventral prefrontal cortex modulation, is highly susceptible to the effects of environmental perturbations and genetic variation. Specifically, environmental stress and select genetic polymorphisms lead to greater amygdala activation and reduced regulatory connectivity with areas in the prefrontal cortex in response to negative stimuli and events (Bogdan, Williamson, & Hariri, 2012; Burghy et al., 2012; Hariri, Tessitore, Mattay, Fera, & Weinberger, 2002b; Maheu et al., 2010; Pezawas et al., 2005; Tottenham et al., 2011; Wiggins et al., 2014a). In healthy development, the general trajectory is for amygdala activation to decrease with age (Gee et al., 2013b; Swartz, Carrasco, Wiggins, Thomason, & Monk, 2014) and for inhibitory connectivity between the amygdala and ventral prefrontal cortex (vPFC) to increase (Gee et al., 2013a), though not all studies find these trends (Thomas et al., 2001b). Untoward environmental and genetic variables can modulate healthy development. Therefore, given its role in emotional states, modulation of amygdala function can potentially shift neural and cognitive resources toward negative events, with corresponding increases in negative affect, including anxiety and depression symptoms.

The chapter is divided into seven sections. First, we describe healthy development of the amygdala and related prefrontal cortex (PFC) structures. The second and third sections detail how environmental events and genetic factors, respectively, impact amygdala and vPFC development. In addition, these two sections also describe how the environmental and genetic variables affect attention to threat. The fourth, fifth, and sixth sections cover three disorders, anxiety, depression, and autism spectrum disorders, focusing on the nature of altered amygdala–vPFC function. The final section provides suggestions for future directions, focusing on novel methodologies, the targeting of a population-based sampling frame, and the acquisition of longitudinal data. This may generate a more complete understanding of the factors that contribute to normal and abnormal amygdala function in health and psychopathology.

Healthy Brain Development

The amygdala and the vPFC form a circuit that is fundamentally involved in the detection, identification, and response to emotional information (Monk et al., 2003; Phan, Wager, Taylor, & Liberzon, 2002). The amygdala and vPFC are densely interconnected (Carmichael & Price, 1995; Ongur & Price, 2000; Ray & Zald, 2012). Activation from the amygdala is associated with assigning emotional significance of stimuli in the environment (Davis & Whalen, 2001; Ghashghaei, Hilgetag, & Barbas, 2007; LeDoux, 2000; Ray & Zald, 2012; Sarter & Markowitsch, 1984). Meanwhile, the vPFC is thought to be involved in modulating activation from the amygdala (Sarter & Markowitsch, 1984).

The dorsal PFC may also modulate amygdala activity. However, since there are few direct connections between the dorsal PFC and the amygdala, dorsal region effects may be mediated through other structures, including the vPFC (Ray & Zald, 2012). Two insightful reviews have highlighted that the model of vPFC regulation of the amygdala is not consistently seen across studies (Crone & Dahl, 2012; Pfeifer & Allen, 2012), emphasizing the need for work on contextual and motivational factors. Moreover, it is also important to identify better the substructures that are involved in various aspects of emotion processing. To date, our knowledge is still crude. Nevertheless, useful frameworks have begun to link brain development to behavior and individual differences (Strang, Chein, & Steinberg, 2013).

Distinct vPFC components may differentially modulate amygdala activation in particular circumstances. The vPFC subregions include the orbitofrontal cortex, the ventromedial PFC, the ventral anterior cingulate cortex, and the ventrolateral PFC. Medial areas, including the ventromedial, subgenual anterior cingulate, and medial orbitofrontal cortices, are involved in automatic emotion processing, as occurs in fear extinction and monitoring of stimulus–reinforcement contingencies (Phillips, Ladouceur, & Drevets, 2008; Ray & Zald, 2012). In contrast, more lateral regions, including the ventrolateral PFC and lateral orbitofrontal cortex, may be more involved in processes that require voluntary control of attention and inhibiting prepotent responses (Phillips et al., 2008; Ray & Zald, 2012). Of note, Myers-Schulz and Koenigs (2012) have suggested that the posterior portion of the ventromedial PFC is involved in amplifying amygdala activation and anterior regions of the ventromedial PFC are involved in inhibiting amygdala activation (Myers-Schulz & Koenigs, 2012). Related to this proposal, a cross-sectional study found positive functional connectivity between the amygdala and medial PFC before age 10, but negative connectivity in older subjects (Gee et al., 2013b). This switch in connectivity was accompanied by a decrease in amygdala activation with age. Taken together, during child and adolescent development, dramatic changes take place in the functioning of the amygdala and vPFC, and it is likely that these changes have an impact on emotional functioning during development (see also Sarro & Sullivan, Chapter 4, this volume).

Environmental Effects

Brain Function

The concept of "allostatic load" describes how stress might impact brain function. Defined as stress-related wear and tear, allostatic load manifests as altered brain and stress hormone function (McEwen & Gianaros, 2010). Specifically, animal work demonstrates that chronic stress leads to three major changes within the amygdala–PFC cortex circuit: (1) an increase in dendrites within the amygdala; (2) an expansion of dendrites in the orbitofrontal cortex; and (3) dendritic retraction and spine loss in the other medial PFC regions (Goldwater et al., 2009). Both the amygdala and orbitofrontal cortex mediate anxiety-related behaviors (Kalin, Shelton, & Davidson, 2007; Kalin et al., 2008). Therefore, stress-related changes to these areas may sculpt neural systems to prioritize threats. Moreover, the medial PFC is involved in cognitive flexibility (Dias-Ferreira et al., 2009;

Liston, McEwen, & Casey, 2009). Thus, reduced dendritic number here may impair the stressed organism's ability to respond flexibly over time.

Studies in humans exposed to environmental stress complement basic science research on allostatic load. Evidence for this comes from work on humans who were exposed to a wide range of adverse environments during development. In a study examining youth who experienced early childhood deprivation because they lived in an institution, adverse rearing conditions were associated with increased amygdala activation in response to emotional faces (Tottenham et al., 2011). Similarly, in another study, children who experienced caregiver deprivation and emotional neglect exhibited greater amygdala activation compared with nondeprived comparisons (Maheu et al., 2010). Another study quantified resting-state functional connectivity in the amygdala–PFC circuit among prospectively followed children experiencing varying levels of stress (Burghy et al., 2012). This study found that early-life stressors in females but not males predict increased cortisol in childhood and decreased connectivity between the amygdala and ventral portion of the medial PFC at age 18. Thus, although there are few studies in humans during development to date, the existing work is broadly consistent with the animal studies and suggests that adverse environmental conditions alter the amygdala and increases activation, while reducing functional connectivity between the amygdala and the medial PFC.

Attention Bias

Are there behavioral manifestations of adverse environments in children and adolescents that might reflect aspects of perturbed amygdala–frontal development? The previously described study of institutionalized children (Tottenham et al., 2011) also found an interesting association with amygdala activation: It correlated with individual differences in reduced eye contact when the same children were engaged in dyadic interactions with another person. Moreover, the association between early adversity and eye contact was also mediated by amygdala activity. Other studies have used a probe detection paradigm (Bradley, Mogg, White, Groom, & de Bono, 1999; Mogg, Bradley, Millar, & White, 1995) to characterize better how adverse environments predict attention to threatening stimuli. To date, however, the precise effects are unclear. Studies indicate that physically abused children exhibited greater attention bias toward threatening faces (Pollak & Tolley-Schell, 2003). However, we found that maltreated children, many with posttraumatic stress disorder (PTSD), showed an attention bias *away* from threat (Pine et al., 2005), consistent with longitudinal research on PTSD in adults (Wald et al., 2013). Finally, in a study of young children between ages 4 and 7, only children who were exposed to violence and had PTSD symptoms exhibited an attention bias to threat

(Swartz, Graham-Bermann, Mogg, Bradley, & Monk, 2011). Children who were exposed to violence but did not have PTSD symptoms did not show the attention bias. Differences in variables, such as the duration of presentation of the threatening stimuli or the age of subjects, may contribute to cross-study differences in the observed associations. It will be important ultimately not only to provide more detailed and longitudinal studies in humans but also to integrate this literature with studies in nonhuman animals where direct experimental perturbations are possible.

Genetic Factors

Brain Function

Considerable attention has focused on the serotonin transporter-linked polymorphic region (*5-HTTLPR*) and how it impacts amygdala function. *5-HTTLPR* has "short" and "long" alleles depending on the number of tandem repeats (Collier et al., 1996), which affects production of the serotonin transporter and hence levels of serotonin during synaptic transmission. There is a single-nucleotide polymorphism (SNP) in the long allele, in which guanine is replaced with adenine. A long allele with adenine (L_A) is related to greater serotonin transporter expression than a long allele with guanine (L_G) or the short allele (Hu et al., 2006).

Studies of adults find that individuals with the lower expressing *5-HTTLPR* variants have greater amygdala activation in response to emotional faces relative to those with higher expressing variants (Hariri et al., 2002a; Munafo, Brown, & Hariri, 2008). Similar findings have been found in youth. Specifically, adolescents with at least one copy of the short (S) or L_G allele demonstrate greater amygdala activation in response to fearful faces relative to adolescents with higher expressing alleles when rating subjective fear (Lau et al., 2009). Similarly, adolescents with the lower expressing polymorphism exhibit greater amygdala activation in response to angry faces (Battaglia et al., 2012). In another study in which sad mood was induced with clips from movies, Furman, Hamilton, Joorman, and Gotlib (2011) showed that the *5-HTTLPR* S allele carriers had greater left amygdala activation in a sample of female children and adolescents. Thus, across ages and fMRI tasks, the lower expressing serotonin allele is associated with greater amygdala activation.

At the same time, a recent study indicates that development may impact *5-HTTLPR*-related findings. Specifically, Wiggins, Swartz, Martin, Lord, and Monk (2014b) found an age × genotype interaction by which the influence of the serotonin transporter genotype only impacted amygdala activation in youth studied in late adolescence. Moreover, an earlier study found that the low-expressing allele is related to decreased connectivity between the amygdala and prefrontal regulatory regions in adults (Pezawas et al., 2005). Similar to the amygdala finding, Wiggins et al. (2014b) also found that the 5-HTTLPR-related connectivity finding did not appear until later in adolescence; therefore, 5-HTTLPR genotype appears to influence the trajectory of brain development, emphasizing the need to consider developmental variables when examining genotype-related brain function.

Another important gene variant is brain-derived neurotrophic factor (BDNF), which is thought to modulate synaptic plasticity and neuronal differentiation (Chen et al., 2006). A functional variant of the gene comprises an SNP with an adenine to guanine substitution (rs6265) in the 5′ prodomain region. This produces either valine or methionine at codon 66 (Val66Met; Bath & Lee, 2006). The Met allele is associated with a decrease in BDNF and is thought to increase vulnerability for affective dysregulation (Chen et al., 2006). In healthy adults, the Met variant is associated with increased amygdala activation in a startle paradigm (Montag, Reuter, Newport, Elger, & Weber, 2008). Interestingly, no BDNF genotype-related differences were found in healthy adolescents using an emotional faces task (Lau et al., 2010). However, in a resting paradigm, Thomason, Yoo, Gover, and Gotlib (2009) reported that Met carriers show increased connectivity between the amygdala, insula, and striatal areas. These seemingly contradictory findings highlight an important issue in neuroimaging research: The task condition (e.g., viewing emotional faces or rest) may heavily influence the types of results that are identified.

Provocative findings are also obtained when researchers examine the effects of both genotype and environment together. Within the exon 2 of the mineralocorticoid receptor gene (NR3C2), a missense polymorphism (rs5522) results in a substitution of an adenine nucleotide for guanine. This changes the amino acid from valine (Val) to isoleucine (Iso). The Val allele is characterized as exhibiting reduced cortisol binding, which has the potential to increase hypothalamic–pituitary–adrenal axis reactivity (DeRijk et al., 2006; van Leeuwen et al., 2010). Indeed, several studies found that the Val allele is also associated with heightened stress reactivity in adults (Bogdan, Perlis, Fagerness, & Pizzagalli, 2010; DeRijk et al., 2006; van Leeuwen et al., 2010). Moreover, in a study of 279 children and adolescents between ages 11 and 15 years, Val carrier status and childhood neglect were each independently associated with increased amygdala activation (Bogdan et al., 2012). Importantly, after accounting for the main effects, there was a significant interaction between mineralocorticoid receptor genotype and childhood neglect. In a study examining the same sample, investigators examined common polymorphisms in the gene for FK506 protein 5 (FKBP5; White et al., 2012). This gene is involved in hypothalamic–pituitary–adrenal axis transcriptional regulation. In addition to a main effect of emotional neglect on the amygdala, an interaction between each SNP and emotional neglect emerged, with risk alleles and higher emotional neglect combining to predict greater amygdala activation. These findings indicate that heightened amygdala activation may mediate the interaction of childhood adversity with genetic variants and increase the risk of psychopathology.

Attention Bias

Just as environmental adversity impacts attention bias to threat, similar results have been found for the relationship between genetic polymorphisms and attention bias. Specifically, Perez-Edgar and colleagues (2010) found that the low expressing variant of the serotonin polymorphism gene was associated with greater attention bias to threatening stimuli; these findings were echoed in a recent meta-analysis (Pergamin-Hight, Bakermans-Kranenburg, van IJzendoorn, & Bar-Haim, 2012). One study found that the low expressing variant of *5-HTTLPR* exhibited greater attention bias in response to fear faces presented subliminally than did their high expressing counterparts, but not when faces were presented supraliminally (Thomason et al., 2010). Further studies of how genetic variants impact attention bias will help investigators to understand better the effect of genes on a precise behavior that is related to various forms of psychopathology. In this way, genetic and environmental influences, as two sets of distal causes, can ultimately be related to both brain function and behavioral bias, permitting a rich understanding of individual differences.

Pediatric Anxiety

Brain Function

Anxiety disorders, including generalized anxiety and social phobia, are consistently linked to increased amygdala activation in response to threats. This has been documented in children, adolescents, and adults (Etkin & Wager, 2007; Guyer et al., 2008; McClure et al., 2007; Monk et al., 2008b; Thomas et al., 2001a). Moreover, analogous to what was described in the previous sections on the environment and genetics, connectivity between the amygdala and vPFC is also affected in anxiety disorders. In particular, Guyer and colleagues (2008) found that adolescents with social anxiety exhibited stronger coupling between the amygdala and ventrolateral PFC while rating desirability of peers. Similarly, in a study in which adolescents viewed briefly presented emotional faces, those with generalized anxiety disorder showed greater connectivity between the amygdala and ventrolateral PFC when the analysis was performed across all conditions (Monk et al., 2008b). However, when a psychophysiological interaction (PPI) analysis was performed specifically to examine connectivity for angry relative to neutral faces, a different pattern emerged: Controls showed stronger negative connectivity compared to the adolescents with generalized anxiety disorder, although this effect only exhibited modest statistical reliability (Monk et al., 2008b). As articulated in the two reviews described earlier (Crone & Dahl, 2012; Pfeifer & Allen, 2012), the relationship between amygdala–prefrontal connectivity and behavioral function is complex. These findings from pediatric anxiety are consistent with that perspective. Part of the problem may be that there are age-related changes in connectivity, as indicated recently (Gee et al., 2013b). In addition, specifics of the task and the connectivity analytic procedures also play a major role in the pattern of findings.

Attention Bias

Examining the role of attention to emotional stimuli, particularly threats, is an area of intense focus. Many studies evaluated attention bias in response to threatening faces in anxious subjects. The impetus for this line of research is that anxiety symptoms may be partly fueled by hyperattention to potential threats, and negative facial expressions represent an important evolutionarily conserved source of threat. Such attention may actually cause or sustain anxiety, based on data in randomized controlled trials in which patients with anxiety disorders were trained to reduce their attention to threatening stimuli (Eldar et al., 2012). In such studies, attention training has been shown to reduce anxiety symptoms significantly in children with anxiety disorders. In addition, Britton and colleagues (2013) found that training subjects to attend to happy faces did not increase patients' response to cognitive-behavioral therapy, based on clinician ratings; nevertheless, those who received training reported decreased anxiety earlier, based on self-report measures, than patients who only received cognitive-behavioral therapy. These clinical trials show that this form of treatment effectively reduces anxiety for those patients who hyperattend to threatening stimuli. Therefore, attention bias to threatening stimuli appears to play a role in anxiety. In terms of the amygdala, we found that the degree of amygdala activation positively correlated with attention bias in response to briefly presented angry faces in a sample of children and adolescents with generalized anxiety disorder (Monk et al., 2008b). In addition, a recent study examined the brain correlates of attention training in a sample of adults with elevated social anxiety symptoms and found that subjects showed reduced bilateral amygdala activation and increased activation of several structures within the PFC following training (Taylor et al., 2014). More work is necessary to understand better how the amygdala and the PFC are involved in biasing attention to or away from threatening stimuli. Taken together, though, these studies suggest that hyperactivation of the amygdala may be involved in the early detection and attention to threat, and that attention training may help to involve the PFC to reduce amygdala activation and modulate the attention bias.

Pediatric Depression

Brain Function

Similar to anxiety, adolescents with depression exhibit greater amygdala activation across multiple types of emotion-based tasks, including reward tasks (Forbes et al., 2006), tasks requiring the viewing of emotional faces (Roberson-Nay et al., 2006), or maintaining an emotional response to negative-valence images (Perlman et al., 2012). In addition, we examined adolescents who were at increased risk for depression based on parental history of the disorder and found that risk for depression also related to greater activation of the amygdala in response to fearful faces when attention was unconstrained (Monk et al., 2008a). Of note, when attention was constrained by task instructions, there were no group differences in activation. These findings suggest that familial depression risk is associated with altered amygdala function when subjects are viewing fearful faces and their attention is not directed. In contrast, directing attention has the capacity to normalize amygdala function temporarily in this at-risk group.

Whereas a growing number of publications examined amygdala function in adolescents with depression, only a few studies have begun to examine the amygdalae in young children with the condition, since depression is relatively rare before puberty. Nevertheless, in an effort to understand early risk markers, researchers have begun to study ever-younger samples, including children diagnosed with depression in preschool. At present, the findings are somewhat mixed. When examining 4- to 6-year-old children, the investigators found that children with depression showed greater amygdala activation in response to emotional faces relative to controls (Gaffrey, Barch, Singer, Shenoy, & Luby, 2013). However, when 7- to 11-year-old children with a history of preschool depression were examined, there were no significant differences in amygdala activation between the patient group and controls (Barch, Gaffrey, Botteron, Belden, & Luby, 2012). These inconsistent findings may be due to differences in the sample or the task. Specifically, some of the participants in the study with older children did not have current depression. In addition, the study with older children induced negative emotion by showing a sad video clip, which was not done in the study of younger children. Moreover, whereas the study with younger children was a block design (i.e., the same emotion was presented multiple times) and subjects pressed a button to indicate that a face was presented, the study with older children was event-related (i.e., different emotions were presented from trial to trial) and subjects pressed a button to identify the gender of the face. Beyond the difference in age in these studies, the differences in the sample and procedures may have accounted for the discrepant findings. More research is necessary to understand amygdala function in young children with depression.

In terms of functional connectivity, youth with depression also evidence differences in coupling between the amygdala and PFC relative to controls. Perlman and colleagues (2012) found that when asked to maintain their emotional reaction to negatively valenced visual stimuli, adolescents with depression showed less connectivity between the amygdala and the medial PFC. Similarly, in a sample of 7- to 11-year-old children, depression was related to weaker connectivity between the amygdala and structures within the PFC (Luking et al., 2011).

Investigations have begun to uncover how genetic variability maps onto heterogeneity in brain function in children and adolescents with depression. Lau and colleagues (2009) found that youth with depression and/or anxiety and controls showed a *5-HTTLPR* genotype × diagnosis interaction for amygdala activation when viewing happy and fearful faces. Consistent with other data in healthy adults (Hariri, Mattay, Tessitore, Fera, & Weinberger, 2003), healthy adolescents with the low expressing genotype demonstrated greater amygdala activation than healthy adolescents with the high expressing genotype. In contrast, depressed and anxious patients with the high expressing genotype showed greater activation in the amygdala compared to patients with the low expressing genotype. Lau and colleagues (2010) also examined the contribution of BDNF genetic variants on amygdala function in adolescent patients with depression and/or anxiety. As stated earlier, no genotype differences were found within the control group. However, within the patient group, the Met allele was associated with greater amygdala activation to emotional faces. These two studies suggest that genotype may modulate between-group differences in amygdala function, possibly identifying subgroups of patients.

Attention Bias

Relative to anxiety, fewer researchers have examined how depression is associated with attention to emotional stimuli and events in children and adolescents. Nevertheless, the few studies that have been done indicate that depression does affect attention function. Specifically, in a relatively large study ($N = 161$) of children and adolescents, depression without anxiety was associated with an attention bias in response to sad faces, depression comorbid with anxiety related to attention bias in response to both sad and angry faces, and anxiety without depression was linked to attention bias in response to angry faces (Hankin, Gibb, Abela, & Flory, 2010).

Moreover, among healthy girls at risk for depression based on maternal history, Joormann, Talbot, and Gotlib (2007) found that the girls at risk for depression attended to the sad but not the happy faces, whereas low-risk girls attended to the happy but not the sad faces following a mood induction procedure. These findings indicate that depression and depression risk is associated with specific cognitive sequelae in the form of a greater attention allocation to sad faces. To date, the brain correlates of this pattern of attention bias are not known. An important next step will be to identify how the amygdala and related structures are involved in attention bias in response to negatively valenced faces in pediatric depression.

Autism Spectrum Disorder

Brain Function

Autism spectrum disorder (ASD) is a neurodevelopmental condition that involves impaired social function, communication difficulties along with repetitive and restrictive behaviors. Similar to anxiety, the amygdala has been the subject of intense focus in ASD, because social impairments are key features of ASD, and the amygdala plays a fundamental role in processing social cues, as well as emotional processes, that so often come with social interactions. Conceptually, one perspective holds that the social deficits in ASD are partly due to an early-appearing lack of interest in the social world. Indirect support for this view comes from many fMRI studies showing that individuals with ASD exhibit reduced amygdala activation compared to control participants (Ashwin, Baron-Cohen, Wheelwright, O'Riordan, & Bullmore, 2007; Critchley et al., 2000; Grelotti et al., 2005; Hadjikhani, Joseph, Snyder, & Tager-Flusberg, 2007; Pelphrey, Morris, McCarthy, & Labar, 2007; Pinkham, Hopfinger, Pelphrey, Piven, & Penn, 2008; Wang, Lee, Sigman, & Dapretto, 2006). Since the amygdala is crucial to processing socioemotional information, reduced activation suggests that such stimuli are less engaging.

At the same time, other studies indicate that individuals with ASD may not lack interest in social stimuli but rather become distressed by such stimuli. Consistent with this perspective, eye tracking research suggests that people with ASD actively avoid looking at the eyes, an area of the face that is a source of rich socioemotional information (Kliemann, Dziobek, Hatri, Steimke, & Heekeren, 2010). In addition, in response to emotional faces, children with ASD evidence greater autonomic arousal than do healthy children (Agam, Joseph, Barton, & Manoach, 2010). Moreover, in contrast to the fMRI studies on participants with ASD described earlier, other studies found that adolescents and adults show increased amygdala activation in response to faces relative to controls (Dalton et al., 2005; Kleinhans et al., 2009; Kliemann, Dziobek, Hatri, Baudewig, & Heekeren, 2012; Monk et al., 2010; Weng et al., 2011). This inconsistency in amygdala findings may be due to a combination of the face presentation duration and attention. Specifically, studies that found that the amygdala was underactive in ASD presented faces for longer periods of time and did not monitor attention to the face or features of the face. Thus, subjects with autism may have spent less time attending to the faces than the control group, since the faces may have caused distress, which led to avoidance and lack of amygdala activation.

To characterize amygdala activation in ASD better, Swartz and colleagues (2013) charted amygdala habituation in children and adolescents. "Habituation" is defined as the decline in activation following initial activation to a stimulus or a class of stimuli (e.g., sad faces) over the course of repeated presentations. Whereas the control group habituated to the faces, the group with ASD did not show amygdala habituation to sad and neutral faces. Indeed, over the course of the face presentation, the ASD group showed increased amygdala activation, a pattern known as "sensitization." Since work from animal models suggests that heightened amygdala activation may index distress (Davis & Shi, 1999; Davis & Whalen, 2001; LeDoux, 2000), the pattern of activation is consistent with the idea that faces induce distress in individuals with ASD.

As for interactions of the amygdala with other structures, youth with ASD have reduced amygdala–ventromedial PFC connectivity relative to controls in response to viewing sad faces (Swartz et al., 2013). Moreover, another group found that the pattern of connectivity between the amygdala and PFC differed depending on the particular structure (Ecker et al., 2012). Specifically, in a task that involved the presentation of emotional faces with interference trials, children with ASD exhibited reduced connectivity between the left amygdala and subgenual anterior cingulate, and increased connectivity between the right amygdala and the pregenual anterior cingulate relative to controls.

Progress is also being made in using genetic variants to better understand heterogeneity in socioemotional function and amygdala activation in ASD. Such work offers the possibility of identifying different etiologies and prognoses for subgroups of individuals with the disorder. Although *5-HTTLPR* variants do not appear to be related to risk for ASD, the lower expressing polymorphisms are related to greater social impairment (Brune et al., 2006; Tordjman et al., 2001). Based on these behavioral findings, as well as the amygdala habituation findings described earlier (Swartz et al., 2013), Wiggins and colleagues (2014b) examined how *5-HTTLPR* genotype impacts amygdala habituation to emotional faces. Specifically, the lack of amygdala habituation to sad faces previously found within the ASD group (Swartz et al., 2013) was driven by the low expressing genotype (Wiggins et al., 2014b). Another gene that is involved in ASD is Met receptor tyrosine kinase (*MET*; Levitt & Campbell, 2009). This gene encodes proteins in the ERK/P13K signaling pathway. The C variant of *MET* leads to reduced expression of *MET* and is linked to ASD (Campbell et al., 2006, 2007; Campbell, Li, Sutcliffe, Persico, & Levitt, 2008; Jackson et al., 2009). In particular, those with the C allele have more severe social and communication impairments (Campbell, Warren, Sutcliffe, Lee, & Levitt, 2010). In an fMRI study of children and adolescents with ASD, as well as controls, the C allele was associated with greater amygdala activation, and this effect was stronger in those with ASD (Rudie et al., 2012). Further work with larger samples are necessary to link the genetic variants and amygdala function to heterogeneity in symptom and severity. Moreover, as described earlier, since the impact of genetic polymorphisms on amygdala activation varies based on age (Wiggins et al., 2014b), it will also be important for future work to consider age and other developmental variables carefully.

Attention Bias

In contrast to brain imaging work, there is little research examining attention to faces and emotion in ASD. One study found that individuals with ASD, as compared with healthy subjects, directed less attention to the eyes in facial photographs (Dalton et al., 2005). Moreover, the same study found that levels of directed gaze to the eyes positively correlated with levels of amygdala activation in ASD. Similarly, as discussed earlier, another eye-tracking study found that individuals with ASD demonstrated an active avoidance of looking to the eyes of the faces (Kliemann et al., 2010). Since the eyes communicate an incredible amount of information concerning the social situation, reduced attention to the eyes represents a missed opportunity for individuals with ASD to comprehend social and emotional cues better. At present, it is unknown why people with ASD evidence reduced gaze to the eyes. As discussed earlier, certain social stimuli, possibly including the eyes, may induce a sense of distress in people with ASD. Further work that combines eye-tracking measures and brain imaging of the amygdala will shed light on the question of what drives people with ASD to avoid attending to the eyes.

Future Directions

The use of fMRI has greatly increased our understanding of the role of the amygdala across multiple forms of psychopathology. Looking ahead, it is important to build on these initial studies. To this end, we propose further emphasis on three approaches: (1) integrating fMRI with other methodologies that will deepen our understanding of potential underlying causes, as well as the effects of the particular profile of amygdala; (2) extending these existing findings to larger and more representative samples that better reflect the population under consideration; and (3) assembling developmental samples that are rich in environmental and genetic variables and follow them longitudinally with fMRI. These three approaches are discussed below.

Integration of Multiple Methodologies

To further understand the causes and consequences of perturbed amygdala activation in specific psychopathologies, it is necessary to acquire multiple types of data. First, since amygdala activation varies with attention and direction of eye gaze (Dalton et al., 2005), it is important to monitor eye gaze. As described earlier, investigators have worked to develop tasks that minimize group differences in attention and eye gaze. Nevertheless, moving forward, it is important to use eye-tracking measures during fMRI acquisition to gain a more thorough understanding of the relationships among attention, amygdala function, and psychopathology. At the same time, MRI-compatible eye-tracking data are difficult to acquire and require a calibration phase. Calibration requires considerable subject cooperation, which can increase anxiety and jeopardize an entire scanning session in some subjects. However, despite these caveats, the simultaneous use of eye-tracking data along with measures of amygdala activation will be important in clarifying the role of attention and amygdala activation in different subject populations.

In addition, including the collection of diffusion tensor imaging (DTI) along with fMRI will provide greater understanding of how amygdala activation is associated with white-matter tracts between the amygdala and other structures, including regions within the PFC. This multimethod approach will aid in increasing the understanding of how other structures influence the amygdala, how the development of connections between these structures impact amygdala activation, and how these trajectories contribute to the emergence of psychopathology.

It will also be important to make progress in understanding the contributions to amygdala function of molecular mechanisms. As detailed earlier, molecular genetics is helping to identify how specific genetic polymorphisms are associated with alterations in amygdala activation. It will be important to extend this to work to epigenetics as well. A major consideration in conducting epigenetic neuroimaging research, however, is that unlike genetic polymorphisms, epigenetic marks may vary across cell types within an individual. Therefore, given that it is not ethically feasible to acquire neurons from living patients, investigators rely on peripheral material (e.g., blood and saliva) to acquire epigenetic marks. However, an epigenetic profile from the periphery may not translate to the brain. Although this may be an acceptable limitation for many areas of investigation (e.g., obesity and cancer), it is less ideal for studying conditions that are thought to involve the brain.

Extension to Larger and More Representative Samples

As detailed in a recent meta-analysis (Button et al., 2013), insufficiently powered studies not only reduce the likelihood of finding true effects but also the likelihood that a statistically significant effect is a true result. Neuroimaging, particularly studies that include difficult-to-recruit samples, such as those with well-characterized forms of psychopathology, are often underpowered. The result is findings that do not replicate. Therefore, to generate reliable, replicable findings, it is important to collect data on larger samples.

A related point is that our clinical samples are often derived from university or government clinics. Similarly, the comparison groups come from Craig's List and other volunteer websites. Thus, as recently articulated, these samples are almost always highly self-selective and, consequently, do not represent the population under consideration (Falk et al., 2013). Moreover, since conditions such as anxiety and depression are underdiagnosed, the participants from the university or government clinic may be particularly unrepresentative of those who suffer from these conditions. The result is that the existing corpus of findings may not be applicable to many groups of individuals. It is not necessary for all studies to recruit representative samples. After all, there is significant value in understanding potential brain mechanisms that mediate psychopathology in samples from clinics, since those are the ones who are and will be seeking treatment. However, it is important for the field to understand brain function related to psychopathology in the broader population as well. To accomplish this, it will be important for neuroscientists to team up with individuals with expertise in recruiting representative samples (Falk et al., 2013).

Longitudinal Studies

Prior structural studies have successfully examined changes in amygdala volume, as well as gray and white matter longitudinally (Barnea-Goraly et al., 2014; Nordahl et al., 2012). In contrast, few fMRI studies have been undertaken to examine longitudinal changes in amygdala function. There are at least three reasons for this. First, the test–retest reliability of fMRI is suboptimal (Britton et al., 2013). Therefore, unlike MRI, an fMRI study of longitudinal change may include a relatively high degree of noise in the analytic models. Second, performing the task during multiple scans may allow for the introduction of practice effects. Third, in a longitudinal design, subjects have multiple opportunities to move. Motion is a major problem in all pediatric neuroimaging research. Multiple scans may make the attrition rate unacceptably high. Fortunately, these issues of reliability of the measure, practice effects, and missing data have been successfully addressed by other disciplines, including psychology, education, and demography. In order to integrate longitudinal designs effectively, it will be important to collaborate with individuals in these fields.

Conclusion

fMRI studies of children and adolescents demonstrate that the amygdala exhibits altered activation across a range of psychopathology, including, anxiety, depression, and autism. Initially, there may have been an expectation that amygdala activation would be specific and diagnostic. That is, one pattern of activation would correspond to one disorder, and another pattern would relate to another disorder. However, as research progresses, it is becoming clear that amygdala activation relates more broadly to many mental health conditions. It may be that amygdala activation indexes an emotional response. Since difficulty in emotion processing is a hallmark of many disorders, including those discussed in this chapter, as well as other conditions such as schizophrenia and bipolar disorder, altered amygdala activation is a common thread. Further work that integrates multiple methodologies, the recruitment of samples that better reflect the population under consideration, and longitudinal neuroimaging studies will further our understanding of the role of the amygdala in the development of psychopathology.

REFERENCES

Agam, Y., Joseph, R. M., Barton, J. J., & Manoach, D. S. (2010). Reduced cognitive control of response inhibition by the anterior cingulate cortex in autism spectrum disorders. *NeuroImage, 52*(1), 336–347.

Ashwin, C., Baron-Cohen, S., Wheelwright, S., O'Riordan, M., & Bullmore, E. T. (2007). Differential activation of the amygdala and the "social brain" during fearful face-processing in Asperger syndrome. *Neuropsychologia, 45*(1), 2–14.

Barch, D. M., Gaffrey, M. S., Botteron, K. N., Belden, A. C., & Luby, J. L. (2012). Functional brain activation to emotionally valenced faces in school-aged children with a history of preschool-onset major depression. *Biological Psychiatry, 72*(12), 1035–1042.

Barnea-Goraly, N., Frazier, T. W., Piacenza, L., Minshew, N. J., Keshavan, M. S., Reiss, A. L., et al. (2014). A preliminary longitudinal volumetric MRI study of amygdala and hippocampal volumes in autism. *Progress in Neuropsychopharmacology and Biological Psychiatry, 48*, 124–128.

Bath, K. G., & Lee, F. S. (2006). Variant BDNF (Val66Met) impact on brain structure and function. *Cognitive, Affective, and Behavioral Neuroscience, 6*(1), 79–85.

Battaglia, M., Zanoni, A., Taddei, M., Giorda, R., Bertoletti, E., Lampis, V., et al. (2012). Cerebral responses to emotional expressions and the development of social anxiety disorder: A preliminary longitudinal study. *Depression and Anxiety, 29*(1), 54–61.

Bogdan, R., Perlis, R. H., Fagerness, J., & Pizzagalli, D. A. (2010). The impact of mineralocorticoid receptor ISO/VAL genotype (rs5522) and stress on reward learning. *Genes, Brain, and Behavior, 9*(6), 658–667.

Bogdan, R., Williamson, D. E., & Hariri, A. R. (2012). Mineralocorticoid receptor Iso/Val (rs5522) genotype moderates the association between previous childhood emotional neglect and amygdala reactivity. *American Journal of Psychiatry, 169*(5), 515–522.

Bradley, B. P., Mogg, K., White, J., Groom, C., & de Bono, J. (1999). Attentional bias for emotional faces in generalized anxiety disorder. *British Journal of Clinical Psychology, 38*(3), 267–278.

Britton, J. C., Bar-Haim, Y., Clementi, M. A., Sankin, L. S., Chen, G., Shechner, T., et al. (2013). Training-associated changes and stability of attention bias in youth: Implications for attention bias modification treatment for pediatric anxiety. *Deveopmental Cognitive Neuroscience, 4*, 52–64.

Brune, C. W., Kim, S. J., Salt, J., Leventhal, B. L., Lord, C., & Cook, E. H., Jr. (2006). *5-HTTLPR* genotype-specific phenotype in children and adolescents with autism. *American Journal of Psychiatry, 163*(12), 2148–2156.

Burghy, C. A., Stodola, D. E., Ruttle, P. L., Molloy, E. K., Armstrong, J. M., Oler, J. A., et al. (2012). Developmental pathways to amygdala–prefrontal function and internalizing symptoms in adolescence. *Nature Neuroscience, 15*(12), 1736–1741.

Button, K. S., Ioannidis, J. P., Mokrysz, C., Nosek, B. A., Flint, J., Robinson, E. S., et al. (2013). Power failure: Why small sample size undermines the reliability of neuroscience. *Nature Reviews Neuroscience, 14*(5), 365–376.

Campbell, D. B., D'Oronzio, R., Garbett, K., Ebert, P. J., Mirnics, K., Levitt, P., et al. (2007). Disruption of cerebral cortex MET signaling in autism spectrum disorder. *Annals of Neurology, 62*(3), 243–250.

Campbell, D. B., Li, C., Sutcliffe, J. S., Persico, A. M., & Levitt, P. (2008). Genetic evidence implicating multiple genes in the MET receptor tyrosine kinase pathway in autism spectrum disorder. *Autism Research, 1*(3), 159–168.

Campbell, D. B., Sutcliffe, J. S., Ebert, P. J., Militerni, R., Bravaccio, C., Trillo, S., et al. (2006). A genetic variant that disrupts MET transcription is associated with autism. *Proceedings of the National Academy of Sciences USA, 103*(45), 16834–16839.

Campbell, D. B., Warren, D., Sutcliffe, J. S., Lee, E. B., & Levitt, P. (2010). Association of MET with social and communication phenotypes in individuals with autism spectrum disorder. *American Journal of Medical Genetics B: Neuropsychiatric Genetics, 153*(2), 438–446.

Carmichael, S. T., & Price, J. L. (1995). Sensory and premotor connections of the orbital and medial prefrontal cortex of macaque monkeys. *Journal of Comparative Neurology, 363*(4), 642–664.

Chen, Z. Y., Jing, D., Bath, K. G., Ieraci, A., Khan, T., Siao, C. J., et al. (2006). Genetic variant BDNF (Val66Met) polymorphism alters anxiety-related behavior. *Science, 314*(5796), 140–143.

Collier, D. A., Stober, G., Li, T., Heils, A., Catalano, M., Di Bella, D., et al. (1996). A novel functional polymorphism within the promoter of the serotonin transporter gene: Possible role in susceptibility to affective disorders. *Molecular Psychiatry, 1*(6), 453–460.

Critchley, H. D., Daly, E. M., Bullmore, E. T., Williams, S. C., Van Amelsvoort, T., Robertson, D. M., et al. (2000). The functional neuroanatomy of social behaviour: Changes in cerebral blood flow when people with autistic disorder process facial expressions. *Brain, 123*(11), 2203–2212.

Crone, E. A., & Dahl, R. E. (2012). Understanding adolescence as a period of social-affective engagement and goal flexibility. *Nature Reviews Neuroscience, 13*(9), 636–650.

Dalton, K. M., Nacewicz, B. M., Johnstone, T., Schaefer, H. S., Gernsbacher, M. A., Goldsmith, H. H., et al. (2005). Gaze fixation and the neural circuitry of face processing in autism. *Nature Neuroscience, 8*(4), 519–526.

Davis, M., & Shi, C. (1999). The extended amygdala: Are the central nucleus of the amygdala and the bed nucleus of the stria terminalis differentially involved in fear versus anxiety? *Annals of the New York Academy of Sciences, 877*, 281–291.

Davis, M., & Whalen, P. J. (2001). The amygdala: Vigilance and emotion. *Molecular Psychiatry, 6*(1), 13–34.

DeRijk, R. H., Wust, S., Meijer, O. C., Zennaro, M. C., Federenko, I. S., Hellhammer, D. H., et al. (2006). A common polymorphism in the mineralocorticoid receptor modulates stress responsiveness. *Journal of Clinical Endocrinology and Metabolism, 91*(12), 5083–5089.

Dias-Ferreira, E., Sousa, J. C., Melo, I., Morgado, P., Mesquita, A. R., Cerqueira, J. J., et al. (2009). Chronic stress causes frontostriatal reorganization and affects decision-making. *Science, 325*(5940), 621–625.

Ecker, C., Suckling, J., Deoni, S. C., Lombardo, M. V., Bullmore, E. T., Baron-Cohen, S., et al. (2012). Brain anatomy and its relationship to behavior in adults with autism spectrum disorder: A multicenter magnetic resonance imaging study. *Archives of General Psychiatry, 69*(2), 195–209.

Eldar, S., Apter, A., Lotan, D., Edgar, K. P., Naim, R., Fox, N. A., et al. (2012). Attention bias modification treatment for pediatric anxiety disorders: A randomized controlled trial. *American Journal of Psychiatry, 169*(2), 213–220.

Etkin, A., & Wager, T. D. (2007). Functional neuroimaging of anxiety: A meta-analysis of emotional processing in PTSD, social anxiety disorder, and specific phobia. *American Journal of Psychiatry, 164*(10), 1476–1488.

Falk, E. B., Hyde, L. W., Mitchell, C., Faul, J., Gonzalez, R., Heitzeg, M. M., et al. (2013). What is a representative brain?: Neuroscience meets population science. *Proceedings of the National Academy of Sciences USA, 110*(44), 17615–17622.

Forbes, E. E., Christopher May, J., Siegle, G. J., Ladouceur, C. D., Ryan, N. D.,

Carter, C. S., et al. (2006). Reward-related decision-making in pediatric major depressive disorder: An fMRI study. *Journal of Child Psychology and Psychiatry and Allied Disciplines, 47*(10), 1031–1040.

Furman, D. J., Hamilton, J. P., Joormann, J., & Gotlib, I. H. (2011). Altered timing of amygdala activation during sad mood elaboration as a function of *5-HTTLPR. Social Cognitive and Affective Neuroscience, 6*(3), 270–276.

Gaffrey, M. S., Barch, D. M., Singer, J., Shenoy, R., & Luby, J. L. (2013). Disrupted amygdala reactivity in depressed 4- to 6-year-old children. *Journal of the American Academy of Child and Adolescent Psychiatry, 52*(7), 737–746.

Gee, D. G., Gabard-Durnam, L. J., Flannery, J., Goff, B., Humphreys, K. L., Telzer, E. H., et al. (2013a). Early developmental emergence of human amygdala-prefrontal connectivity after maternal deprivation. *Proceedings of the National Academy of Sciences USA, 110*(39), 15638–15643.

Gee, D. G., Humphreys, K. L., Flannery, J., Goff, B., Telzer, E. H., Shapiro, M., et al. (2013b). A developmental shift from positive to negative connectivity in human amygdala–prefrontal circuitry. *Journal of Neuroscience, 33*(10), 4584–4593.

Ghashghaei, H. T., Hilgetag, C. C., & Barbas, H. (2007). Sequence of information processing for emotions based on the anatomic dialogue between prefrontal cortex and amygdala. *NeuroImage, 34*(3), 905–923.

Goldwater, D. S., Pavlides, C., Hunter, R. G., Bloss, E. B., Hof, P. R., McEwen, B. S., et al. (2009). Structural and functional alterations to rat medial prefrontal cortex following chronic restraint stress and recovery. *Neuroscience, 164*(2), 798–808.

Grelotti, D. J., Klin, A. J., Gauthier, I., Skudlarski, P., Cohen, D. J., Gore, J. C., et al. (2005). fMRI activation of the fusiform gyrus and amygdala to cartoon characters but not to faces in a boy with autism. *Neuropsychologia, 43*(3), 373–385.

Guyer, A. E., Lau, J. Y., McClure-Tone, E. B., Parrish, J., Shiffrin, N. D., Reynolds, R. C., et al. (2008). Amygdala and ventrolateral prefrontal cortex function during anticipated peer evaluation in pediatric social anxiety. *Archives of General Psychiatry, 65*(11), 1303–1312.

Hadjikhani, N., Joseph, R. M., Snyder, J., & Tager-Flusberg, H. (2007). Abnormal activation of the social brain during face perception in autism. *Human Brain Mapping, 28*(5), 441–449.

Hankin, B. L., Gibb, B. E., Abela, J. R., & Flory, K. (2010). Selective attention to affective stimuli and clinical depression among youths: Role of anxiety and specificity of emotion. *Journal of Abnormal Psychology, 119*(3), 491–501.

Hariri, A. R., Mattay, V. S., Tessitore, A., Fera, F., & Weinberger, D. R. (2003). Neocortical modulation of the amygdala response to fearful stimuli. *Biological Psychiatry, 53*(6), 494–501.

Hariri, A. R., Mattay, V. S., Tessitore, A., Kolachana, B., Fera, F., Goldman, D., et al. (2002a). Serotonin transporter genetic variation and the response of the human amygdala. *Science, 297*(5580), 400–403.

Hariri, A. R., Tessitore, A., Mattay, V. S., Fera, F., & Weinberger, D. R. (2002b). The amygdala response to emotional stimuli: A comparison of faces and scenes. *NeuroImage, 17*(1), 317–323.

Hu, X. Z., Lipsky, R. H., Zhu, G., Akhtar, L. A., Taubman, J., Greenberg, B. D., et al. (2006). Serotonin transporter promoter gain-of-function genotypes are linked to obsessive–compulsive disorder. *American Journal of Human Genetics, 78*(5), 815–826.

Jackson, P. B., Boccuto, L., Skinner, C., Collins, J. S., Neri, G., Gurrieri, F., et al. (2009). Further evidence that the rs1858830 C variant in the promoter region of the MET gene is associated with autistic disorder. *Autism Research, 2*(4), 232–236.

Joormann, J., Talbot, L., & Gotlib, I. H. (2007). Biased processing of emotional information in girls at risk for depression. *Journal of Abnormal Psychology, 116*(1), 135–143.

Kalin, N. H., Shelton, S. E., & Davidson, R. J. (2007). Role of the primate orbitofrontal cortex in mediating anxious temperament. *Biological Psychiatry, 62*(10), 1134–1139.

Kalin, N. H., Shelton, S. E., Fox, A. S., Rogers, J., Oakes, T. R., & Davidson, R. J. (2008). The serotonin transporter genotype is associated with intermediate brain phenotypes that depend on the context of eliciting stressor. *Molecular Psychiatry, 13*(11), 1021–1027.

Kleinhans, N. M., Johnson, L. C., Richards, T., Mahurin, R., Greenson, J., Dawson, G., et al. (2009). Reduced neural habituation in the amygdala and social impairments in autism spectrum disorders. *American Journal of Psychiatry, 166*(4), 467–475.

Kliemann, D., Dziobek, I., Hatri, A., Baudewig, J., & Heekeren, H. R. (2012). The role of the amygdala in atypical gaze on emotional faces in autism spectrum disorders. *Journal of Neuroscience, 32*(28), 9469–9476.

Kliemann, D., Dziobek, I., Hatri, A., Stcimke, R., & Heekeren, H. R. (2010). Atypical reflexive gaze patterns on emotional faces in autism spectrum disorders. *Journal of Neuroscience, 30*(37), 12281–12287.

Lau, J. Y., Goldman, D., Buzas, B., Fromm, S. J., Guyer, A. E., Hodgkinson, C., et al. (2009). Amygdala function and *5-HTT* gene variants in adolescent anxiety and major depressive disorder. *Biological Psychiatry, 65*(4), 349–355.

Lau, J. Y., Goldman, D., Buzas, B., Hodgkinson, C., Leibenluft, E., Nelson, E., et al. (2010). BDNF gene polymorphism (Val66Met) predicts amygdala and anterior hippocampus responses to emotional faces in anxious and depressed adolescents. *NeuroImage, 53*(3), 952–961.

LeDoux, J. E. (2000). Emotion circuits in the brain. *Annual Review of Neuroscience, 23*, 155–184.

Levitt, P., & Campbell, D. B. (2009). The genetic and neurobiologic compass points toward common signaling dysfunctions in autism spectrum disorders. *Journal of Clinical Investigation, 119*(4), 747–754.

Liston, C., McEwen, B. S., & Casey, B. J. (2009). Psychosocial stress reversibly disrupts prefrontal processing and attentional control. *Proceedings of the National Academy of Sciences USA, 106*(3), 912–917.

Luking, K. R., Repovs, G., Belden, A. C., Gaffrey, M. S., Botteron, K. N., Luby, J. L., et al. (2011). Functional connectivity of the amygdala in early-childhood-onset depression. *Journal of the American Academy of Child and Adolescent Psychiatry, 50*(10), 1027–1041.

Maheu, F. S., Dozier, M., Guyer, A. E., Mandell, D., Peloso, E., Poeth, K., et al.

(2010). A preliminary study of medial temporal lobe function in youths with a history of caregiver deprivation and emotional neglect. *Cognitive, Affective, and Behavioral Neuroscience, 10*(1), 34–49.

McClure, E. B., Monk, C. S., Nelson, E. E., Parrish, J. M., Adler, A., Blair, R. J., et al. (2007). Abnormal attention modulation of fear circuit function in pediatric generalized anxiety disorder. *Archives of General Psychiatry, 64*(1), 97–106.

McEwen, B. S., & Gianaros, P. J. (2010). Central role of the brain in stress and adaptation: Links to socioeconomic status, health, and disease. *Annals of the New York Academy of Sciences, 1186*, 190–222.

Mogg, K., Bradley, B. P., Millar, N., & White, J. (1995). A follow-up study of cognitive bias in generalized anxiety disorder. *Behaviour Research and Therapy, 33*(8), 927–935.

Monk, C. S., Klein, R. G., Telzer, E. H., Schroth, E. A., Mannuzza, S., Moulton, J. L., III, et al. (2008a). Amygdala and nucleus accumbens activation to emotional facial expressions in children and adolescents at risk for major depression. *American Journal of Psychiatry, 165*(1), 90–98.

Monk, C. S., McClure, E. B., Nelson, E. E., Zarahn, E., Bilder, R. M., Leibenluft, E., et al. (2003). Adolescent immaturity in attention-related brain engagement to emotional facial expressions. *NeuroImage, 20*(1), 420–428.

Monk, C. S., Telzer, E. H., Mogg, K., Bradley, B. P., Mai, X., Louro, H. M., et al. (2008b). Amygdala and ventrolateral prefrontal cortex activation to masked angry faces in children and adolescents with generalized anxiety disorder. *Archives of General Psychiatry, 65*(5), 568–576.

Monk, C. S., Weng, S. J., Wiggins, J. L., Kurapati, N., Louro, H. M., Carrasco, M., et al. (2010). Neural circuitry of emotional face processing in autism spectrum disorders. *Journal of Psychiatry and Neuroscience, 35*(2), 105–114.

Montag, C., Reuter, M., Newport, B., Elger, C., & Weber, B. (2008). The BDNF Val66Met polymorphism affects amygdala activity in response to emotional stimuli: Evidence from a genetic imaging study. *NeuroImage, 42*(4), 1554–1559.

Munafo, M. R., Brown, S. M., & Hariri, A. R. (2008). Serotonin transporter (5-HTTLPR) genotype and amygdala activation: A meta-analysis. *Biological Psychiatry, 63*(9), 852–857.

Myers-Schulz, B., & Koenigs, M. (2012). Functional anatomy of ventromedial prefrontal cortex: implications for mood and anxiety disorders. *Molecular Psychiatry, 17*(2), 132–141.

Nordahl, C. W., Scholz, R., Yang, X., Buonocore, M. H., Simon, T., Rogers, S., et al. (2012). Increased rate of amygdala growth in children aged 2 to 4 years with autism spectrum disorders: A longitudinal study. *Archives of General Psychiatry, 69*(1), 53–61.

Ongur, D., & Price, J. L. (2000). The organization of networks within the orbital and medial prefrontal cortex of rats, monkeys and humans. *Cerebral Cortex, 10*(3), 206–219.

Pelphrey, K. A., Morris, J. P., McCarthy, G., & Labar, K. S. (2007). Perception of dynamic changes in facial affect and identity in autism. *Social Cognitive and Affective Neuroscience, 2*(2), 140–149.

Perez-Edgar, K., Bar-Haim, Y., McDermott, J. M., Gorodetsky, E., Hodgkinson, C.

A., Goldman, D., et al. (2010). Variations in the serotonin-transporter gene are associated with attention bias patterns to positive and negative emotion faces. *Biological Psychology, 83*(3), 269–271.

Pergamin-Hight, L., Bakermans-Kranenburg, M. J., van IJzendoorn, M. H., & Bar-Haim, Y. (2012). Variations in the promoter region of the serotonin transporter gene and biased attention for emotional information: A meta-analysis. *Biological Psychiatry, 71*(4), 373–379.

Perlman, G., Simmons, A. N., Wu, J., Hahn, K. S., Tapert, S. F., Max, J. E., et al. (2012). Amygdala response and functional connectivity during emotion regulation: A study of 14 depressed adolescents. *Journal of Affective Disorders, 139*(1), 75–84.

Pezawas, L., Meyer-Lindenberg, A., Drabant, E. M., Verchinski, B. A., Munoz, K. E., Kolachana, B. S., et al. (2005). 5-HTTLPR polymorphism impacts human cingulate-amygdala interactions: A genetic susceptibility mechanism for depression. *Nature Neuroscience, 8*(6), 828–834.

Pfeifer, J. H., & Allen, N. B. (2012). Arrested development?: Reconsidering dual-systems models of brain function in adolescence and disorders. *Trends in Cognitive Sciences, 16*(6), 322–329.

Phan, K. L., Wager, T., Taylor, S. F., & Liberzon, I. (2002). Functional neuroanatomy of emotion: a meta-analysis of emotion activation studies in PET and fMRI. *NeuroImage, 16*(2), 331–348.

Phillips, M. L., Ladouceur, C. D., & Drevets, W. C. (2008). A neural model of voluntary and automatic emotion regulation: Implications for understanding the pathophysiology and neurodevelopment of bipolar disorder. *Molecular Psychiatry, 13*(9), 829, 833–857.

Pine, D. S., Mogg, K., Bradley, B. P., Montgomery, L., Monk, C. S., McClure, E., et al. (2005). Attention bias to threat in maltreated children: Implications for vulnerability to stress-related psychopathology. *American Journal of Psychiatry, 162*(2), 291–296.

Pinkham, A. E., Hopfinger, J. B., Pelphrey, K. A., Piven, J., & Penn, D. L. (2008). Neural bases for impaired social cognition in schizophrenia and autism spectrum disorders. *Schizophrenia Research, 99*(1–3), 164–175.

Pollak, S. D., & Tolley-Schell, S. A. (2003). Selective attention to facial emotion in physically abused children. *Journal of Abnormal Psychology, 112*(3), 323–338.

Ray, R. D., & Zald, D. H. (2012). Anatomical insights into the interaction of emotion and cognition in the prefrontal cortex. *Neuroscience and Biobehavioral Reviews, 36*(1), 479–501.

Roberson-Nay, R., McClure, E. B., Monk, C. S., Nelson, E. E., Guyer, A. E., Fromm, S. J., et al. (2006). Increased amygdala activity during successful memory encoding in adolescent major depressive disorder: An fMRI study. *Biological Psychiatry, 60*(9), 966–973.

Rudie, J. D., Shehzad, Z., Hernandez, L. M., Colich, N. L., Bookheimer, S. Y., Iacoboni, M., et al. (2012). Reduced functional integration and segregation of distributed neural systems underlying social and emotional information processing in autism spectrum disorders. *Cerebral Cortex, 22*(5), 1025–1037.

Sarter, M., & Markowitsch, H. J. (1984). Collateral innervation of the medial and lateral prefrontal cortex by amygdaloid, thalamic, and brain-stem neurons. *Journal of Comparative Neurology, 224*(3), 445–460.

Strang, N. M., Chein, J. M., & Steinberg, L. (2013). The value of the dual systems model of adolescent risk-taking. *Frontiers in Human Neuroscience, 7*, 223.

Swartz, J. R., Carrasco, M., Wiggins, J. L., Thomas, M. E., & Monk, C. S. (2014). Age-related changes in the structure and function of prefrontal cortex–amygdala circuitry in children and adolescents: A multi-modal imaging approach. *NeuroImage, 86*, 212–220.

Swartz, J. R., Graham-Bermann, S. A., Mogg, K., Bradley, B. P., & Monk, C. S. (2011). Attention bias to emotional faces in young children exposed to intimate partner violence. *Journal of Child and Adolescent Trauma, 4*, 109–122.

Swartz, J. R., Wiggins, J. L., Carrasco, M., Lord, C., & Monk, C. S. (2013). Amygdala habituation and prefrontal functional connectivity in youth with autism spectrum disorders. *Journal of the American Academy of Child and Adolescent Psychiatry, 52*(1), 84–93.

Taylor, C. T., Aupperle, R. L., Flagan, T., Simmons, A. N., Amir, N., Stein, M. B., et al. (2014). Neural correlates of a computerized attention modification program in anxious subjects. *Social Cognitive and Affective Neuroscience, 9*(9), 1379–1387.

Thomas, K. M., Drevets, W. C., Dahl, R. E., Ryan, N. D., Birmaher, B., Eccard, C. H., et al. (2001a). Amygdala response to fearful faces in anxious and depressed children. *Archives of General Psychiatry, 58*(11), 1057–1063.

Thomas, K. M., Drevets, W. C., Whalen, P. J., Eccard, C. H., Dahl, R. E., Ryan, N. D., et al. (2001b). Amygdala response to facial expressions in children and adults. *Biological Psychiatry, 49*(4), 309–316.

Thomason, M. E., Henry, M. L., Paul Hamilton, J., Joormann, J., Pine, D. S., Ernst, M., et al. (2010). Neural and behavioral responses to threatening emotion faces in children as a function of the short allele of the serotonin transporter gene. *Biological Psychology, 85*(1), 38–44.

Thomason, M. E., Yoo, D. J., Glover, G. H., & Gotlib, I. H. (2009). BDNF genotype modulates resting functional connectivity in children. *Frontiers in Human Neuroscience, 3*, 55.

Tordjman, S., Gutknecht, L., Carlier, M., Spitz, E., Antoine, C., Slama, F., et al. (2001). Role of the serotonin transporter gene in the behavioral expression of autism. *Molecular Psychiatry, 6*(4), 434–439.

Tottenham, N., Hare, T. A., Millner, A., Gilhooly, T., Zevin, J. D., & Casey, B. J. (2011). Elevated amygdala response to faces following early deprivation. *Developmental Science, 14*(2), 190–204.

van Leeuwen, N., Kumsta, R., Entringer, S., de Kloet, E. R., Zitman, F. G., DeRijk, R. H., et al. (2010). Functional mineralocorticoid receptor (MR) gene variation influences the cortisol awakening response after dexamethasone. *Psychoneuroendocrinology, 35*(3), 339–349.

Wald, I., Degnan, K. A., Gorodetsky, E., Charney, D. S., Fox, N. A., Fruchter, E., et al. (2013). Attention to threats and combat-related posttraumatic stress symptoms: Prospective associations and moderation by the serotonin transporter gene. *JAMA Psychiatry, 70*(4), 401–408.

Wang, A. T., Lee, S. S., Sigman, M., & Dapretto, M. (2006). Developmental changes in the neural basis of interpreting communicative intent. *Social Cognitive and Affective Neuroscience, 1*(2), 107–121.

Weng, S. J., Carrasco, M., Swartz, J. R., Wiggins, J. L., Kurapati, N., Liberzon, I., et al. (2011). Neural activation to emotional faces in adolescents with autism spectrum disorders. *Journal of Child Psychology and Psychiatry and Allied Disciplines, 52*(3), 296–305.

White, M. G., Bogdan, R., Fisher, P. M., Munoz, K. E., Williamson, D. E., & Hariri, A. R. (2012). FKBP5 and emotional neglect interact to predict individual differences in amygdala reactivity. *Genes, Brain, and Behavior, 11*(7), 869–878.

Wiggins, J. L., Bedoyan, J. K., Carrasco, M., Swartz, J. R., Martin, D. M., & Monk, C. S. (2014a). Age-related effect of serotonin transporter genotype on amygdala and prefrontal cortex function in adolescence. *Human Brain Mapping, 35*(2), 646–658.

Wiggins, J. L., Swartz, J. R., Martin, D. M., Lord, C., & Monk, C. S. (2014b). Serotonin transporter genotype impacts amygdala habituation in youth with autism spectrum disorders. *Social Cognitive and Affective Neuroscience, 9*(6), 832–838.

Epilogue

DAVID G. AMARAL
RALPH ADOLPHS

One of the joys of editing a multidisciplinary book like this is the opportunity to see consistent threads of findings and perspectives wend their way through the various chapters representing different types of research. By way of closing this book, we highlight just a few of these that seem particularly prominent to us and conclude with a few comments related to future directions for behavioral research on the amygdaloid complex. We have organized this epilogue through a series of conclusions that have emerged from the chapters.

The amygdala is a danger detector and mediates the behavioral response of fear. But there appear to be several fear systems, and some do not require amygdala participation.

During the 1950s, due largely to knowledge obtained from the important patient H. M., who underwent bilateral medial temporal lobectomy in an effort to control his epilepsy, our understanding of memory went through a process of fractionation and neuroanatomical specialization. H. M. was not able to encode new information about episodes of his life into long-term memory. But memories that had been encoded years prior to his surgery were largely intact. And his ability to retain information for brief periods of time (minutes), as well as his ability to learn and retain new skills, suggested that different brain regions mediated these different forms of memory. Subsequently, memory has been broadly schematized as having a declarative component that is mediated by the hippocampus and other parts of the medial temporal lobe memory system and a procedural component that is mediated by a variety of structures including the amygdala, basal ganglia, and cerebellum (Squire & Wixted, 2011; Squire & Dede, 2015).

One gets the sense that fear is also distributed across different brain systems. Patient S. M., for example, described by Feinstein, Adolphs, and Tranel (Chapter 1) and by Adolphs (Chapter 10) demonstrates very blunted fear responses to exteroceptive signals such as snakes or fearful faces. However, she is able to demonstrate a full-blown panic attack when the stimulus is interoceptive, such as excessive levels of CO_2 in inhaled air. Similarly, the work from the Amaral laboratory (summarized by Bliss-Moreau, Moadab, & Amaral, Chapter 6), in which the amygdala is lesioned in 2-week-old monkeys, demonstrates that the monkeys without an amygdala show a very minimal emotional response to external stimuli such as novel objects, including species-specific fear elicitors such as snakes. On the other hand, these young animals demonstrated enhanced levels of fear responses such as facial grimaces and vocalizations, when they engaged in social behavior. This was particularly unusual, since the animals actually engaged in greater levels of social behavior.

The conclusion that not all fear is gone when the amygdala is removed immediately raises the question as to which other brain regions play an important role in mediating other forms or components of fear. The bed nucleus of the stria terminalis, which is intimately connected with the amygdala, has been suggested, but the extent to which it relies on amygdala circuitry for its function is not clear (Adhikari, 2014; Avery, Clauss, & Blackford, 2015). Another region is the dorsal periaqueductal gray, which is known to mediate fear responses to unconditioned stimuli through reciprocal connectivity with the amygdala (Kim et al., 2013). Possibly, structures such as this are sufficient to mediate fear responses to interoceptive stimuli also in the case of humans and monkeys (Mobbs et al., 2007, 2009).

The behavioral consequences of living without an amygdala depend on whether the loss happens early or later in development.

Many of the chapters in this book emphasize that the behavioral alterations seen in individuals living without an amygdala may be due to compensatory changes following damage to the amygdala. There is no documented case of a human subject who is born with selective loss of the amygdala. All of the patients with Urbach–Wiethe disease have a progressive loss of amygdala function with an uncertain onset but perhaps occurring as late as adolescence. One could argue that the behavioral impairments observed in these subjects identify key functions that are highly dependent on the amygdala. Thus, aspects of danger detection and mobilization of whole-body responses to external threats are consistently observed in all species studied after loss of amygdala function. Other functions associated with the amygdala, such as contributing to normal species-specific social behavior or memory modulation, do not appear to be as obviously impaired after loss of the amygdala. In the nonhuman primate studies summarized by Bliss-Moreau et al. (Chapter 6) and Bachevalier, Sanchez, Raper, Stephens, and Wallen (Chapter 7), one of the consistent observations is that even in animals in which the amygdala was removed near birth, their complex social behavior is nearly intact—at least initially. In these studies, it is clear that the behavior of the animals does change throughout life, presumably as the brain continues to adapt to the loss of the amygdala and to face new behavioral challenges in adolescence and adulthood.

The chapter by Patin and Hurlemann (Chapter 11) about the monozygotic twins A. M. and B. G. with Urbach–Wiethe disease is strong testimony to the fact that not only is there substantial functional brain plasticity but also even in individuals with identical genetics and very similar upbringing, the extent and quality of this plasticity can be strikingly different. Twin A.M. appears to have a much more normal response to fearful stimuli than does B.G. Neuroimaging studies indicate that brain regions such as the left inferior frontal operculum and superior temporal gyrus appear to be recruited to mediate these compensatory amygdala functions. Since B. G. does not show the same behavioral or brain functional responses, one wonders what are the triggers for functional compensation? What life circumstance affected A. M. and not B. G? They may be subtle and potentially highly idiosyncratic! Van Honk, Terburg, Thornton, Stein, and Morgan (Chapter 12) suggest that some behavioral functions may be enhanced without amygdala function. They found in some of their patients with Urbach–Wiethe disease that working memory function was facilitated, and they ascribe this to decreased environmental vigilance. Equally interesting is the apparent hypersensitivity to fear stimuli seen in some of these patients, possibly related to lesions of the amygdala that are incomplete and primarily involve the basolateral nucleus. Perhaps even more interesting, these authors emphasize that the behavioral sequelae of lack of amygdala function may be importantly related to the socioeconomic status of the individual who is evaluated. Clearly, there are a whole host of different expectations and experiences for someone who is at the top of the social strata compared to someone near the bottom. How the brain adapts to the loss of amygdala function appears to be heavily affected by these different societal influences.

The amygdala is involved in many behavioral and cognitive functions beyond fear.

If functional magnetic resonance imaging (MRI) studies have taught us anything about how the brain works, it is that all brain regions participate in complex distributed networks. Moreover, while these networks can partially be predicted based on classic neuroanatomy, there is no strict correspondence between regions that have monosynaptic connections and those that have correlated brain activity (Honey et al., 2009). Resting state MRI studies of the amygdala, for example, show that there is very high correlation between activation in the left and right amygdala (Roy et al., 2009). However, there are no monosynaptic commissural connections of the amygdala in the primate brain. The take-home message is that disruption of the function of a single brain region may have complex and potentially subtle influences on a complex network of brain regions. It is not surprising, therefore, that chapters in this book have highlighted a bevy of behavioral and cognitive functions ranging from fear to salience, to sensory perception and learning and memory. The challenge for the future will be to determine the precise computational contributions to each of these functions. In other words, what neural computations have the unique intrinsic organization and network interactions of the amygdala evolved to carry out, and how do these contribute to the various functions attributed to the amygdala. This type of understanding will naturally lead to implications for the emergence of psychopathology when the amygdala is not functioning properly.

It is valuable to make comparisons and to consider subjective experience.

The chapters in this book also demonstrate the value of making comparisons: across species, ages, and methods. Although the focus of this volume is on what happens when amygdala function is disrupted, it should be clear that a full understanding of what the amygdala does will require a highly multimodal approach. Lesion studies need to be combined with functional MRI studies, and even with electrophysiological studies.

Comparisons across species also raise a perennial question highlighted by several chapters: What is the role of the amygdala in the conscious experience of fear? In patient S. M., the abolition specifically of the experience of fear was striking. Do monkeys or rodents with amygdala lesions also not experience fear? Which other components of the network are required to experience fear? Answers to these questions will require continued close collaborations between those studying the amygdala in humans, and in nonhuman animals; and it will require continued development of measures to assay the experience of fear. This is, of course, the most important aspect of anxiety disorders (see Monk and Pine, Chapter 14), since it is the subjective experience of patients that ultimately matters the most. The first and last chapters of this book therefore frame one of the largest questions: How does the amygdala contribute to our conscious experience of fear in health and disease?

Conclusions

The chapters in this book have highlighted some of the benefits and many of the disadvantages of the lesion technique for behavioral neuroscience. It is likely that the era of permanent lesions is, if not over, rapidly coming to an end. The clear and substantial compensatory changes that the rest of the brain undergoes following a lesion limits what can be said about the function of the lesioned structure. However, the fact that many of the chapters in this book have highlighted the process of compensatory changes points to the fact that we really do not understand the limits of brain reorganization after selectively lesioning a structure such as the amygdala. Given the advances of MRI technology, it is now possible to follow the time course of functional brain reorganization following selective lesioning. The studies of patients with Urbach–Wiethe disease in which various neuroimaging modalities and intensive behavioral analyses are carried out provide an exciting and important window into the processes of brain reorganization following amygdala damage. These studies suffer, however, from the lack of knowledge concerning the onset of amygdala pathology. If parallel studies are carried out in an appropriate animal model, answers to questions related to the differences in brain compensation following early versus late lesions could be addressed. The functional limits of brain plasticity could also be probed. If fear can migrate from a structure such as the amygdala to cortical regions such as inferior frontal cortex, what are the limits in "reeducating" the brain?

As in most areas of behavioral neuroscience, the function of the amygdala will increasingly be probed by transient activation and inactivation strategies. Techniques such as optogenetics (Johansen et al., 2010) allow selective and transient activation or inhibition of regions or cell types in the amygdala. Even the nonhuman primate amygdala can be transiently influenced by pharmacogenomic manipulations such as designer receptors exclusively activated by designer drugs (DREADDs; Lee, Giguere, & Roth, 2014). Since these manipulations are short lasting, they are much less likely to trigger the compensatory brain machinery that is put in place following lesions. It will be interesting to see the extent to which these techniques confirm notions about amygdala function based on the lesion technique and to clarify areas where this technique and its faults have led us astray.

REFERENCES

Adhikari, A. (2014). Distributed circuits underlying anxiety. *Frontiers in Behavioral Neuroscience, 8*, 112.

Avery, S. N., Clauss, J. A., & Blackford, J. U. (2015, June 24). The human BNST: Functional role in anxiety and addiction. *Neuropsychopharmacology.* [Epub ahead of print]

Honey, C. J., Sporns, O., Cammoun, L., Gigandet, X., Thiran, J. P., Meuli, R., et al. (2009). Predicting human resting-state functional connectivity from structural connectivity. *Proceedings of the National Academy of Sciences USA, 106*, 2035–2040.

Johansen, J. P., Hamanaka, H., Monfils, M. H., Behnia, R., Deisseroth, K., Blair, H. T., et al. (2010). Optical activation of lateral amygdala pyramidal cells instructs associative fear learning. *Proceedings of the National Academy of Sciences USA, 107*, 12692–12697.

Kim, E. J., Horovitz, O., Pellman, B. A., Tan, L. M., Li, Q., Richter-Levin, G., & Kim, J. J. (2013). Dorsal periaqueductal gray–amygdala pathway conveys both innate and learned fear responses in rats. *Proceedings of the National Academy of Sciences USA, 110*, 14795–14800.

Lee, H. M., Giguere, P. M., & Roth, B. L. (2014). DREADDs: Novel tools for drug discovery and development. *Drug Discovery Today, 19*, 469–473.

Mobbs, D., Marchant, J. L., Hassabis, D., Seymour, B., Tan, G., Gray, M., et al. (2009). From threat to fear: The neural organization of defensive fear systems in humans. *Journal of Neuroscience, 29*, 12236–12243.

Mobbs, D., Petrovic, P., Marchant, J. L., Hassabis, D., Weiskopf, N., Seymour, B., et al. (2007). When fear is near: Threat imminence elicits prefrontal-periaqueductal gray shifts in humans. *Science, 317*, 1079–1083.

Roy, A. K., Shehzad, Z., Margulies, D. S., Kelly, A. M., Uddin, L. Q., Gotimer, K., et al. (2009). Functional connectivity of the human amygdala using resting state fMRI. *NeuroImage, 45*, 614–626.

Squire, L. R., & Dede, A. J. (2015). Conscious and unconscious memory systems. *Cold Spring Harbor Perspectives in Biology, 7*(3), a021667.

Squire, L. R., & Wixted, J. T. (2011). The cognitive neuroscience of human memory since H. M. *Annual Review of Neuroscience, 34*, 259–288.

Index

Note: *b* following a page number indicates a box;
f indicates a figure; *n* indicates a note; *t* indicates a table